Wang Ang's Collected and Analyzed Medical Formulas

醫方集解
(Yi Fang Ji Jie)

Translated by Joungeun Lee

Preface

Wang Ang (汪昂, 1615 - ?) is a distinguished doctor in the Qing Dynasty in China. He re cords six or seven hundreds of formulas that are used commonly and extracted from vario us books. He classified these formulas according to the character of them; Supplementing, Exterior-Effusing Releasing, Ejection, Interior-Attacking, Exterior-Interior, Harmonizing, Qi-Rectifying, Blood-Rectifying, Wind-Dispelling, Cold-Dispelling, Summerheat-Cleari ng, Dampness Rectifying, Dryness-Moistening, Fire-Draining, Phlegm-Eliminating, Disp ersing and Abducting, Contracting and Astringing, The Eyes Brightening, Welling-Absce sses and Sores, and Menstruation and Childbirth.

Table of Contents

6

Chapter 5. Exterior-Interior Formulas. *表裏之劑 120*

9

Chapter 11. Summerheat-Clearing Formulas. 清暑之劑 254

Chapter 13. Dryness-Moistening Formulas. *潤燥之劑* 298

Chapter 15. Phlegm-Eliminating Formulas. 除痰之劑 *359*

17

Chapter 20. Oral Formulas for Welling-Abscesses and Sores. *癰瘍之劑 430*

21

Chapter 1. Supplementing Formulas. 補養之劑

1. Liu Wei Di Huang Wan. Six-Ingredient Pill with Rehmannia. 六味地黃丸

·**ACTIONS**：supplements true yin and eliminates every disease (one hundred disease). Qian Yi (錢乙: a doctor in the Song dynasty) removes Gui Zhi and Fu Zi from Ba Wei Wan to treat child. Child belongs to pure yang, therefore Gui Zhi and Fu Zi are not used. Nowadays this formula generally treats not only child but also adult.

·**COMPOSITION**：Shu Di Huang. Fu Ling. Mu Dan Pi. Shan Zhu Yu. S han Yao. Ze Xie.

·**INDICATIONS**：

      (1) Live-Kidney insufficiency, true yin depletion, essence-blood desiccation, hardness and emaciation.

      (2) lumbar pain and aching foot, spontaneous sweating and night sweating, phlegm due to water flood, heat effusion with cough.

      (3) dizziness and dizzy vision, tinnitus and deafness, seminal emi ssion and hematochezia, wasting-thirst and strangury.

      (4) loss of blood and voice, dry tongue and sore throat, toothache due to vacuity fire.

      (5) heel pain, sore and ulcer in the lower part, etc.

·**MODIFICATIONS**：

      (1) in case of blood vacuity and yin debilitation, Shu Di Huang is used as a sovereign.

      (2) with seminal emission and dizziness, Shan Zhu Yu is used as a sovereign.

      (3) when urination is copious or scant, and red or white, Fu Ling is used as a sovereign.

      (4) with strangury, Ze Xie is used as sovereign.

      (5) if vacuity fire is exuberant and there is static blood, Mu Dan Pi is used as a sovereign.

      (6) with the weakness of Spleen and Stomach and the dryness of the skin and flesh, Shan Yao is used as a sovereign.

·**CHANNELS ENTERED**：The foot lesser yin and reverting yin channel

s. [The kidney and liver]

·THE MEANING ON THE FORMULA

(1) Shu Di Huang nourishes yin, supplements the kidney, and en genders blood and essence.

(2) Shan Zhu Yu warms the liver and expels wind, astringes esse nce and secures qi.

(3) Mu Dan Pi drains the latent fire of the heart and liver, cools b lood and drains bone-steaming fever.

(4) Shan Yao clears vacuity heat in the lung and spleen, supplem ents the spleen and secures the kidney.

(5) Fu Ling drains damp heat in the spleen, and lets the kidney a nd heart interact.

(6) Ze Xie drains the water evil of the bladder, improves hearing and vision.

(7) this formula treats all of the six channels but mainly has an ef fect in the kidney and liver. This is not biased toward cold and dry and also sup plements qi and blood, if one can often eat the formula, it is hard to say every e ffects of it.

·RELATED FORMULA :

(1) When this formula is taken as a decoction, this is called Liu Wei Di Huang Tang. The therapeutic action is same with Liu Wei Di Huang W an.

(2) When Fu Zi and Rou Gui are added to this pills, this is called Gui Fu Ba Wei Wan and treats the insufficiency of ministerial fire, weakness, a nd shortage of qi.

Wang Bing says that the origin of boosting fire is on dispersing yin. It is a ppropriate to use to whom with the weak pulse in cubit.

(3) When Huang Bai and Zhi Mu (two liang respectively) are ad ded to this pills, this is called Zhi Bai Ba Wei Wan, treats yin vacuity stirring fi re, bone wilting, and marrow desiccation.

Wang Bing says that invigorating water controls sunlight (yang guang). It is appropriate to use to whom with the pulse that is strong in cubit.

(4) If rou gui (one liang) is added, this is called Qi Wei Di Huan g Wan, induces the rootless fire to turn down back into the origin.

(5) If Wu Wei Zi (three liang) is added, this is called Dao Qi Wa n, treats taxation cough.

(6) If Wu Wei Zi (two liang) and Mai Men Dong (three liang) are added, this is called Ba Xian Chang Shou Wan, if Zi He Che is added again, this treats vacuity detriment and taxation heat.

(7) If Du Zhong (stir-bake with sheng jiang) and Niu Xi(clean with wine) (respectively two liang) are added, treats aching pain in aching lumbus and knees due to kidney vacuity.

(8) If Ze Xie is removed and Yi Zhi Ren (three liang) is added, treats frequent urination.

(9) If Shu Di Huang (two liang), Shan Yao, Shan Zhu Yu, Mu Dan Pi, Dang Gui Wei, Wu Wei Zi, and Chai Hu (five qian respectively), Fu Shen and Ze Xie (two qian five fen respectively) are made into pills by honey, this is called Yi Yin Shen Qi Wan, treats blurred vision due to kidney vacuity.

(10) If Che Qian Zi and Niu Xi is added to Gui Fu Ba Wei Wan, this is called Shen Qi Wan, treats gu distention.

1. 六味地黃丸
·總結：補眞陰，除百病. 錢氏仲陽因仲景八味丸減去桂附，以治小兒，以小兒純陽，故減桂附，今用通治大小證.
·組成：熟地黃　茯苓　丹皮　山茱肉　山藥　澤瀉
·主治：(1)治肝腎不足，眞陰虧損，精血枯竭，憔悴羸弱.
　　　　(2)腰痛足酸，自汗盜汗，水泛爲痰，發熱欬嗽.
　　　　(3)頭暈目眩，耳鳴耳聾，遺精便血，消渴淋瀝.
　　　　(4)失血失音，舌燥喉痛，虛火牙痛.
　　　　(5)足跟作痛，下部瘡瘍等證.
·加減：(1)血虛陰衰…熟地爲君.
　　　　(2)精滑頭昏…山茱爲君.
　　　　(3)小便或多或少，或赤或白…茯苓爲君.
　　　　(4)小便淋瀝…澤瀉爲君.
　　　　(5)心虛火盛及有瘀血…丹皮爲君.
　　　　(6)脾胃虛弱，皮膚乾濇…山藥爲君.
　　　　→言爲君者，其分用八兩，地黃只用臣分兩.
·歸經：足少陰厥陰藥
·方義：(1)熟地…滋陰補腎，生血生精.
　　　　(2)山茱…溫肝逐風，濇精秘氣.
　　　　(3)牡丹…瀉君相之伏火，涼血退蒸.
　　　　(4)山藥…清虛熱于肺脾，補脾固腎.

(5)茯苓…滲脾中濕熱, 而通腎交心.

(6)澤瀉…瀉膀胱水邪, 而聰耳明目.

(7)六經備治. 而功專腎肝, 寒燥不偏, 而補兼氣血, 苟能常服, 其功未易殫述也.

·變化方：(1)本方煎服…名六味地黃湯…治同

(2)本方加「附子, 肉桂」各一兩…名桂附八味丸→治相火不足, 虛羸少氣.

王冰所謂「益火之原以消陰翳也」. 尺脈弱者宜之.

(3)本方加「黃柏, 知母」各二兩…名知藥八味丸→治陰虛火動, 骨痿髓枯.

王冰所謂「壯水之主以制陽光也」. 尺脈旺者宜之.

(4)本方加「桂」一兩→名七味地黃丸. 引無根之火, 降而歸元.

(5)本方加「五味」三兩, 名都氣丸→治勞嗽.

(6)本方加「五味」二兩, 麥冬三兩→名八仙長壽丸. 再加紫河車一具, 並治虛損勞熱.

(7)本方加「杜仲(薑炒), 牛膝(酒洗)」各二兩→治腎虛腰膝酸痛.

(8)本方「去澤瀉, 加益智仁」三兩→治小便頻數.

(9)本方用「熟地二兩, 山藥, 山茱, 丹皮, 歸尾, 五味, 柴胡各五錢. 茯神, 澤瀉各二錢半」, 蜜丸, 硃砂爲衣→名益陰腎氣丸→治腎虛目昏.

(10)桂附八味丸, 加「車前, 牛膝」名腎氣丸→治蠱脹.

2. Qi Bao Mei Ran Dan. Seven-Treasure Special Pill for Beautiful Whiskers. 七寶美髯丹

·**ACTIONS**：supplements the liver and kidney

·**COMPOSITION**：He Shou Wu, Po Gu Zhi, Bai Fu Ling, Tu Si Zi, Gou Qi, Niu Xi, Dang Gui

·**INDICATIONS**：(1) qi and blood insufficiency, emaciation and generalized impediment, and subfertility due to kidney vacuity.

(2) wasting-thirst and strangury, seminal emission, metrorrhagia and leukorrhargia, welling abscess, sore, hemorrhoid, swelling, and so on.

28

·**CHANNELS ENTERED**：The foot lesser yin and reverting yin channel. [The kidney and liver]

·**Analysis of Formula**：(1) He Shou Wu astringes essence and secures qi, supplements the liver and consolidates the kidney, acts as a sovereign.

(2) Fu Ling makes the heart and kidney interact and drains spleen damp.

(3) Niu Xi strengthens sinew and bone, boosts the lower burner.

(4) Dang Gui tonifies blood with pungent and warm

(5) Gou Qi supplements water with sweet and cold

(6) Tu Si Zi boosts three yin and strengthens the defense qi.

(7) Bu Gu Zhi assists life fire and warms cinnabar field.

(8) This formula which secures the root, makes the construction and defense harmonize and water and fire interact, then qi and blood become harmonious and every disease gets disappear.

·**Original Source**：Shao Ying Jie

2. 七寶美髯丹
　·總結：補肝腎
　·組成：何首烏，破故紙，白茯苓，菟絲子，枸杞，牛膝，當歸
　·主治：(1)治氣血不足，羸弱周痺，腎虛無子.
　　　　　(2)消渴淋瀝，遺精崩帶，癭瘤痔腫等證.
　·歸經：足少陰厥陰藥
　·方義：(1)何首烏...澀精固氣，補肝堅腎→爲君.
　　　　　(2)茯苓...交心腎而滲脾濕.
　　　　　(3)牛膝...強筋骨而益下焦.
　　　　　(4)當歸...辛溫以養血.
　　　　　(5)枸杞...甘寒而補水.
　　　　　(6)菟絲子...益三陰而強衛氣.
　　　　　(7)補骨脂...助命火而暖丹田.
　　　　　(8)此皆固本之藥，使榮衛調適，水火相交，則氣血太和，而
諸疾自己也.
　·來源：邵應節

3. Huan Shao Dan. Return to Youth Pills. 還少丹

·**ACTIONS**∶ pacifies and supplements yin and yang.

·**COMPOSITION**∶ Da Zao, Du Zhong, Niu Xi, Yuan Zhi, Shi Chang Pu, Rou Cong Rong, Ba Ji Tian, Xiao Hui Xiang, Shan Zhu Yu, Wu Wei Zi子, Fu Ling, Shan Yao, Shu Di Huang, Gou Qi Zi, Chu Shi

·**INDICATIONS**∶ (1) spleen-kidney vacuity cold, blood-qi emaciation, and no though of food and drink.

　　　　(2) loss of strength, heat effusion, night sweating, seminal emission and white turbidity, toothache with swelling, etc.

·**CHANNELS ENTERED**∶ The hand and foot lesser yin and the foot greater yin channels. [The heart, kidney, and spleen]

·**Analysis of Formula**∶ Life fire which is between the kidneys is the true yang of earlier heaven and on which people depends when living daily life. When this fire is weak, there will be no motive power to steam the spleen and stomach, taking of food and drink decreases, and essence qi gets weak daily.

　　　　(1) Rou Cong Rong and Ba Ji Tian enters the blood part of the kidney channel. Xiao Hui Xiang enters the qi part of the kidney channel. These can supplement insufficient life gate ministerial fire, exuberant fire strengthens earth, and then the spleen can transport the essence of food and water well.

　　　　(2) Shu Di Huang and Gou Qi are herbs to supplement water, when [kidney] water is sufficient, heart yin can be saved, which makes the heart fire not to be hyperactive.

　　　　(3) Du Zhong and Niu Xi supplement lumbus and knees by assisting the kidney.

　　　　(4) Fu Ling and Shan Yao drain damp by assisting the spleen.

　　　　(5) Shan Zhu Yu and Wu Wei Zi engender Lung Humor and secure essence.

　　　　(6) Yuan Zhi and Shi Chang Pu make the heart qi and kidney interact.

　　　　(7) Da Zao supplements qi and boosts blood, moistens the lung and strengthens the spleen.

　　　　(8) Chu Shi assists yang and supplements vacuity, fills the flesh and invigorates bone.

This regulates water and fire neutrally, makes the spleen and kidney intera

30

ct, and supplements the spleen and kidney.

·**RELATED FORMULA**：1) Dan Xi eliminates Chu Shi from this formula, this is called Zi Yin Da Bu Yin Wan (Nourish Yin and Great Tonify Pill).

·**Original Source**：Yang Shi

3．還少丹

·總結：陰陽平補

·組成：大棗，杜仲，牛膝，遠志，石菖蒲，肉蓯蓉，巴戟天，小茴香，山茱肉，五味子，茯苓，山藥，熟地黃，枸杞，楮實

·主治：(1)治脾腎虛寒，血氣羸乏，不思飲食．

(2)肌體瘦弱，發熱盜汗，遺精白濁，牙齒浮痛等證．

·歸經：手足少陰（心，腎）足太陰（脾）藥也．

·方義：兩腎中間有命火，乃先天之真陽，人之日用云為，皆此火也，此火衰微，則無以薰蒸脾胃，飲食減少，而精氣日衰矣．

(1)蓯蓉，巴戟…能入腎經血分；茴香…能入腎經氣分，兩者可同補命門相火之不足，火旺則土強而脾能健運矣．

(2)熟地，枸杞…補水之藥，水足則有以濟火，而不亢不害矣．

(3)杜仲，牛膝…補腰膝以助腎．

(4)茯苓，山藥…滲濕以助脾．

(5)山茱，五味…生肺液而固精．

(6)遠志，菖蒲…通心氣以交腎．

(7)大棗…補氣益血，潤肺強脾．

(8)楮實…助陽補虛，充肌壯骨．

此水火平調，脾腎交補之劑也．

·變化方：丹溪去「楮實」→更名滋陰大補丸．

·又附方：一方茯苓換茯神，加川續斷，名打老兒丸．

·來源：楊氏

4. Hei Di Huang Wan. Black Rehmannia Pills. 黑地黃丸

·**ACTIONS**：fortifies the spleen and supplements the kidney

·**COMPOSITION**：Cang Zhu, Shu Di Huang, Wu Wei Zi, Gan Jiang, Da Zao.

·**INDICATIONS**：(1) Spleen and Kidney insufficiency, sexual vacuity an

31

d detriment, emaciation, bluish and yellow complexion.

        (2) enduring hemorrhoids due to blood vacuity.

·**CHANNELS ENTERED**：The foot greater yin and lesser yin channels. [The spleen and kidney]

·**Analysis of Formula**：喻嘉言 says that ：

        (1) In this formula, Cang Zhu is sovereign, Di Huang is minister, Wu Wei Zi is assistant, and Gan Jiang is courier.

        (2) This formula treats the vacuity of both Spleen and Kidney, and eliminates Spleen Damp and Kidney Dryness.

        (3) Formulas about supplementing both Spleen and Kidney which are made by posterior are too miscellaneous, compared to those, this formula is very good.

4. 黑地黃丸
　·總結：健脾補腎
　·組成：蒼朮, 熟地黃, 五味子, 乾薑, 棗肉
　·主治：(1)治脾腎不足, 房室虛損, 形瘦無力, 面色青黃.
　　　　　(2)亦治血虛久痔.
　·歸經：足太陰少陰藥.
　·方義：喻嘉言曰：
　　　　　(1)此方以蒼朮爲君, 地黃爲臣, 五味爲佐, 乾薑爲使.
　　　　　(2)治脾腎兩臟之虛, 而去脾濕, 除腎燥, 兩擅其長, 超超元箸.

　　　　　(3)視後人之脾腎雙補, 藥味龐雜者, 相去不遠耶?

5. Hu Qian Wan. Hidden Tiger Pill from the Analytic Collection. 虎潛丸

·**ACTIONS**：supplements yin

·**COMPOSITION**：Huang Bai, Zhi Mu, Shu Di Huang, Dang Gui, Shao Yao, Niu Xi, Gui Ban, Hu Jing Gu, Suo Yang, Chen Pi, Gan Jiang, Yang Rou (mutton)

·**INDICATIONS**：essence-blood insufficiency, wilting and weakness of sinew and bone, failing to stand on foot, steaming bone and taxation heat.

·**MODIFICATIONS**：in winter, add Gan Jiang.

·**CHANNELS ENTERED**：The lesser yin channel. [The kidney]

·**Analysis of Formula**：(1) Huang Bai, Zhi Mu, and Shu Di Huang invigorate kidney Water and nourish yin.

(2) Dang Gui, Shao Yao, and Niu Xi supplement Liver Vacuity and nourish blood.

(3) Niu Xi can induce every medicinal to descend, invigorates sinew and bone, and treats both Liver and Kidney.

(4) Gui Ban is the animal that is supplied with yin qi strongly, therefore this supplements yin and acts as a sovereign.

(5) Hu Gu is the animal supplied with yin qi strongly, therefore this fortifies bone and acts as assistant. The reason of using the shinbone of the tiger is because even though a tiger gets die, it won't fall down and tries to stand, and the power is generally in the anterior shinbone, therefore using it to enter directly the lower limbs and supplement the legs.

(6) Suo Yang boosts essence and invigorates yang, nourishes sinew and moistens dryness.

(7) most of herbs in this formula belong to blood herbs, therefore Chen Pi is added to disinhibit qi, Gan Jiang is used to free yang.

(8) Yang Rou (mutton) is sweet and heat, this is related with fire and supplements greatly, and also the flavor supplements essence, makes qi and blood to interact and yin and yang to help each other.

·**RELATED FORMULA**：(1) Dan Xi adds Gan Jiang, Bai Zhu, Fu Ling, Gan Cao, Wu Wei Zi, Tu Si Zi, and Zi He Che to this formula, this is called Bu Yi Wan (Tonifying and Augmenting Pills) and treats wilting disease.

(2) In another formula, Long Gu is added to this formula, this is called Long Hu Ji Yin Dan (Dragon and Tiger Help Yin Pills), treats seminal emission.

5. 虎潛丸
 ·總結：補陰
 ·組成：黃柏, 知母, 熟地, 當歸, 芍藥, 牛膝, 龜板, 虎脛骨, 瑣陽, 陳皮, 乾薑, 羊肉
 ·主治：治精血不足, 筋骨痿弱, 足不任地, 及骨蒸勞熱.
 ·加減：冬加「乾薑」一兩.
 ·歸經：足少陰藥（腎）也.

·方義：⑴黃柏，知母，熟地…所以壯腎水而滋陰.

⑵當歸，芍藥，牛膝…所以補肝虛而養血.

⑶牛膝…又能引諸藥下行，以壯筋骨，蓋肝腎同一治也.

⑷龜版…得陰氣最厚，故以補陰而爲君.

⑸虎骨…得陰氣最強，故以健骨而爲佐. 用脛骨者，虎雖死猶立不仆，其氣力皆在前脛，故用以入足，從其類也.

⑹瑣陽…益精壯陽，養筋潤燥.

⑺然數者皆血藥，故又加「陳皮」以利氣；加「乾薑」以通陽.

⑻羊肉…甘熱屬火而大補，亦以味補精，以形補形之義，使氣血交通，陰陽相濟也.

·變化方：⑴丹溪加「乾薑，白朮，茯苓，甘草，五味，菟絲，紫河車」…名補益丸 ⇒治瘻.

⑵一方加龍骨…名龍虎濟陰丹⇒治遺洩.

6. Tai Zhen Wan. Great True Pills. 太眞丸

·**ACTIONS**：supplements qi and blood

·**COMPOSITION**：Ren Shen, Yang Rou (mutton), Rou Cong Rong, Shan Yao, Dang Gui, Huang Qi, Tian Men Dong, Bai Zhu

·**INDICATIONS**：(1) All kinds of blood collapse, emaciation, lack of appetite, efflux diarrhea, depletion of fluids.

(2) Long-term use of this pills engenders blood and boosts qi, and warms the stomach and makes face look young.

·**CHANNELS ENTERED**：The hand and foot greater yin channels. [The lung and spleen]

·**Analysis of Formula**：(1) 喻嘉言 says this formula is good at supplementing.

(2) Ren Shen and Yang Rou (mutton) have same effect.

(3) Rou Cong Rong and Shan Yao supplement the superior article of man.

(4) combined with Dang Gui nourishes the construction, Huang Qi boosts the defense. Tian Men Dong preserves the lung. Bai Zhu fortifies the spleen.

(5) The composition strategy in making this formula is very exquisite and this formula is the major one of supplementing.

34

6. 太眞丸

·總結：補氣血

·組成：人參, 羊肉, 蓯蓉, 山藥, 當歸, 黃耆, 天冬, 白朮

·主治：(1)治一切亡血過多, 形槁肢羸, 飲食不進, 腸胃滑泄, 津液枯竭.

      (2)久服生血益氣, 暖胃駐顏.

·歸經：手足太陰藥

·方義：(1)喻嘉言曰：「此方可謂長于用補矣.」

      (2)人參, 羊肉…同功.

      (3)蓯蓉, 山藥…爲男子之佳珍.

      (4)合之：當歸…養榮；黃耆…益衛；天冬…保肺；白朮…健脾.

      (5)其製法尤精, 允爲補方之首.

7. San Cai Feng Sui Wan. Heaven, Earth, Human, and Seal up Marrow Pills. 三才封髓丸

·**ACTIONS**：supplements the spleen, lung, and kidney

·**COMPOSITION**：Tian Men Dong, Ren Shen, Shu Di Huang, Huang Bai, Sha Ren, Gan Cao

·**INDICATIONS**：descends heart fire, boosts kidney water, enriches yin and tonifies blood, moistens without drying.

·**CHANNELS ENTERED**：The hand and foot greater yin and the foot lesser yin channels. [The lung, spleen, and kidney]

·**Analysis of Formula**：(1) Tian Men Dong supplements the lung and engenders water. Ren Shen supplements the spleen and boosts qi. Shu Di Huang supplements Kidney and nourishes yin.

      (2) 喻嘉言 says that：Huang Bai enters the kidney to enrich yin, Sha Ren enter s the spleen to move stagnation, Gan Cao weakens a little the bitter of Tian Men Dong and Huang Bai and helps Ren Shen tonifying the middle qi, through this, the action of ascending and descending of the lung and kidney works well.

·**RELATED FORMULA**：(1) without Huang Bai, Sha Ren, and Gan Cao in this formula, this is called San Cai Tang, this treats cough due to the vacuous vexation of the spleen and lung. .

      (2) without Tian Men Dong, Ren Shen, and Shu Di Huang in this

35

formula, this is called Feng Sui Dan, treats heart fire exuberant, kidney essence insecurity, and seminal emission occurred often.

7. 三才封髓丸
　·總結：補脾肺腎
　·組成：天冬, 人參, 熟地, 黃柏, 砂仁, 甘草
　·主治：降心火, 益腎水, 滋陰養血, 潤而不燥.
　·歸經：手足太陰足少陰藥
　·方義：(1)天冬：以補肺生水, 人參：以補脾益氣, 熟地：以補腎滋陰.
　(2)喻嘉言曰：加黃柏以入腎滋陰, 加砂仁以入脾行滯, 加甘草以少變天冬, 黃柏之苦 ⇒ 俾合「人參」建立中氣, 以伸參兩之權, 殊非好爲增益成方之比也.
　·變化方：(1)除後三味等分煎⇒名三才湯, 治脾肺虛勞欬嗽.
　　　　　(2)除前三味⇒名鳳髓丹, 治心火旺盛, 腎精不固, 易于施泄.

8. Da Zao Wan. Great Creation Pill. 大造丸

·**ACTIONS**：vacuity detriment of the lung and kidney

·**COMPOSITION**：Zi He Che, Huang Bai, Gui Ban, Niu Xi, Du Zhong, Di Huang, Ren Shen, Mai Men Dong, Tian Men Dong

·**INDICATIONS**：vacuity detriment and taxation damage, cough and tidal heat effusion.

·**MODIFICATIONS**：in summer, add Wu Wei Zi.

In case of women, eliminate Gui Ban and add Dang Gui.

·**CHANNELS ENTERED**：The hand greater yin and the lesser yin channels. [The lung and kidney]

·**Analysis of Formula**：(1) Zi He Che is originally the place where the blood and qi of the body engenders, can supplement qi and blood, and acts as a sovereign.

(2) Gui Ban is supplied with yin qi perfectly, Huang Bai is supplied with yin qi strongly, thus they nourish yin and supplement water and act as a minister.

(3) Du Zhong moistens the kidney and supplements lumbus.

(4) Niu Xi strengthens sinew and invigorates bone.

(5) Shu Di Huang nourishes yin and abates heat, is restrained by Fu Ling and Sha Ren, enters the lesser yin, and boosts kidney essence.

36

(6) Tian Men Dong and Mai Men Dong descend fire and clear metal, with Ren Shen and Wu Wei Zi, can engender vessel and supplement lung qi.

This formula is based on the theory that metal and water are the source of engendering and transformation, therefore the composition of this formula is concentrated on supplementing the lung and kidney.

·**Original Source**：Wu Qiu

8. 大造丸

  ·總結：肺腎虛損

  ·組成：紫河車，黃柏，敗龜板，牛膝，杜仲，地黃，人參，麥冬，天冬

  ·主治：治虛損勞傷，欬嗽潮熱.

  ·加減：夏…加五味子.

      女人…去龜板，加當歸(乳煮糊丸).

  ·歸經：手太陰足少陰藥

  ·方義：(1)紫河車…本血氣所生，大補氣血爲君

      (2)敗龜板…陰氣最全；黃柏…稟陰氣最厚⇒滋陰補水爲臣

      (3)杜仲…潤腎補腰.

      (4)牛膝…強筋壯骨.

      (5)熟地黃…養陰退熱，製以「茯苓，砂仁」→入少陰而益腎精.

      (6)天冬，麥冬…降火清金，合之「人參，五味」→能生脈而補肺氣.

      大要以金水爲生化之原，合補之以成大造之功也

  ·煎服法：酒米糊丸，鹽湯下，冬酒下.

  ·來源：吳球

9. Bu Tian Wan. Tonify Heaven Pills. 補天丸

·**ACTIONS**：kidney detriment

·**COMPOSITION**：Huang Bai, Gui Ban, Du Zhong, Niu Xi, Zi He Che, Chen Pi

·**INDICATIONS**：emaciation of qi and blood, Six Pulse are fine and rapid, the pattern of vacuity taxation.

·**MODIFICATIONS**：In winter, add Gan Jiang (five qian). In summer, add Wu Wei Zi (one liang, stir-bake)

·**CHANNELS ENTERED**：The lesser yin channel. [The kidney]

·**Analysis of Formula**：(1) Huang Bai and Gui Ban enrich the kidney. Du Zhong and Niu Xi are the herbs invigorating lumbus and knee, and supplement Kidney and strengthen yin.

(2) Zi He Che is called Hun Dun Pi (the skin of chaos). Zi He Che is the place where blood and qi engender. By using blood and qi, it supplements qi and blood, as later heaven helps earlier heaven, therefore this is called Bu Tian Wan. (Tonify Heaven Pills).

(3) Chen Pi is added to regulate qi during supplementing blood.

(4) In winter the weather is cold, add Gan Jiang to assist yang. In summer, exuberant fire burns metal, add Wu Wei Zi to preserve the lung.

·**Original Source**：Dan Xi

9. 補天丸

　·總結：腎損

　·組成：黃柏，龜板，杜仲，牛膝，河車，陳皮

　·主治：治氣血衰弱，六脈細數虛勞之證.

　·加減：冬加乾薑五錢. 夏加炒五味子一兩.

　·歸經：足少陰藥也

　·方義：(1)黃柏，龜板…滋腎之藥；杜仲，牛膝…腰膝之藥；皆以補腎而強陰也.

(2)紫河車，名曰混沌皮…用氣血以補氣血，假後天以濟先天，故曰補天.

(3)加「陳皮」者…于補血之中而兼調其氣也

(4)冬月寒水用事，故加乾薑以助陽. 夏月火旺爍金，故加五味以保肺.

　·來源：丹溪

10. Ren Shen Gu Ben Wan. Ginseng Decoction Guard the Root Pills. 人參固本丸

·**ACTIONS**：　lung taxation

·**COMPOSITION**：Tian Men Dong, Mai Men Dong, Shu Di Huang, Sheng Di Huang, Ren Shen

·**INDICATIONS**：　lung taxation and vacuous heat effusion.

·**CHANNELS ENTERED**：The hand greater yin and the foot lesser yin.

[The lung and kidney]

·**Analysis of Formula**：(1) The lung controls qi which is rooted to cinnabar field, therefore the lung and kidney are in the relationship of mother and son, sufficient kidney water can constrain heart fire and then fire is unable to punish metal.

(2) Tian Men Dong and Mai Men Dong clears lung heat.

(3) Shu Di Huang and Sheng Di Huang boosts kidney water.

(4) Ren Shen greatly supplements source qi. Qi is the mother of water, Ren Shen can be used variously, it leads qi herbs to supplement yang and blood herbs to supplement yin.

10. 人參固本丸

·總結：肺勞

·組成：天冬, 麥冬, 熟地, 生地, 人參

·主治：治肺勞虛熱.

·歸經：手太陰足少陰藥

·方義：(1)肺主氣, 而氣根于丹田, 故肺腎爲子母之臟, 必水能制火, 而後火不刑金也.

(2)二冬...清肺熱.

(3)二地...益腎水.

(4)人參...大補元氣. 氣者水之母也, 且人參之用, 無所不宜, 以氣藥引之則補陽, 以血藥引之亦補陰也.

11. Shen Ru Wan. Ginseng and Breast Milk Pills. 參乳丸

·**ACTIONS**：supplements qi and blood.

·**COMPOSITION**：Ren Shen, breast milk.

·**INDICATIONS**：greatly supplements qi and blood.

·**CHANNELS ENTERED**：The hand and foot greater yin and the foot reverting yin channel. [The lung, spleen, and liver]

·**Analysis of Formula**：(1) Ren Shen greatly supplements source qi.

(2) Breast milk is originally transformed from blood, with Ren Shen supplements qi and blood.

11. 參乳丸

·總結：氣血交補

·組成：人參, 人乳

39

·主治：大補氣血.

·歸經：手足太陰足厥陰藥也

·方義：⑴人參…大補元氣.

　　　　⑵人乳…本血液化成, 用之以交補氣血, 實平淡之神奇也.

·煎服法：頓乳取粉法：取無病年少婦人乳, 用銀瓢或錫瓢, 傾乳少許, 浮滾水上頓, 再浮冷水上立乾, 刮取粉用, 如攤粉皮法.

12. Tian Wang Bu Xin Dan. Emperor of Heaven's Special Pill to Tonify the heart. 天王補心丹

·**ACTIONS**：supplements the heart

·**COMPOSITION**：Jie Geng, Tian Men Dong, Mai Men Dong, Ren Shen, Fu Ling, Sheng Di Huang, Yuan Shen, Zao Ren, Wu Wei Zi, Yuan Zhi, Bai Zi Ren, Dan Shen, Dang Gui, Honey, Zhu Sha

·**INDICATIONS**：(1) excessive thinking, insufficiency of heart blood, fearful throbbing with forgetfulness, and profuse sweating.

(2) constipation or sloppy stool, sore of the mouth and tongue, etc.

·**CHANNELS ENTERED**：The hand lesser yin channel. [The heart]

·**Analysis of Formula**：(1) Sheng Di Huang and Yuan Shen belong to herbs of kidney, supplement water to constrain fire, this makes the heart and kidney to help each other.

(2) Dan Shen and Dang Gui engender heart blood.

(3) Blood engenders from qi, Ren Shen and Fu Ling boosts heart qi.

(4) The combination of Ren Shen, Mai Men Dong, and Wu Wei Zi is Sheng Mai San, the heart controls vessels, the lung is the florid canopy of the heart and the most of blood vessels meet in the lung, this supplements the lung and engenders vessel, therefore this formula makes heaven qi [lung qi] to descend.

(5) The bitter of Tian Men Dong enters the heart and the cold drains fire, with Mai Men Dong enriches water and moistens dryness.

(6) Yuan Zhi, Zao Ren, and Bai Zi Ren nourish heart spirit.

(7) The sour of Zao Ren and Wu Wei Zi has a astringent character, this collects the consumed heart qi.

(8) Jie Geng clears the lung and disinhibits the diaphragm, and le

ads every herbs upward to turn back to the heart, therefore this acts as a courier.

(9) The color of Zhu Sha is red, enters the heart, cold drains heat and quiets spirit.

(10) One who read books often should frequently take this pills.

12. 天王補心丹

·總結：補心

·組成：桔梗, 天冬, 麥冬, 人參, 茯苓, 生地, 元參, 棗仁, 五味, 遠志, 柏仁, 丹參, 當歸, 蜜, 硃砂

·主治：(1)治思慮過度, 心血不足, 怔忡健忘. 心口多汗.

(2)大便秘或溏, 口舌生瘡等證.

·歸經：手少陰藥

·方義：(1)生地, 元參, 北方之藥, 補水所以制火, 取既濟之義也.

(2)丹參, 當歸, 所以生心血.

(3)血生于氣, 人參, 茯苓所以益心氣.

(4)人參合麥冬, 五味, 又爲生脈散. 蓋心主脈, 肺爲心之華蓋而朝百脈, 補肺生脈, 所以使天氣下降也.

(5)天冬, 苦入心而寒瀉火, 與麥冬同爲滋水潤燥之劑.

(6)遠志, 棗仁, 柏仁, 所以養心神.

(7)而棗仁, 五味, 酸以收之, 又以斂心氣之耗散也.

(8)桔梗, 清肺利膈取其載藥上浮而歸于心, 故以爲使.

(9)硃砂, 色赤入心, 寒瀉熱而重寧神.

(10)讀書之人, 所當常服.

13. Kong Sheng Zhen Zhong Dan. Sagely Confucius' Pillow Elixir. 孔聖枕中丹

·**ACTIONS**：supplements the heart and kidney

·**COMPOSITION**：Yuan Zhi, Shi Chang Pu, Gui Ban, Long Gu

·**INDICATIONS**：tendency to forget what reading, enduring Long-term taking of this makes people bright.

·**CHANNELS ENTERED**：The hand and foot lesser yin channel. [The heart and kidney]

·**Analysis of Formula**：(1) Gui Ban is the top of Crustacea and is a mystical yin character animal. Long Gu is the top in the animal with squama and is a mystical yang character animal, with the yin and yang animals, this supplement s human's yin and yang, and with the mystical qi of these, assists spirit qi of the heart in human.

(2) Human's essence and mind are stored in the kidney, when kid ney essence is insufficiency, mind qi gets weak and is unable to free upward to the heart, forgetfulness frequently occurs.

(3) The bitter of Yuan Zhi drains heat and the pungent disperses congestion and is able to free to kidney qi and reaches upward to the heart, ther efore it strengthens mind and boosts wisdom.

(4) The pungent of Shi Chang Pu disperses the liver and the aro ma soothes the spleen, thus it opens heart pore and disinhibits nine pores, and e liminates damp and phlegm.

(5) Gui Ban can supplement the kidney, Long Gu can settle the li ver, they makes phlegm fire dispersed and the heart and liver quieted, therefore memory becomes better.

·**Original Source**：Tian Jin Yao Fang

13. 孔聖枕中丹
　·總結：補心腎
　·組成：遠志, 菖蒲, 敗龜板, 龍骨
　·主治：治讀書善忘, 久服令人聰明.
　·歸經：手足少陰藥
　·方義：(1)龜者介蟲之長, 陰物之至靈者也；龍者鱗蟲之長, 陽物之至靈者也, 借二物之陰陽, 以補吾身之陰陽, 假二物之靈氣, 以助吾心之靈氣者.

(2)又人之精與志, 皆藏于腎, 腎精不足, 則志氣衰, 不能上通於心, 故迷惑善忘也.

(3)遠志, 苦洩熱而辛散鬱...能通腎氣上達于心, 强志益智.

(4)菖蒲, 辛散肝而香舒脾...能開心孔而利九竅, 去濕除痰.

(5)又龜能補腎, 龍能鎮肝, 使痰火散而心肝寧, 則聰明開而記憶强矣.
　·來源：千金

14. Da Bu Yin Wan Great. Tonify the Yin Pill. 大補陰丸

·**ACTIONS**：supplements yin

·**COMPOSITION**：Huang Bai, Zhi Mu, Shu Di Huang, Gui Ban

·**INDICATIONS**：(1) water depletion and fire flaming, tinnitus and deafness, counterflow cough due to vacuity heat.

(2) when the pulse in the kidney part is surging and large, one cannot use supplementing treatment strongly.

·**CHANNELS ENTERED**：The foot lesser yin channel. [The kidney]

·**Analysis of Formula**：(1) Huang Bai, Zhi Mu, Shu Di Huang, and Gui Ban nourish yin and supplement Kidney. They supplement water to descend fire, in other word, invigorating water restrains yang exasperation.

(2) the reason of adding the marrow of pig is because the marrow frees to the kidney, bone enters bone and marrow supplements marrow.

·**Original Source**：Dan Xi

14. 大補陰丸

·總結：補陰

·組成：黄柏, 知母, 熟地黄, 敗龜板

·主治：(1)治水虧火炎, 耳鳴耳聾, 欬逆虛熱.

(2)腎脈洪大, 不能受峻補者.

·歸經：足少陰藥也

·方義：(1)四者皆滋陰補腎之藥, 補水卽所以降火, 所謂壯水之主以制陽光是也.

(2)加脊髓者, 取其通腎命, 以骨入骨, 以髓補髓也.

·來源：丹溪

15. Zi Yin Wan. Nourish Yin Pills to. 滋腎丸

·**ACTIONS**：supplements water

·**COMPOSITION**：Huang Bai, Zhi Mu, Rou Gui

·**INDICATIONS**：(1) steaming heat effusion due to kidney vacuity, lack of strength in the legs and knees, yin wilting and yin sweating, thoroughfare vessel surging upward with panting.

(2) evil heat in the lower burner, absence of thirsty with inhibited urination.

·**CHANNELS ENTERED**：The foot lesser yin channel. [The kidney]

·**Analysis of Formula**：(1) When water fails to overcome fire, one should invigorate water to restrain yang exasperation.

(2) The bitter, cold, and mild pungent of Huang Bai drains the bladder and ministerial fire, supplements insufficiency of kidney water, and enters the blood part in the kidney channel. The pungent, bitter, and cold of Zhi Mu clears lung metal and descends fire in the upper part, and moistens kidney dryness and nourishes yin and enters the qi part in the kidney channel, therefore Huang Bai and Zhi Mu reinforce each other's action with moving, and are good herbs at supplementing water.

(3) The pungent and heat of Rou Gui is used as a counteracting assistant [of huang bai and zhi mu] and leads them to the foot lesser yin channel. Small amount of heat herb is added as a counteracting assistant.

·**RELATED FORMULA**：(1) When Rou Gui is eliminated, this is called Liao Shen Zi Ben Wan, treats blurred vision due to kidney vacuity.

(2) When Rou Gui is eliminated and Huang Lian is added, this is called Huang Bai Zi Shen Wan, treats upper heat and lower cold, heart vexation due to depleted water.

(3) When only one herb of Huang Bai is used, this is called Da Bu Wan, treats vacuity heat of the kidney and bladder, pain in the lumbus and leg and heat in the soles.

(4) When only one herb of huang bai (powder) is taken with ginger juice, this is called Qian Xing San, treats gout and deep multiple abscess below lumbus.

·**Original Source**：Li Dong Yuan

15. 滋腎丸
·總結：補水
·組成：黃柏, 知母, 桂
·主治：(1)治腎虛蒸熱, 脚膝無力, 陰痿陰汗, 衝脈上衝而喘.

(2)及下焦邪熱, 口不渴而小便秘.
·歸經：足少陰藥
·方義：(1)水不勝火, 法當壯水以制陽光.

(2)黃柏, 苦寒微辛瀉膀胱相火, 補腎水不足, 入腎經血分；知母, 辛苦寒滑, 上清肺金而降火, 下潤腎燥而滋陰, 入腎經氣分, ⇒故二藥每相須而行, 爲補水之良劑.

(3)肉桂, 辛熱, 假以反佐, 爲少陰引經, 寒因熱用也.
·變化方：(1)去桂...名療腎滋本丸, 治腎虛目昏.

(2)去桂加黃連...名黃柏滋腎丸, 治上熱下冷, 水衰心煩.

(3)單黃柏一味...名大補丸, 治腎膀胱虛熱, 腰股痛而足心熱.

44

(4)爲末, 薑汁酒調服...名潛行散, 治痛風腰以下濕熱流注.

·來源：東垣

16. Ban Long Wan. Striped Dragon Pill. 斑龍丸

·**ACTIONS**：supplements yang

·**COMPOSITION**：Lu Jiao Jiao, Lu Jiao Shuang, Tu Si Zi, Shu Di Huang , Bai Zi Ren

·**INDICATIONS**：treats vacuity detriment, controls one hundred disease, keeps one young and makes one live a long life.

·**CHANNELS ENTERED**：The hand and foot lesser yin channel. [The heart and kidney]

·**Analysis of Formula**：(1) Lu Jiao Shuang, Tu Si Zi, and Shu Di Huang are the herbs entering the blood part of kidney channel and greatly supplement essence and marrow.

(2) Bai Zi Ren enters the heart and nourishes heart qi, and also enters the kidney and moistens kidney dryness, makes the heart and kidney interact. When heart mind is exuberant, spirit and ethereal soul are quiet, when essence and marrow are sufficient, sinew and bone get invigorated, this eliminates disease and makes one live a long life.

16. 斑龍丸

·總結：補陽

·組成：鹿角膠, 鹿角霜, 菟絲子, 熟地黃, 柏子仁

·主治：治虛損, 理百病, 駐顏益壽.

·歸經：手足少陰藥

·方義：(1)鹿角霜, 菟絲, 熟地...皆腎經血藥也, 大補精髓.

(2)柏子仁...入心而養心氣, 又能入腎而潤腎燥, 使心腎相交. 心志旺而神魂安, 精髓充而筋骨壯, 去病益壽, 不亦宜乎.

·又附方：一方加補骨脂. 一方加鹿茸, 肉蓯蓉, 陽起石, 附子, 黃耆, 當歸, 棗仁炒, 辰砂, 亦名斑龍丸.

·煎服法：等分爲末. 酒化膠爲丸.

45

17. Gui Lu Er Xian Gao. Tortoise Shell and Deer Antler Paste. 龜鹿二仙膏

·**ACTIONS**：supplements qi and blood

·**COMPOSITION**：Gui Ban, Lu Jiao, Ren Shen, Gou Qi

·**INDICATIONS**：emaciation, shortage of qi, dream emission, seminal emission, poor eyesight, the pattern of essence collapse.

·**CHANNELS ENTERED**：The foot lesser yin channel. [The kidney]

·**Analysis of Formula**：(1) Gui Ban is the top of Crustacea and is supplied with yin qi perfectly.

(2) Lu Jiao takes off Cornu at the summer solstice, is supplied with pure yang, before two months passes, the Cornu grows to the height of ten or twenty Jin, the growth of bone is not so fast as this, therefore it can greatly supplement qi and blood. The Qi and blood in Gui Ban and Lu Jiao are used to supplement qi and blood in body.

(3) Ren Shen greatly supplements source qi.

(4) Gou Qi nourishes yin and assists yang.

(5) This formula supplements all of blood, qi, yin, and yang. When qi is sufficient, essence is secured and seminal emission will not occur. When blood is sufficient, vision and hearing are clear. Enduring Long-term use of this makes one live a long life, how does it treat only disease?

17. 龜鹿二仙膏

·總結：補氣血

·組成：龜板，鹿角，人參，枸杞

·主治：治瘦弱少氣，夢遺洩精，目視不明，精極之證.

·歸經：足少陰藥

·方義：(1)龜，爲介蟲之長，得陰氣最全.

(2)鹿角，遇夏至卽解，稟純陽之性，且不兩月，長至一，二十斤，骨之速生無過於此者，故能峻補氣血. 兩者皆用氣血以補氣血，所謂補之其類也.

(3)人參...大補元氣.

(4)枸杞...滋陰助陽.

(5)此血氣陰陽交補之劑，氣足則精固不遺，血足則視聽明了，久服可以益壽，豈第已疾而已哉.

18. Bu Hup Wan. Tonify Fire Pills. 補火丸

·**ACTIONS**：supplements the kidney and life fire

·**COMPOSITION**：Shi Liu Huang, Zhu Da Chang (pig's large intestine)

·**INDICATIONS**：cold taxation, desiccation of qi and blood, flesh emaciation and falling out of teeth, fatigued cumbersome limbs and lack of strength in speaking.

·**CHANNELS ENTERED**：The foot lesser yin kidney and life gate.

·**Analysis of Formula**：(1) Liu Huang is the essence of fire. This is also called 'General' and is used to supplement fire.

(2) Liu Huang is great heat and toxin, therefore pig's large intestine is used to resolve and moderate the heat and toxin character. Mundane doctors fear to use it so that just uses a little, they don't know that Liu Huang can break evil and make right qi to return, eliminate stagnation and make clear qi to come back, disperse yin evil and make origin yang to return, and transform corporeal soul and engender ethereal soul.

18. 補火丸

·總結：補腎命火

·組成：石硫黃，豬大腸

·主治：治冷勞，氣血枯竭，肉瘠齒落，肢倦言微.

·歸經：足少陰命門藥

·方義：(1)硫黃：火之精也，亦號將軍…故用之以補火.

(2)以其大熱有毒，故用豬腸爛煮以解之. 庸俗之人，忌而罕用，蓋不知其有破邪歸正，返滯還清，消陰回陽，化魄生魂之力也.

19. Tang Zheng Xiang Guo Fang. Tang Premier Zheng's Folrmula. 唐鄭相國方

·**ACTIONS**：supplements the lung and kidney

·**COMPOSITION**：Po Gu Zhi, Hu Tao Rou

·**INDICATIONS**：treats vacuity cold with panting and cough, aching lumbus and legs.

·**CHANNELS ENTERED**：The hand greater yin and foot lesser yin channel. [The lung and kidney]

·**Analysis of Formula**：(1) Po Gu Zhi belongs to fire, enters pericardium and life g ate, can supplement ministerial fire to free sovereign fire, warm cinnabar field, and invigorate origin yang.

⑵ Hu Tao Rou belongs to wood, can free life gate, disinhibit the triple burner, warm the lung, moisten intestines, and supplement and nourish qi and blood. This formula has the meaning of wood engendering fire. When qi is sufficient, the lung is not vacuous cold, when blood is sufficient, the kidney is not desiccated. Long-term use of this formula is benefit to the body, this formula not only treats panting and cough in the upper part but also strengthens lumbus and legs.

·**RELATED FORMULA**：⑴ When Du Zhong (one Jin) and Sheng Jiang (stir-bake with garlic, four Liang) are added, this is called Qing E Wan, treats lumbar pain due to vacuous kidney. Again when Niu Xi, Huang Bai, and Chuan Bi Xie are added, this teats same things.

⑵ When Du Zhong, Hu Lu Ba, Xiao Hui Xiang, and Bi Xie are added, this is called He Qi Wan, treats mounting(shan) pain which spreads to lumbus.

19. 唐鄭相國方
·總結：補肺腎
·組成：破故紙，胡桃肉
·主治：治虛寒喘嗽，腰腳酸痛.
·歸經：手太陰足少陰藥
·方義：⑴破故紙，屬火，入心包命門，能補相火以通君火，暖丹田，壯元陽.

⑵胡桃，屬木，能通命門，利三焦，溫肺潤腸，補養氣血，有木火相生之妙. 氣足則肺不虛寒，血足則腎不枯燥，久服利益甚多，不獨上療喘嗽，下強腰腳而已也.

·變化方：⑴本方加杜仲一斤，生薑炒蒜四兩…名青娥丸，治腎虛腰痛. 再加牛膝，黃柏，川萆薢，蜜丸…治同.

⑵本方加杜仲，胡盧巴，小茴香，萆薢…名喝起丸，治小腸氣痛引腰.

20. Er Zhi Wan. Two-Ultimate Pill. 二至丸

·**ACTIONS**：supplement s the kidney

·**COMPOSITION**：Han Lian Cao, Dong Qing Zi (Nu Zhen Zi)

·**INDICATIONS**：supplements lumbus and knees, invigorates sinew and bone, strengthens yin kidney, and blackens the hair and beard.

·**CHANNELS ENTERED**：The foot lesser yin channel. [The kidney]

·**Analysis of Formula**：(1) Nu Zhen Zi is sweet and neutral, the color is blue with black, boosts the liver and supplements the kidney.

(2) Han Lian Cao is sweet and cold, this enters the kidney and supplements essence, therefore this can boost the lower part and nourish the upper part, and strengthen yin and blacken hair and beard.

20. 二至丸

　　·總結：補腎
　　·組成：旱蓮草, 冬青子(卽女貞子)
　　·主治：補腰膝, 壯筋骨, 強陰腎, 烏髭髮, 價廉而功大.
　　·歸經：足少陰藥
　　·方義：(1)女貞甘平, 少陰之精, 隆冬不凋, 其色青黑, 益肝補腎.
　　　　　　(2)旱蓮甘寒, 汁黑入腎補精, 故能益下而榮上, 強陰而黑髮

也.

21. Fu Sang Wan. Mulberry Leaf and Sesame Pill. 扶桑丸

·**ACTIONS**：eliminates wind-damp and moistens five viscera.

·**COMPOSITION**：(tender) Sang Ye, Hei Zhi Ma, Honey

·**INDICATIONS**：eliminates wind-damp, recovers from emaciation, blackens hair and beard, eliminates disease, and makes one live ling life.

·**CHANNELS ENTERED**：The foot lesser yin and the hand and foot yang brightness channels. [The kidney, large intestine, and stomach].

·**Analysis of Formula**：(1) A mulberry tree disinhibits joints, nourishes the liquid and humor, Sang Ye is sweet and cold, enters the hand and foot yang brightness to cool blood, dry damp, and eliminate wind.

(2) Hei Zhi Ma is sweet and neutral, the color is black. This boosts the kidney, supplements the liver, moistens the organs and bowels, and replenishes essence marrow.

(3) Generally when wind-damp are eliminated, sinew and bone get strong, when essence and marrow are charged, complexion is good, disease is eliminated, and hair and beard become black.

49

·**Original Source**：Hu Seng

21. 扶桑丸
　·總結：除風濕潤五臟
　·組成：嫩桑葉，巨勝子(卽黑脂麻)，白蜜
　·主治：除風濕，起羸尫，烏髭髮，卻病延年.
　·歸經：足少陰手足陽明藥
　·方義：(1)桑乃箕星之精，其木利關節，養津液，其葉甘寒，入手足陽明，涼血燥濕而除風.
　　　　　(2)巨勝，甘平，色黑…益腎補肝，潤臟腑，填精髓.
　　　　　(3)夫風溼去則筋骨強，精髓充則容顏澤，卻病烏髭，不亦宜乎?
　·來源：胡僧

22. Shen Ling Bai Zhu San. Ginseng, Poria, and Atractylodes Macrocephala Powder. 參苓白朮散

·**ACTIONS**：supplements the spleen

·**COMPOSITION**：Ren Shen, Bai Zhu, Fu Ling, Gan Cao, Lian Rou, Shan Yao, Bian Dou, Yi Yi Ren, Sha Ren, Chen Pi, Jie Geng

·**INDICATIONS**：treats weak spleen and stomach, non-dispersion of food and drink, or vomiting, or diarrhea.

·**CHANNELS ENTERED**：The foot greater yin and yang brightness channels. [The spleen and stomach]

·**Analysis of Formula**：(1) when treating the spleen and stomach, one should supplement vacuity, eliminate damp, move stagnation, and regulate qi.

　　　　(2) Ren Shen, Bai Zhu, Fu Ling, Gan Cao, Shan Yao, Yi Yi Ren, Bian Dou, and Lian Rou supplement the spleen channel.

　　　　(3) Fu Ling, Shan Yao, and Yi Yi Ren rectify the spleen and also can drain damp.

　　　　(4) Sha Ren and Chen Pi regulate qi and move stagnation. Ren Shen, Bai Zhu, Fu Ling, and Gan Cao warm the stomach and can supplement the middle.

　　　　(5) Jie Geng is bitter and sweet. This enters the lung. This can conduct every herb to the upper part, and also can free heaven qi to earth qi. When qi ascends and descends normally, qi is boosted and harmonious, and this pre

serves the lung and makes the dry herbs not to attack the upper part.

22. 參苓白朮散
　·總結：補脾
　·組成：人參，白朮，茯苓，甘草，蓮肉，山藥，扁豆，薏仁，砂仁，陳皮，桔梗
　·主治：治脾胃虛弱，飲食不消，或吐或瀉.
　·歸經：足太陰陽明藥
　·方義：(1)治脾胃者...補其虛，除其濕，行其滯，調其氣而已：
　　　　　(2)人參，白朮，茯苓，甘草，山藥，薏仁，扁豆，蓮肉...皆補脾之藥也.
　　　　　(3)茯苓，山藥，薏仁...理脾而兼能滲濕.
　　　　　(4)砂仁，陳皮...調氣行滯之品也. 然合「參，朮，苓，草」，暖胃而又能補中.
　　　　　(5)桔梗苦甘入肺...能載諸藥上浮，又能通天氣于地道，使氣得升降而益和，且以保肺，防燥之上僭也.

23. Miao Xiang San. Beautiful Aucklandia Powder. 妙香散

·**ACTIONS**：seminal emission and fright palpitations
·**COMPOSITION**：Shan Yao, Jie Geng, Mu Xiang, Yuan Zhi, Fu Ling, Fu Shen, Gan Cao, Dan Sha, She Xiang, Ren Shen, Huang Qi
·**INDICATIONS**：treats dream emission, consumption of essence, right p alpitations, and depression.
·**CHANNELS ENTERED**：The hand and foot lesser yin. [The heart and kidney]
·**Analysis of Formula**：(1) The heart is sovereign fire, if sovereign fire move s once, ministerial fire follows, ministerial fire entrusts to the liver and gall bl adder. When kidney yin is vacuous, essence is unable to be stored. If liver ya ng is excessive, qi fails to secure, therefore collapse of essence and dreaming of intercourse occur.

(2) Shan Yao boosts yin and clears heat, and also can contract es sence, therefore this acts as sovereign.

(3) Ren Shen and Huang Qi secure qi. Yuan Zhi, Fu Ling, and Z hu Ling quiet spirit. When spirit is quiet and qi is secure, essence spontaneousl y preserves the position.

51

(4) Fu Ling and Zhu Ling move downward and disinhibit water, and also drain the evil fire of the kidney.

(5) Jie Geng clears the lung and disperses stagnation.

(6) Mu Xiang courses the liver and harmonizes the spleen.

(7) Dan Sha settles the heart and quiets spirit. She Xiang frees orifices and resolves depression. Dan Sha and She Xiang also can expel evil and treat disease contracted evil.

(8) Gan Cao is used to harmonize the middle.

·**Original Source**：Wang Jing Gong

23. 妙香散

·總結：遺精驚悸

·組成：山藥，桔梗，木香，遠志，茯苓，茯神，甘草，丹砂，麝香，人參，黃耆

·主治：治夢遺失精，驚悸鬱結.

·歸經：手足少陰藥

·方義：⑴心君火也，君火一動，相火隨之，相火寄于肝膽. 腎之陰虛，則精不藏. 肝之陽強，則氣不固，故精脫而成夢矣.

⑵山藥...益陰清熱，兼能濇精，故以爲君.

⑶人參，黃耆...所以固其氣；遠志，二茯...所以寧其神，神寧氣固，則精自守其位矣.

⑷且二茯...下行利水，又以泄腎中之邪火也.

⑸桔梗...清肺散滯.

⑹木香...疏肝和脾.

⑺丹砂...鎮心安神；麝香...通竅解鬱，二藥又能辟邪，亦所以治其邪感也.

⑻加甘草者...用以交和乎中，猶黃婆之媒嬰妊也.

·來源：王荆公

24. Yu Ping Feng San. Jade Windscreen Powder. 玉屏風散

·**ACTIONS**：supplements exterior.

·**COMPOSITION**：Huang Qi, Bai Zhu, Fang Feng

·**INDICATIONS**：treats incessant spontaneous sweating, qi vacuity and exterior weakness, often contraction to wind and cold.

52

·**CHANNELS ENTERED**：The foot greater yang and the hand and foot greater yin channels [The bladder, lung, and spleen]

·**Analysis of Formula**：(1) Huang Qi supplements qi, only secures flesh exterior, therefore acts as sovereign.

(2) Bai Zhu boosts the spleen, the spleen governs the flesh, therefore acts as minister.

(3) Fang Feng eliminates wind and belongs to wind herb, Huang Qi fears it, therefore it acts as courier.

·**RELATED FORMULA**：(1) When this formula is boiled with an equal division, this is called Huang Qi Tang, Jie Gu uses this formula instead of Gui Zhi Tang, treats heat effusion and sweating in spring and summer, the pulse that is faint and weak, aversion to wind and cold, if aversion to wind is severe, add Gui Zhi.

(2) Chuan Xiong, Cang Zhu, Qiang Huo is boiled with an equal division, this is called Chuan Xiong Tang, this is used instead of Ma Huang Tang, treats heat effusion, absence of sweating in autumn and winter, and aversion to wind and cold, if aversion to cold is severe, add Ma Huang.

24. 玉屏風散
    ·總結：補表
    ·組成：黃耆, 白朮, 防風
    ·主治：治自汗不止, 氣虛表弱, 易感風寒.
    ·歸經：足太陽手足太陰藥也
    ·方義：(1)黃耆...補氣, 專固肌表, 故以爲君.
        (2)白朮...益脾, 脾主肌肉, 故以爲臣.
        (3)防風...去風, 爲風藥卒徒, 而黃耆畏之, 故以爲使.
    ·變化方：(1)前藥等分煎...名黃耆湯, 潔古用代「桂枝湯」, 治春夏發熱有汗, 脈微弱, 惡風寒者. 惡風甚...加桂枝.
        (2)又用川芎, 蒼朮, 羌活等分...名川芎湯, 以代「麻黃湯」. 治秋冬發熱無汗, 惡風寒者. 惡寒甚...加麻黃.

25. Si Jun Zi Tang. Four-Gentlemen Decoction. 四君子湯

·**ACTIONS**：supplements yang and boosts qi

·**COMPOSITION**：Ren Shen, Bai Zhu, Fu Ling, Gan Cao, Sheng Jiang, Da Zao

·**INDICATIONS** ∶ all kinds of yang vacuity and qi weakness, spleen emaciat ion and lung detriment, little thought of food and drink, emaciation with yello w complexion, the cracked skin and loss of hair. The pulse is fine and soft wh en coming.

·**CHANNELS ENTERED** ∶ The hand and foot greater yin and foot yang brightness channels [the lung, spleen, and stomach]

·**Analysis of Formula** ∶ (1) The sweet and warm of Ren Shen greatly supp lements source qi and acts as a sovereign

(2) The bitter and warm of Bai Zhu dries the spleen and supplem ents qi, acts as a minister.

(3) The sweet and bland of Fu Ling drains damp and drains heat, acts as an assistant

(4) The sweet and neutral of Gan Cao harmonizes the middle and boosts earth, acts as a courier. When qi is sufficient, the spleen transports qi, di et increases, the other organ can be nourished, complexion becomes better, and the body gets stronger.

(5) Chen Pi rectifies qi and disperses counterflow. Ban Xia dries damp and eliminates phlegm, when Chen Pi and Ban Xia are added, this is call ed Liu Jun Zi Tang.

·**RELATED FORMULA** ∶ (1) When Chen Pi is added, this is called Yi G ong San (Extraordinary Merit Powder), regulates and rectifies Spleen and Stom ach.

(2) When Ban Xia is again added to Yi Gong San, this is called Liu Jun Zi Tang, treats qi vacuity with phlegm and tympanites due to spleen vacuit y.

(3) When Xiang Fu and Sha Ren are again added to Liu Jun Zi T ang, this is called Xiang Sha Liu Jun Zi Tang, treats stomach pain due to vacuit y cold or abdominal pain or diarrhea.

(4) Liu Jun Zi Tang with Mai Men Dong and Zhu Li treats inabil ity to raise limbs.

(5) Liu Jun Zi Tang with Chai Hu, Ge Gen, Huang Qin, and Bai Shao Yao, this is called Shi Wei Ren Shen San, treats vacuity heat, tidal heat ef fusion, and fatigue.

(6) Liu Jun Zi Tang with Wu Mei, Cao Dou Kou, Sheng Jiang, a nd Da Zao, this is called Si Shou yin, treats qi vacuity of five viscera, seven em otions damaging person, phlegm transformed by depressed water and damp, ma laria, and miasmic malaria.

(7) When Huang Qi and Shan Yao are added to this formula, this

54

is also called Liu Jun Zi Tang, this regulates and rectifies the condition after dis ease, and assists the spleen to make one eat more.

(8) When Sheng Jiang and Suan Zao Ren are added, this treats p alpitations and inability to sleep.

(9) When Zhu Li and juice of Sheng Jiang are added, this treats h emiplegia, which is in left, this belongs to qi vacuity. This also treats phlegm sy ncope.

(10) When Mu Xiang, Huo Xiang, and Ge Gen (dry) are added, th is is called Qi Wei Bai Zhu San, treats spleen vacuity with flesh heat, diarrhea, thirst due to vacuity heat.

(11) When Wu Wei Zi and Chai Hu are added, this treats wasting-thirst and inability to eat.

(12) When Ren Shen is eliminated and Bai Shao Yao is added, thi s is called San Bai Tang, treats vacuity vexation or diarrhea or thirst, regulates and rectifies interior damage, and is good formula for external contraction.

(13) When Fu Ling is eliminated and Gan Jiang is added, this is c alled Si Shun Tang, this also can be made into pill with Honey, treats yin patter n with the pulse that is sunken and absence of heat effusion, no desire to see su n, abdominal pain, and diarrhea.

(14) When Shan Yao, Bian Dou, Sheng Jiang, and Da Zao, this is called Liu Shen San, treats heat effusion after exterior heat has gone in child.

(15) The combination of Si Jun Zi Tang and Si Wu Tang is called Ba Zhen Tang, treats the vacuity detriment of the heart and lung, both qi and bl ood vacuity, the detriment of the stomach, and flesh emaciation in spite of eatin g.

(16) If severe damage causes interior exhaustion of true yin, vacui ty yang which is stirred in the exterior, and the uprising of every pattern, then H uang Qi should be added to Si Jun Zi Tang with Si Wu Tang to assist yang and secure exterior, and add Rou Gui to lead fire to turn back to the origin, this is ca lled Shi Quan Da Bu Tang.

(17) In Shi Quan Da Bu Tang, Chuan Xiong is eliminated and Ch en Pi is added, this is called Wen Jing Yi Yuan San, treats dizziness after sweat ing, heart palpitations, muscular twitching and cramp, or incessant sweating, in cessant diarrhea after precipitation, and generalized pain.

(18) when Fang Feng (sovereign), Qiang Huo, Fu Zi, Du Zhong, a nd Niu Xi are added to Shi Quan Da Bu Tang, this is called Da Fang Feng Tan g, treats cran's knee wind.

25. 四君子湯

·總結：補陽益氣

·組成：人參, 白朮, 茯苓, 甘草, 生薑, 大棗

·主治：治一切陽虛氣弱, 脾衰肺損, 飲食少思, 體瘦面黃, 皮聚毛落. 脈來細軟.

·歸經：手足太陰足陽明藥

·方義：(1)人參甘溫...大補元氣, 爲君

(2)白朮苦溫...燥脾補氣, 爲臣

(3)茯苓甘淡...滲濕瀉熱, 爲佐

(4)甘草甘平...和中益土, 爲使也 ⇒ 氣足脾運, 飲食倍進, 則餘臟受蔭, 而色澤身強矣.

(5)再加陳皮, 以理氣散逆；半夏, 以燥濕除痰, 名曰六君.

·變化方：(1)加陳皮...名異功散, 調理脾胃.

(2)異功散再加半夏, 名六君子湯, 治氣虛有痰, 脾虛鼓脹.

(3)六君子再加香附, 砂仁...名香砂六君子湯, 治虛寒胃痛, 或腹痛泄瀉.

(4)六君子加麥冬, 竹瀝, 治四肢不舉.

(5)六君子加柴胡, 葛根, 黃芩, 白芍...名十味人參散, 治虛熱潮熱, 身體倦怠.

(6)六君子加烏梅, 草蔻等分, 薑, 棗煎...名四獸飲, 治五臟氣虛, 七情兼併, 結聚痰飲, 與衛氣相搏, 發爲瘧疾. 亦治瘴癘.

(7)本方加黃耆, 山藥亦名六君子湯, 亦名六君子湯爲病後調理, 助脾進食之劑.

(8)加生薑, 酸棗仁, 治振悸不得眠.

(9)加竹瀝, 薑汁, 治半身不遂, 在右者屬氣虛. 亦治痰厥暴死.

(10)加木香, 藿香, 乾葛, 名七味白朮散, 治脾虛肌熱, 泄瀉, 虛熱作渴.

(11)楊仁齋再加五味子, 柴胡, 治消渴不能食.

(12)除人參, 加白芍...名三白湯, 治虛煩. 或泄或渴, 爲調理內傷外感之奇方.

(13)除茯苓, 加乾薑...名四順湯；亦可蜜丸, 治陰證脈沉無熱, 不欲見光, 腹痛不和.

(14)加山藥, 扁豆, 薑, 棗煎...名六神散, 治小兒表熱去後又發熱者.

⒂四君合四物名八珍湯治心肺虛損，氣血兩虛，及胃損飲食不爲肌膚(血氣充，然後肌肉長).

⒃若傷之重者，眞陰內竭，虛陽外鼓，諸證蜂起，則于四君四物之中，又加黃耆以助陽固表，加肉桂以引火歸元，名十全大補湯.

⒄十全大補去川芎，加陳皮…名溫經益元散…治汗後頭眩心悸，筋惕肉潤，或汗出不止，及下後下利不止，身體疼痛.

⒅十全大補加防風爲君，再加羌活，附子，杜仲，牛膝…名大防風湯，治鶴膝風.

26. Si Wu Tang. Four-Substance Decoction. 四物湯

See number 1 in chapter 8. Blood-Rectifying Formulas.

27. Bu Zhong Yi Qi Tang. Tonify the Middle and Augment the Qi Decoction. 補中益氣湯

See number 1 in chapter 8. Qi-Rectifying Formulas.

28. Sheng Yang Yi Wei Tang. Raise the Yang and Augment the stomach Decoction. 升陽益胃湯

·**ACTIONS**：raises yang and boosts the stomach.

·**COMPOSITION**：Shao Yao, Huang Lian, Ren Shen, Bai Zhu, Fu Ling, Gan Cao, Chen Pi, Ban Xia, Ze Xie, Huang Qi, Qiang Huo, Du Huo, Fang Feng, Chai Hu, Sheng Jiang, Da Zao

·**INDICATIONS**：⑴ The weakness of Spleen and Stomach, fatigue and a tendency to lie down.

⑵ This disease often occurs when the season is autumn in which the qi of dryness works and the qi of damp with heat is about to retreat, there is generalized heaviness and joint pain, bitter taste in the mouth and dry tongue, no desire to eat, eating without knowing the taste, unregulated defecation and frequent urination.

⑶ When lung disease is combined with, there is huddled aversion to cold, a feeling of sadness without pleasure, this is because yang qi fails to ascend.

·**CHANNELS ENTERED**： The foot greater yin and yang brightness ch

57

annels. [The spleen and stomach]

·**Analysis of Formula**：(1) Liu Jun Zi Tang in this formula assists yang, boosts the stomach, and supplements Spleen and Stomach. Huang Qi supplements the lung and secures Defense. Shao Yao restrains yin and regulates Construction. Qiang Huo, Du Huo, Fang Feng, and Chai Hu eliminate pain due to damp and raise clear yang. Fu Ling and Ze Xie drain damp heat and descend turbid yin. A small amount of Huang Lian acts as assistant and retreats yin fire.

(2) This formula disperses evil during supplementing the middle and restrains yin during dispersing, this makes qi sufficient and yang raise, then the right qi gets effulgent and evil gets to subside.

· **RELATED FORMULA**　：When Shen Qu (fried) and Huang Qin are added to Bu Zhong Yi Qi tang, this is also called Sheng Yang Yi Wei Tang, treats menstruation with clot, sudden uterine blood clot bleeding, water diarrhea due to spleen vacuity.

·**Original Source**：Li Dong Yuan

28. 升陽益胃湯

·總結：升陽益胃

·組成：芍藥, 黃連, 人參, 白朮, 茯苓, 甘草, 陳皮, 半夏, 澤瀉, 黃耆, 羌活, 獨活, 防風, 柴胡, 生薑, 大棗

·主治：(1)治脾胃虛弱, 怠惰嗜臥.

(2)時值秋燥令行, 濕熱方退, 體重節痛, 口苦舌乾, 心不思食, 食不知味, 大便不調, 小便頻數.

(3)兼見肺病, 灑淅惡寒, 慘慘不樂, 乃陽氣不升也.

·歸經：足太陰陽明藥也

·方義：(1)六君子：助陽益胃, 補脾胃之上藥也. 加黃耆, 以補肺而固衛；芍藥, 以斂陰而調榮；羌活, 獨活, 防風, 柴胡, 以除濕痛而升清陽；茯苓, 澤瀉, 以瀉濕熱而降濁陰. 少佐黃連, 以退陰火.

(2)補中有散, 發中有收, 使氣足陽升, 則正旺而邪服矣.

·又附方：又補中益氣湯加炒麴, 黃芩-亦名益胃升陽湯, 治婦人經候凝結, 血塊暴下, 脾虛水瀉.

·來源：東垣

29. Bu Pi Wei Xie Yin Huo Sheng Yang Tang. Tonify the Lung and stomach, Drain Yin Fire, and Raise the Yang

Decoction. 補脾胃瀉陰火升陽湯

·**ACTIONS**：supplements the spleen, raises yang, and drains fire

·**COMPOSITION**：Huang Qin, Huang Lian, Shi Gao, Chai Hu, Sheng Ma, Qiang Huo, Ren Shen, Cang Zhu, Huang Qi, Gan Cao

·**INDICATIONS**： damaged stomach due to diet, damaged spleen due to taxation fatigue, excessive fire evil generating great heat. The pulse in the right bar is moderate with weak, or string like, of floating with rapid.

·**CHANNELS ENTERED**：The foot greater yin, yang brightness, and lesser yang channels [The spleen, stomach, and gall bladder]

·**Analysis of Formula**：(1) Chai Hu, Sheng Ma, Qiang Huo assist yang and boost the stomach by raising clear qi.

(2) Ren Shen, Cang Zhu, Huang Qi, and Gan Cao boost qi and eliminate damp through supplementing Spleen and Stomach .

(3) Huang Qin, Huang Lian, and Shi Gao cool the heart and clear the stomach through draining yin fire.

·**Original Source**：Li Dong Yuan

29. 補脾胃瀉陰火升陽湯
　·總結：補脾升陽瀉火
　·組成：黃芩, 黃連, 石膏, 柴胡, 升麻, 羌活, 人參, 蒼朮, 黃耆, 甘草
　·主治：治飲食傷胃, 勞倦傷脾, 火邪乘之而生大熱. 右關脈緩弱, 或弦, 或浮數.
　·歸經：足太陰陽明少陽藥
　·方義：(1)柴胡, 升麻, 羌活...助陽益胃以升清氣.
　　　　　(2)人參, 蒼朮, 黃耆, 甘草...益氣除濕以補脾胃.
　　　　　(3)黃芩, 黃連, 石膏...涼心清胃以瀉陰火.
　·來源：東垣

30. Gui Pi Tang. Restore the Spleen Decoction. 歸脾湯

See number 3 in chapter 8. Blood-Rectifying Formulas.

59

31. Yang Xin Tang. Nourish the Heart Decoction. 養心湯

See number 4 in chapter 8. Blood-Rectifying Formulas.

32. Ren Shen Yang Ying Tang. Ginseng Decoction to Nourish the Nutritive Qi. 人參養榮湯

See number 5 in chapter 8. Blood-Rectifying Formulas.

33. Bu Fei Tang. Tonify the Lung Decoction. 補肺湯

·**ACTIONS**：supplements the lung and suppresses cough

·**COMPOSITION**：Ren Shen, Huang Qi, Wu Wei Zi, Shu Di Huang, Sang Bai Pi, Zi Wan

·**INDICATIONS**：cough due to lung vacuity.

·**CHANNELS ENTERED**：　the hand greater yin and foot lesser yin channel [the lung and kidney]

·**Analysis of Formula**

　　　　(1) In lung vacuity, Ren Shen and Huang Qu are used, the spleen is the mother of the lung, and qi is the mother of water. Shu Di Huang is used, the kidney is the son of the lung, when son is in vacuity, son will nourish himself through stealing mother qi, therefore herb associated with the kidney is used to enrich the water in advance, and Shu Di Huang is also good at transforming phlegm. Cough means the damage of qi, the sour and warm of the Wu Wei Zi restrains lung qi. When cough occurs due to fire exuberant, the sweet and cold of Sang Pi drains lung fire. The pungent of Zi Wan moistens the lung and the warm supplements vacuity.

　　　　⑶ This formula makes metal effulgent and water generate, then cough gets to stops spontaneously.

33. 補肺湯

　·總結：補肺止嗽

　·組成：人參, 黃耆, 五味子, 熟地黃, 桑白皮, 紫菀

　·主治：治肺虛欬嗽.

　·歸經：肺

　·方義：⑴此手太陰足少陰藥也.

　　　　　⑵肺虛而用參, 耆者, 脾爲肺母, 氣爲水母也. 用熟地者, 腎

60

爲肺子，子虛必盜母氣以自養，故用腎藥先滋其水，且熟地亦化痰之妙品也. 欬則氣傷，五味酸溫，能斂肺氣. 欬由火盛，桑皮甘寒，能瀉肺火. 紫菀辛能潤肺，溫能補虛.

　　　(3)合之而名曰補肺，蓋金旺水生，欬嗽自止矣.

34. Bu Fei E Jiao San. Tonify the Lung Decoction with Ass-Hide Gelatin. 補肺阿膠散

·**ACTIONS**：supplements the lung and clears fire

·**COMPOSITION**：E Jiao, Xing Ren, Ma Dou Ling, Gan Cao, Geng Mi, Niu Bang Zi

·**INDICATIONS**：lung vacuity with fire, cough without fluids and breath being blocked.

·**CHANNELS ENTERED**：The hand greater yin channel. [The lung]

·**Analysis of Formula**：(1) This formula is associated with the hand great er yin.

　　　(2) Ma Dou Ling clears heat and descends fire. Niu Bang Zi disinhibits diaphragm and lubricates phlegm. Xing Ren moistens dryness, disperses wind, descends qi, and suppresses cough. E Jiao clears the lung, enriches the kidney, boosts blood, and supplements yin. When qi is in normal, breath being blocked won't occur, when humors are supplemented, fluids will generate, when fire retreats, cough gets quieted. Earth is the mother of metal, therefore Gan Cao and Geng Mi are added to boost Spleen and Stomach.

·**Original Source**：Qian Yi

34. 補肺阿膠散

　·總結：補肺清火

　·組成：阿膠, 杏仁, 馬兜鈴, 甘草, 粳米, 牛蒡子

　·主治：治肺虛有火, 嗽無津液而氣哽者.

　·歸經：肺經

　·方義：(1)此手太陰藥也.

　　　(2)馬兜鈴清熱降火. 牛蒡子利膈滑痰. 杏仁潤燥散風, 降氣止欬. 阿膠清肺滋腎, 益血補陰, 氣順則不哽, 液補則津生, 火退而嗽寧矣. 土爲金母, 故加甘草, 粳米以益脾胃.

　·來源：錢乙

35. Sheng Mai San. Generate the Pulse Powder. 生脈散

See number 3 in chapter 11. Summerheat-Clearing Formulas.

36. Bai He Gu Jin Tang. Lily Bulb Decoction to Preserve the Metal. 百合固金湯

·**ACTIONS**：preserves the lung

·**COMPOSITION**：Bai He, sheng Di Huang, Shu Di Huang, Mai Men Dong, Bei Mu, Dang Gui, Shao Yao, Yuan Shen, Jie Geng, Sheng Gan Cao

·**INDICATIONS**：lung damage and sore throat, panting with cough and phlegm blood.

·**CHANNELS ENTERED**：The hand greater yin and the foot lesser yin. [The lung and kidney]

·**Analysis of Formula**：(1) When metal fails to generate water, fire gets to flam and water gets to dry, therefore Sheng Di Huang and Shu Di Huang assist the kidney, enrich water, abate heat, and act as a sovereign. Bai He preserves the lung and quiets spirit. Mai Men Dong clears heat and moistens dryness. Yuan Shen assists Sheng Di Huang and Shu Di Huang by generating water. Bei Mu disperses the depressed lung and eliminates phlegm. Dang Gui and Shao Yao nourish blood and stable the liver. Gan Cao and Jie Geng clear metal and have an effect in the throat.

(2) Generally sweet and cold bank up the origin of kidney water and clear the root of lung heat, having a desire not to use bitter and cold not to damage the generating qi.

·**Original Source**：Zhao Ji An

36. 百合固金湯

·總結：保肺

·組成：百合, 生地黃, 熟地黃, 麥冬, 貝母, 當歸, 芍藥, 元參, 桔梗, 生甘草

·主治：治肺傷咽痛, 喘嗽痰血.

·歸經：手太陰足少陰藥也.

·方義：(1)金不生水, 火炎水乾, 故以二地助腎滋水退熱爲君. 百合保肺安神. 麥冬清熱潤燥. 元參助二地以生水. 貝母散肺鬱而除痰. 歸芍養血以平肝. 甘, 桔清金, 成功上部.

(2)皆以甘寒培元清本, 不欲以苦寒傷生發之氣也.

37. Zi Wan Tang. Aster Decoction. 紫菀湯

·**ACTIONS**：lung taxation and qi exhaustion

·**COMPOSITION**：Zi Wan, E Jiao, Zhi Mu, Bei Mu, Jie Geng, Ren Shen, Fu Ling, Gan Cao, Wu Wei Zi

·**INDICATIONS**：(1) Lung damage and qi exhaustion, taxation heat with enduring cough, and vomiting of phlegm and blood.

(2) Welling abscess which is transformed from lung wilting.

·**CHANNELS ENTERED**：The hand greater yin channel. [The lung]

·**Analysis of Formula**：(1) Taxation and enduring cough due to lung vacuity, heat pattern due to vacuity fire. .

(2) Wang Hai Zang devised this formula to mainly preserve the lung, therefore Zi Wan and E Jiao are used as a sovereign. Clearing fire is the next, therefore Zhi Mu and Bei Mu are used as a minister.

(3) Ren Shen and Fu Ling act as an assistant, and support earth resulting in generating metal. Gan Cao and Jie Geng act as a courier and lead other herbs to ascend upward to the spleen and lung.

(4) Wu Wei Zi enriches water in kidney insufficiency, restrains the lung, one with enduring cough should be restrained with wu wei zi.

·**Original Source**：Wang Hai Zang

37. 紫菀湯

·總結：肺勞氣極

·組成：紫菀, 阿膠, 知母, 貝母, 人參, 茯苓, 甘草, 五味子

·主治：(1)治肺傷氣極, 勞熱久嗽, 吐痰吐血.

(2)及肺痿變癰.

·歸經：手太陰藥.

·方義：(1)勞而久嗽, 肺虛可知, 即有熱證, 皆虛火也.

(2)海藏以保肺爲君, 故用紫菀, 阿膠. 以清火爲臣, 故用知母, 貝母.

(3)以參, 苓爲佐者, 扶土所以生金. 以甘, 桔爲使者, 載藥上行脾肺.

(4)五味子滋腎家不足之水, 收肺家耗散之金, 久嗽者所必收也.

38. Qing Hao Fe Lei Tang. Artemisia Annua Decoction to Aid Emaciation. 秦艽扶羸湯

·**ACTIONS**： Lung Taxation

·**COMPOSITION**：Chai Hu, Qin Jiao, Dang Gui, Ban Xia, Ren Shen, Gan Cao (mix fried), Zi Wan, Bie Jia, Di Gu Pi, Sheng Jiang, Da Zao

·**INDICATIONS**：(1) Lung wilting and steaming bone.

(2) Aversion to cold or heat effusion, which is transformed to lung taxation, cough and hoarseness, vacuity constitution and spontaneous sweating, fatigued cumbersome limbs.

·**CHANNELS ENTERED**：The hand greater yin and the foot lesser yang. [The lung and gall bladder].

·**Analysis of Formula**：(1) Chai Hu and Qin Jiao disperse exterior evil and clear interior heat, Bie Jia and Di Gu Pi nourish yin and blood and make steaming bone retreat. Ren Shen and Gan Cao supplement qi. Dang Gui harmonizes blood. Zi Wan rectifies phlegm cough. Ban Xia makes sound come out.

·**Original Source**：Zhi Zhi

38. 秦艽扶羸湯

·總結：肺勞

·組成：柴胡, 秦艽, 當歸, 半夏, 人參, 炙甘草, 紫菀, 鱉甲, 地骨皮, 生薑, 大棗

·主治：(1)治肺痿骨蒸.

(2)或寒或熱成勞, 咳嗽聲嗄不出, 體虛自汗, 四肢倦怠.

·歸經：手太陰足少陽藥也.

·方義：(1)柴胡, 秦艽, 散表邪兼清裏熱, 鱉甲, 地骨, 滋陰血而退骨蒸. 參, 草補氣. 當歸和血. 紫菀理痰嗽. 半夏發音聲.

·來源：直指

39. Huang Qi Jiao Bie Jia San. Astragalus and Soft-shelled Turtle Shell Powder. 黃耆鱉甲散.

·**ACTIONS**：taxation heat

64

·**COMPOSITION**：Bie Jia, Zhi Mu, Shao Yao, Tian Men Dong, Sheng Di Huang, Rou Gui, Fu Ling, Gan Cao(mix fried), Ren Shen, Huang Qi, Chai Hu, Sang Pi, Jie Geng, Qin Jiao, Di Gu Pi, Ban Xia, Zi Wan

·**INDICATIONS**：(1) Vacuity taxation and visiting heat in man and woman, vexing heat in the chest, palms and soles, and fatigued cumbersome limbs.

(2) Cough and dry throat, spontaneous sweating and decrease in diet, sometimes heat effusion in the afternoon.

·**MODIFICATIONS**：In Wei Sheng Bao Jian, Rou Gui, Shao Yao, and Di Gu Pi are eliminated, this is called Ren Shen Huang Qi San, the treat is same.

·**CHANNELS ENTERED**：The hand and foot greater yin and the foot lesser yang channels. [The lung, spleen, gall bladder]

·**Analysis of Formula**：(1) Bie Jia, Tian Men Dong, Shao Yao, Sheng Di Huang, and Zhi Mu enrich kidney water, drain the fire of the lung and liver, and nourish yin.

(2) Huang Qi, Ren Shen, Rou Gui, Fu Ling, and Gan Cao secure defense qi, supplement the vacuity of the spleen and lung, and assist yang.

(3) Sang Pi and Jie Geng drain lung heat. Ban Xia and Zi Wan rectify phlegm cough. Qin Jiao and Di Gu Pi disperse interior heat and eliminate steaming heat.

(4) Chai Hu resolves flesh heat and ascends yang upward.

(5) This formula treats qi and blood of interior and exterior.

·**Original Source**：Qian Fu

39. 黃耆鱉甲散
·總結：勞熱
·組成：鱉甲，知母，芍藥，天冬，生地黃，肉桂，茯苓，炙甘草，人參，黃耆，柴胡，桑皮，桔梗，秦艽，地骨皮，半夏，紫菀
·主治：(1)治男女虛寒客熱，五心煩熱，四肢怠惰.
(2)欬嗽咽乾，自汗食少，或日晡發熱.
·加減：衛生減桂，芍，地骨，名人參黃耆散. 治同.
·歸經：手足太陰足少陽藥也.
·方義：(1)鱉甲，天冬，芍，地，知母，滋腎水而瀉肺肝之火，以養陰也.
(2)黃耆，人參，桂，苓，甘草，固衛氣而補脾肺之虛，以助陽也.
(3)桑皮，桔梗，以瀉肺熱. 半夏，紫菀，以理痰嗽. 秦艽，地

65

骨, 以散內熱而除蒸.

　　　　(4)柴胡以解肌熱而升陽.

　　　　(5)此表裏氣血交治之劑也.

　·來源：謙甫

40. Qin Jiao Bie Jia San. Gentiana Macrophylla and Soft-shelled Turtle Shell Powder. 秦艽鱉甲散

·**ACTIONS**：Wind Taxation

·**COMPOSITION**：Di Gu Pi, Zhi Mu, Qing Hao, Wu Mei, Bie Jia, Chai Hu, Qin Jiao, Dang Gui

·**INDICATIONS**：Wind Taxation and steaming bone, invigorating heat effusion in the afternoon, cough with flesh emaciation, red complexion and night sweating, the pulse that is fine and rapid.

·**MODIFICATIONS**：if sweating is copious, then add Huang Qi more.

·**CHANNELS ENTERED**：The foot lesser yang and reverting yin. [The gall bladder and liver].

·**Analysis of Formula**：(1) Wind generates heat and heat generates wind, without Chai Hu and Qin Jiao, it is impossible to expel wind evil to outward.

　　　　(2) Bie Jia belongs to yin, this formula uses a carapace, this means that bone is used to treat bone.

　　　　(3) The sour and astringent of Wu Mei leads every herbs to enter bone and restrains heat.

　　　　(4) The bitter and cold of Qing Hao leads every herbs to enter flesh and resolves steaming heat. Zhi Mu nourishes yin.

　　　　(5) Dang Gui harmonizes blood. Di Gu Pi disperses exterior evil and clears interior heat, and also checks sweating and eliminates steaming heat.

·**Original Source**：Qian Fu

40. 秦艽鱉甲散

　·總結：風勞

　·組成：地骨皮, 知母, 青蒿, 烏梅, 鱉甲, 柴胡, 秦艽, 當歸

　·主治：治風勞骨蒸, 午後壯熱, 咳嗽肌瘦, 煩赤盜汗, 脈來細數.

　·加減：汗多倍黃耆.

　·歸經：足少陽厥陰藥也.

　·方義：(1)風生熱而熱生風, 非柴胡, 秦艽不能驅風邪使外出.

(2)鱉陰類，用甲者，骨以及骨之義.

(3)烏梅酸澀，能引諸藥入骨而斂熱.

(4)青蒿苦寒，能從諸藥入肌而解蒸. 知母滋陰.

(5)當歸和血. 地骨散表邪兼清裏熱，又止汗除蒸之上品也.

·來源：謙甫

41. Yi Qi Cong Ming Tang. Augment the Qi and Increase Acuity Decoction. 益氣聰明湯

·**ACTIONS**：increases hearing acuity and improves vision

·**COMPOSITION**：Huang Qi, Ren Shen, Bai Shao Yao, Huang Bai, Ge Gen, Sheng Ma, Man Jing Zi, Gan Cao (mix fried)

·**INDICATIONS**：cataract and blurred vision, tinnitus and deafness.

·**CHANNELS ENTERED**：The greater yin, yang brightness, lesser yin and reverting yin channels. [The spleen, stomach, kidney, and liver]

·**Analysis of Formula**：(1) All of the qi of clear yang of the twelve channels ascend upward to the head and runs the orifices, owing to diet, taxation, and labor, if Spleen and Stomach get damaged, this causes heart fire to be exuberant, then all of vessels become boiled, evil gets to damage orifices.

(2) The sweet and warm of Ren Shen and Huang Qi supplement Spleen and Stomach. The sweet of Gan Cao harmonizes Spleen and Stomach. Ge Gen (dry), Sheng Ma, and Man Jing Zi are light and tend to ascend and disperse, and enter yang brightness, inspire stomach qi, and ascend upward to the head and eyes. The middle qi in sufficiency clears yang and ascends upward, then frees and disinhibits nine orifices, and then hearing and vision get clear.

(3) Bai Shao Yao restrains yin and harmonizes blood, Huang Bai supplements Kidney and generates water, the eye is the orifice of the liver and the ear is the orifice of the kidney, therefore the two herbs calm the liver and enrich the kidney.

·**Original Source**：Li Dong Yuan

41. 益氣聰明湯

·總結：聰耳明目

·組成：黃者, 人參, 白芍, 黃柏, 葛根, 升麻, 蔓荊子, 炙甘草

·主治：治內障目昏, 耳鳴耳聾.

·歸經：足太陰陽明少陰厥陰藥也.

·方義：⑴十二經清陽之氣，皆上于頭面而走空竅，因飲食勞役，脾胃受傷，心火太盛，則百脈沸騰，邪害空竅矣.

⑵參，耆甘溫，以補脾胃．甘草甘緩，以和脾胃．乾葛，升麻，蔓荊，輕揚升發，能入陽明，鼓舞胃氣，上行頭目．中氣旣足，清陽上升，則九竅通利，耳聰而目明矣.

⑶白芍斂陰和血，黃柏補腎生水，蓋目爲肝竅，耳爲腎竅，故又用二者，平肝滋腎也.

·來源：東垣

42. Yang Rou Tang. Mutton Decoction. 羊肉湯

·**ACTIONS**：yang collapse and loss of blood

·**COMPOSITION**：Bai Shao Yao, Dang Gui, Gui Zhi, Fu Zi, Sheng Jiang, Mu Li, Long Gu, Yang Rou (mutton)

·**INDICATIONS**：⑴ Excessive sweating or precipitation in cold damage, yang collapse and loss of blood, no desire to see person and fatigue, a periodic shiver as malaria.

⑵ Excessive bleeding during childbirth.

·**CHANNELS ENTERED**：The foot lesser yin channel. [The kidney]

·**Analysis of Formula**：⑴ Dang Gui and Shao Yao supplement yin.

⑵ Fu Zi, Sheng Jiang, and Gui Zhi restore yang.

⑶ Long Gu and Mu Li collect the desertion.

⑷ Yang Rou (mutton) greatly supplements and generates qi and blood.

·**Original Source**：Han Qi He

42. 羊肉湯

·總結：亡陽失血

·組成：白芍，當歸，桂枝，附子，生薑，牡蠣，龍骨，羊肉

·主治：⑴治傷寒汗下太過，亡陽失血，惡人踡臥，時戰如瘧.

⑵及產脫血虛.

·歸經：足少陰藥也.

·方義：⑴當歸，芍藥，以補其陰.

⑵附子，薑，桂，以復其陽.

⑶龍骨，牡蠣，以收其脫.

⑷羊肉大補，以生其氣血.

·來源：韓祇和

Chapter 2. Exterior-Releasing Formulas. 發表之劑

1. Ma Huang Tang. Ephedra Decoction. 麻黃湯

·**ACTIONS**： cold damaging construction, release the exterior.

·**COMPOSITION**：Ma Huang, Gui Zhi, Xing Ren, Gan Cao

·**INDICATIONS**：(1) Cold damage greater yang pattern, evil qi in the exterior, heat effusion, headache, generalized pain, lumbar pain, bone and joints pain, the stiffness of the nape and back, aversion to cold and aversion to wind, absence of sweating with panting, and the pulse that is floating and tight.

(2) The combination disease of greater yang and yang brightness, panting and thoracic fullness.

(3) Wheezing.

·**CHANNELS ENTERED**：The foot greater yang channel. [The bladder]

·**Analysis of Formula**：(1) ① The inner part of Ma Huang is empty, the character is pungent, warm, and light. This is the herb for the lung and enters greater yang, opens the flesh, and disperses cold.

② Gui Zhi is pungent and warm, leads the evil in construction part to reach flesh exterior. Xing Ren is bitter and sweet, disperses cold and descends qi.

③ Gan Cao is sweet and neutral, disperses, and harmonizes the middle.

(2) Nei Jing says that when cold stays interior, this should be treated with sweet with heat and assisted with bitter with pungent.

·**RELATED FORMULA**：(1) When in this formula Gui Zhi is eliminated and Shi Gao is added, this is called Ma Huang Xing Ren Gan Cao Shi Gao Tang, treats that after promotion of sweating or precipitation, Gui Zhi Tang can be used again, but there is sweating with panting, absence of great heat effusion. And also treats warm malaria with aversion to cold after heat effusion.

(2) When Bai Zhu is added to this formula, this is called Ma Huang Jia Zhu Tang, treats one who has usually damp with generalized vexation and pain, sweating should be promoted.

(3) When in this formula Gui Zhi and Xing Ren are eliminated and Fu Zi is added, this is called Ma Huang Fu Zi Tang, treats the pulse that is sunken and abdominal vacuous distention, this is called qi water and belongs to lesser yin, if sweating is promoted, the sweat will pause.

(4) When Gui Zhi and Xing Ren are eliminated, this is called Ga

n Cao Ma Huang Tang, treats interior water.

⑸ When Gui Zhi is eliminated, and then Ma Huang, Xing Ren, and Gan Cao are used, this combination is called San Ao Tang, treats contraction to wind cold and cough with nasal congestion.

·**Original Source**：Zhong Jing

1. 麻黃湯
 ·總結：寒傷營，發表
 ·組成：麻黃，桂枝，杏仁，甘草
 ·主治：⑴治傷寒太陽證，邪氣在表，發熱頭痛，身痛腰痛，骨節痛，項背強，惡寒惡風，無汗而喘，脈浮而緊.
  ⑵亦治太陽陽明合病，喘而胸滿.
  ⑶亦治哮證.
 ·歸經：足太陽藥
 ·方義：⑴①麻黃中空，辛溫氣薄，肺家專藥而走太陽，能開腠散寒.
    ②桂枝辛溫，能引營分之邪，達之肌表. 杏仁苦甘，散寒而降氣.
    ③甘草甘平，發散而和中.
  ⑵經曰：『寒淫于內，治以甘熱，佐以苦辛.』是也.
 ·變化方：⑴本方除桂枝，加石膏，名麻黃杏仁甘草石膏湯，治汗下後不可更行桂枝湯，汗出而喘，無大熱者. 亦治溫瘧先熱後寒.
  ⑵本方加白朮名麻黃加朮湯，治溼家身體煩痛，宜發汗.
  ⑶本方去桂枝，杏仁，加附子，名麻黃附子湯，治脈沉虛脹者爲氣水，屬少陰，發其汗卽止.
  ⑷本方除桂枝，杏仁，名甘草麻黃湯，治裏水，重覆取汗.
  ⑸本方去桂，用麻黃，杏仁，甘草，名三拗湯，治感冒風寒，欬嗽鼻塞.
 ·來源：仲景

2. Gui Zhi Tang. Cinnamon Twig Decoction. 桂枝湯

 ·**ACTIONS**：wind damaging Defense, releases the flesh
 ·**COMPOSITION**：Gui Zhi, Bai Shao Yao, Da Zao, Sheng Jiang, Gan Cao
 ·**INDICATIONS**：⑴ when in greater yang wind strike, the pulse that is f

71

loating in yang part and weak in yin part, there is heat effusion, headache, spontaneous sweating, aversion to wind, aversion to cold, noisy nose, and dry retching.

(2) When in yang brightness disease, the pulse is slow, there is copious sweating, and mild aversion to cold, this means that the exterior has not resolved, it is inappropriate to promote sweating.

·**CHANNELS ENTERED** : The foot greater yang channel. [The bladder]

·**Analysis of Formula** : (1) Zhong Jing uses promotion of sweating at severe case and releasing the flesh at slight case, wind strike cannot be treated with greatly promotion of sweating, if sweating is too excessive, instead this stirs construction and blood, even though there is exterior evil, this should be treated with releasing the flesh, therefore Gui Zhi Tang can mildly harmonize this.

(2) Nei Jing says that wind evil is predominant, pungent with cool should be used to calm, bitter with sweet to assistant, sweet to relax, and sour to restrain.

(3) The pungent with sweet of Gui Zhi disperses and belongs to yang. The sour of Shao Yao restrains yin as minister, the sweet and neutral of Gan Cao makes yin qi not to drain and acts as assistant.

The pungent and warm of Sheng Jiang disperses the exterior, the sweet and warm of Da Zao harmonizes the other herbs. The action of this formula is in not only dispersing the exterior but also moving the fluid and humor of the spleen to harmonize Construction and Defense.

(4) Ma Huang Tang acts only on dispersing the exterior, therefore this does not use Sheng Jiang and Da Zao, the aim of this formula is for the fluid and humor to free.

·**RELATED FORMULA** : (1) When in this formula Bai Zhu, Chuan Xiong, Qiang Huo, Fang Feng, and Yi Tang are added, this is called Shu Xie Shi Biao Tang, treats same thing with Gui Zhi Tang.

(2) When Shao Yao and Sheng Jiang are eliminated, this is called Gui Zhi Gan Cao Tang, treats that after excessive sweating, there is the hands crossed over the heart, precipitation below the heart, with a desire for pressure.

(3) When Fu Zi is added, this is called Gui Zhi Jia Fu Zi Tang, treats that when in greater yang disease, sweating is promoted and then gives way to incessant leaking, the person is averse to cold, has difficult urination, the limbs are slightly tensed so that they bend and stretch with difficulty,

(4) When Shao Yao is eliminated and Fu Zi is added, this is called Gui Zhi Fu Zi Tang, treats that when cold damage has lasted eight or nine days, and wind and damp contend with each other, there is generalized vexing pain, inabil

72

ity to turn sides, absence of retching, absence of thirst, and a pulse that is floating, vacuous and rough.

(5) When Shao Yao and Sheng Jiang (respectively one liang), and Ren Shen (three liang) are added, this is called Gui Zhi Xin Jia Tang, treats that when after the promotion of sweating in cold damage, there is generalized pain, and a pulse that is sunken and slow,

(6) Gan Cao decrease by one half and same amount of Shao Yao is added, this is called Gui Zhi Jia Shao Yao Tang, treats that after precipitation erroneously in greater yang, there is abdominal pain belonging to greater yin pattern.

(7) When Da Huang is added, this is called Gui Zhi Jia Da Huang Tang, treats exterior pattern after precipitation erroneously and great deplete pain in the abdomen.

(8) When Gui Zhi is eliminated and Fu Ling and Bai Zhu are added, this is called Gui Zhi Qu Gui Jia Fu Ling Bai Zhu Tang, treats that when Gui Zhi Tang is taken, or precipitation is used and there is still stiffness and pain of the head and nape, feather-warm heat effusion, absence of sweating, fullness below the heart with slight pain, and inhibited urination.

(9) When Hou Po and Xing Ren are added, this is called Gui Zhi Jia Hou Po Xing Ren Tang, treats that when in greater yang disease, there is mild panting following precipitation, it means that the exterior has not resolved.

(10) When Shao Yao and Sheng Jiang are eliminated and Fu Ling is added, this is called Fu Ling Gui Zhi Gan Cao Da Zao Tang, treats that after sweating has been promoted, the person has precipitation below the umbilicus about to become running piglet.

(11) When Ma Huang Tang is combined with this formula, this is called Gui Ma Ge Ban Tang, treats that in greater yang disease, resembling malaria, in which there is heat effusion and aversion to cold (with the heat effusion more pronounced than the aversion to cold).

(12) When this formula (two fen) is combined with Ma Huang Tang (one fen), this is called Gui Zhi Er Ma Huang Yi Tang, treats that when in greater yang disease sweating has already promoted, there is the disease resembling malaria which occurs twice a day.

(13) The combination of this formula (two fen) and Yue Bi Tang (one fen), this is called Gui Zhi Er Yue Bi Tang, treats that when in greater yang disease there is heat effusion, aversion to cold (with the heat effusion more pronounced than the aversion to cold), and the pulse is faint and weak, this means there is absence of yang, it is impossible to promote sweating.

⒁ When the same amount of Shao Yao and Yi Tang are added, this is called Xiao Jian Zhong Tang. Huang Qi is added to Xiao Jian Zhong Tang, this is called Huang Qi Jian Zhong Tang. When Yi Tang is eliminated, this is called Gui Zhi Jia Huang Qi Tang, treats yellow sweating, heat effusion, both leg coldness, generalized pain and heaviness, sweating above lumbus, absence of sweating below lumbus, and inhibited urination.

⒂ When Dang Gui is added to Xiao Jian Zhong Tang, this is called Dang Gui Jian Zhong Tang, treats emaciation and depletion after childbirth, abdominal pain leading to lumbus and back, lower abdominal cramp.

If there is incessant flooding, add Di Huang and E Jiao.

⒃ When Gan Cao is eliminated and Huang Qi (three liang) is added, this is called Gui Zhi Wu Wu Tang, treats blood impediment.

⒄ When Gua Lou Gen is added, this is called Gua Lou Gui Zhi Tang, treats that in greater yang pattern, there is generalized stiffness and the pulse that is sunken and slow. This means convulsive disease.

⒅ When Long Gu and Mu Li are added, this is called Gui Zhi Jia Long Gu Mu Li Tang, treats consumption of essence in man, dreaming of intercourse in women.

⒆ When Ge Gen and Ma Huang are added, this is called Ge Gen Tang.

·**Original Source**：Zhong Jing

2. 桂枝湯
　·總結：風傷衛, 解肌
　·組成：桂枝, 白芍, 大棗, 生薑, 甘草
　·主治：⑴治太陽中風, 陽浮而陰弱, 發熱頭痛, 自汗, 惡風惡寒, 鼻鳴乾嘔.

⑵及陽明病脈遲, 汗出多, 微惡寒者, 表末解也, 可發汗.
　·歸經：足太陽藥也.
　·方義：⑴仲景以發汗爲重, 解肌爲輕, 中風不可大汗, 汗過則反動營血, 雖有表邪, 只可解肌, 故桂枝湯少和之也.

⑵經曰：「風淫所勝, 平以辛涼, 佐以苦甘, 以甘緩之, 以酸收之.」

⑶桂枝辛甘發散爲陽. 臣以芍藥之酸收. 佐以甘草之甘平, 不令泄陰氣也.

薑辛溫能散, 棗甘溫能和, 此不專于發散, 又以行脾之津液

74

而和營衛者也.

　　(4)麻黃湯專于發散, 故不用薑, 棗, 而津液得通矣.

　·變化方：(1)本方加白朮, 川芎, 羌活, 防風, 飴糖, 名疏邪實表湯治同.

　　(2)本方去芍藥, 生薑, 名桂枝甘草湯, 治發汗過多, 叉手冒心, 心下悸欲得按者.

　　(3)本方加附子, 名桂枝加附子湯, 治太陽病發汗, 遂漏不止, 惡風, 小便難, 四肢微急.

　　(4)本方去芍藥, 加附子, 名桂枝附子湯, 治傷寒八九日, 風溼相搏, 身體痛煩, 不能轉側, 不嘔不渴, 脈浮虛而濇.

　　(5)本方加芍藥, 生薑各一兩, 人參三兩, 名桂枝新加湯, 治傷寒汗後身痛, 脈來沉遲.

　　(6)本方減甘草一半, 加芍藥一倍, 名桂枝加芍藥湯, 治太陽誤下, 腹痛屬太陰證.

　　(7)本方加大黃, 名桂枝加大黃湯, 治表證誤下, 大實痛者.

　　(8)本方去桂枝, 加茯苓, 白朮, 名桂枝去桂加茯苓白朮湯, 治服桂枝湯, 或下之, 仍頭項強痛, 發熱無汗, 心滿微痛, 小便不利.

　　(9)本方加厚朴, 杏仁, 名桂枝加厚朴杏仁湯, 治太陽病下之微喘, 表未解也.

　　(10)本方芍藥, 生薑, 加茯苓, 名桂枝甘草大棗湯, 甘瀾水煎, 治汗後臍下悸, 欲作奔豚.

　　(11)本方合麻黃湯, 名桂麻各半湯, 治太陽證如瘧狀, 熱多寒少.

　　(12)本方二分合麻黃湯一分, 名桂枝二麻黃一湯, 治太陽病已大汗, 形如瘧, 日再發.

　　(13)本方二分合越婢一分, 名桂枝二越婢一湯, 治太陽病發熱惡寒, 熱多寒少, 脈微弱者. 此無陽也, 不可發汗.

　　(14)本方倍芍藥, 加飴糖, 名小建中湯. 再加黃耆, 名黃耆建中湯. 除飴糖, 名桂枝加黃耆湯, 治黃汗發熱, 兩脛自冷, 身痛身重, 腰上有汗, 腰下無汗, 小便不利.

　　(15)小建中加當歸, 名當歸建中湯, 治婦人產後虛羸不足, 腹中痛引腰背, 小腹拘急.

　　若崩傷不止, 加地黃, 阿膠.

　　(16)本方除甘草, 加黃耆三兩, 名桂枝五物湯, 治血痺.

　　(17)本方加栝蔞根, 名栝蔞桂枝湯, 治太陽證備, 身強几几,

脈反沉遲，此爲痙.

⒅本方加龍骨，牡蠣，名桂枝加龍骨牡蠣湯，治男子失精，女子夢交.

⒆本方加葛根，麻黃，名葛根湯.

·來源：仲景

3. Da Qing Long Tang. Major Bluegreen Dragon Decoction. 大青龍湯

·**ACTIONS**：releases both wind and cold

·**COMPOSITION**：Ma Huang, Gui Zhi, Xing Ren, Gan Cao, Shi Gao, Sheng Jiang, Da Zao

·**INDICATIONS**：(1) in greater yang wind strike, the pulse is floating and tight, there is generalized pain, heat effusion, aversion to cold, absence of sweating, and vexation and agitation.

(2) in cold damage, the pulse is floating and moderate, and there is no generalized pain, only generalized heaviness, with sudden periods of lightness, and there is no lesser yin pattern

·**CHANNELS ENTERED**：The foot greater yang channel [the bladder].

·**Analysis of Formula**：(1) Cheng Wu Ji says that Gui Zhi Tang controls wind strike, Ma Huang Tang does cold damage. Then, now both wind and cold are damaged, one tries to use Gui Zhi Tang to release the flesh and expel wind, but this cannot treat the cold, on the other hand, one tries to use Ma Huang Tang to promote sweating and disperse cold, but this cannot expel the wind, thus Zhong Jing made Da Qing Long Tang to resolve both cold and wind.

(2) Ma Huang is sweet and warm and Gui Zhi is pungent and heat. Cold damages Construction, thus sweet relaxes it, wind damages Defense, thus pungent disperses it, therefore Ma Huang acts as sovereign and Gui Zhi acts as minister.

The sweet and neutral of Gan Cao and the sweet and bitter of Xing Ren assist Ma Huang to disperse the exterior. The sweet and warm of Da Zao and the pungent and warm of Sheng Jiang assist Gui Zhi to release the flesh.

(3) When all of Construction, Defense, yin, and yang are damaged, this cannot be treated with only herbs which are light. Both heavy and light herbs are needed to release and disperse the exterior, and then wind and cold evil

can be eliminated and Construction and Defense become harmonious.

        Shi Gao is pungent, sweet, mild cold, and heavy. This reaches fl esh exterior, acting as courier.

  ·**Original Source**：Zhong Jing

3. 大青龍湯

  ·總結：風寒兩解

  ·組成：麻黃，桂枝，杏仁，甘草，石膏，生薑，大棗

  ·主治：⑴治太陽中風，脈浮緊，身疼痛，發熱惡寒，不汗出而煩躁.

        ⑵又治傷寒脈浮數，身不痛，但重，乍有輕時，無少陰證者.

  ·歸經：足太陽藥

  ·方義：⑴成氏曰：「桂枝主中風，麻黃主傷寒. 今風寒兩傷，欲以桂枝解肌驅風，而不能已其寒；欲以麻黃發汗散寒，而不能去其風，仲景所以處青龍而兩解也.」

        ⑵麻黃甘溫，桂枝辛熱. 寒傷營，以甘緩之；風傷衛，以辛散之. 故以麻黃爲君，桂枝爲臣.

        甘草甘平，杏仁甘苦，佐麻黃以發表. 大棗甘溫，生薑辛溫，佐桂枝以解肌.

        ⑶營衛陰陽俱傷，則非輕劑所能獨解，必須重輕之劑同散之，乃得陰陽之邪俱已，營衛俱和.

        石膏辛甘微寒，質重而又專達肌表爲使也.

  ·來源：仲景

4. Xiao Qing Long Tang. Minor Bluegreen Dragon Decoction. 小青龍湯

  ·**ACTIONS**：moves water and promotes sweating.

  ·**COMPOSITION**：Ma Huang, Gui Zhi, Bai Shao Yao, Gan Jiang, Xi Xin, Ban Xia, Wu Wei Zi, Gan Cao

  ·**INDICATIONS**：⑴ When in cold damage the exterior has not resolved, there is water qi below the heart, dry retching, heat effusion, and cough. ⑵Or dysphagia, or panting, or thirst, or disinhibited urination, or inhibited urination, lesser abdominal fullness, and shortness of breath with inability to lie down.

  ·**MODIFICATIONS**：⑴ for thirst, eliminate Ban Xia and add Tian Hua

Fen.

　　　　　(2) for panting, eliminate Ma Huang and add Xing Ren.

　　　　　(3) for edema, eliminate Ma Huang.

　　　　　(4) for dysphagia, eliminate Ma Huang and add Fu Zi.

　　　　　(5) for inhibited urination, eliminate Ma Huang and add Fu Ling.

·**CHANNELS ENTERED**：The foot greater yang channel. [The bladder]

·**Analysis of Formula**：(1) The exterior has not resolved, so Ma Huang promotes sweating and acts as sovereign, Gui Zhi and Gan Cao assist Ma Huang to release exterior and act as assistant. Cough with dyspnea means counterflow lung qi, therefore the cold and sour of Shao Yao and the sour and warm of Wu Wei Zi are used to restrain. When water stays below the heart, the kidney gets dry, the pungent and warm of Xi Xin and Gan Jiang can moisten the kidney and move water.

　　　　　The pungent and warm of Ban Xia can restrain counterflow qi and disperse water rheum, and acts as courier.

　　　　　(2) When sweating is promoted in the exterior and water moves in the interior, the evil of exterior and interior gets to disperse.

·**RELATED FORMULA**：When Shi Gao is added to this formula, this is called Xiao Qing Long Tang Jia Shi Gao Tang, treats lung distention, cough with dyspnea, vexation and agitation, panting, water qi below the heart, and the pulse that is floating.

·**Original Source**：Zhong Jing

4. 小青龍湯

　·總結：行水發汗

　·組成：麻黃, 桂枝, 白芍, 乾薑, 細辛, 半夏, 五味子, 甘草

　·主治：(1)治傷寒表不解, 心下有水氣, 乾嘔發熱而欬.

　　　　　(2)或噎, 或喘, 或渴, 或利, 或小便不利, 少腹滿, 短氣不得臥.

　·加減：(1)渴去半夏, 加花粉.

　　　　　(2)喘去麻黃加杏仁.

　　　　　(3)形腫亦去麻黃.

　　　　　(4)噎去麻黃, 加附子.

　　　　　(5)小便祕去麻黃, 加茯苓.

　·歸經：足太陽藥也.

　·方義：(1)表不解, 故以麻黃發汗爲君, 桂枝, 甘草佐之, 解表爲佐.

欬喘, 肺氣逆也, 故用芍藥酸寒, 五味酸溫以收之. 水停心下則腎躁, 細辛, 乾薑辛溫, 能潤腎而行水.

半夏辛溫, 能收逆氣, 散水飲, 爲使也.

(2)外發汗, 內行水則表裏之邪散矣.

·變化方：本方加石膏, 名小青龍加石膏湯, 治肺脹欬而上氣, 煩躁而喘, 心下有水, 脈浮.

·來源：仲景

5. Ge Gen Tang. Kudzu Decoction. 葛根湯

·ACTIONS：promotes sweating and releases the flesh.

·COMPOSITION：Ge Gen, Ma Huang, Gui Zhi, Bai Shao Yao, Gan Cao, Da Zao, Sheng Jiang

·INDICATIONS：(1) In greater yang disease, there is disease with stretched stiff nape and back, absence of sweating, and aversion to wind.

(2) The combination disease of greater yang and yang brightness.

·CHANNELS ENTERED：The foot greater yang channel. [The bladder]

·Analysis of Formula：Cheng Wu Ji says that something light can eliminate repletion. Ge Gen and Ma Huang belong to the light herb. This pattern is wind strike exterior repletion, therefore Ma Huang and Ge Gen are added to Gui Zhi Tang.

·RELATED FORMULA：(1) When Ma Huang is eliminated, this is called Gui Zhi Jia Ge Gen Tang, treats the above pattern with sweating and aversion to wind.

(2) When Ban Xia is added, this is called Ge Gen Jia Ban Xia Tang, treats the combination disease of greater yang and yang brightness, absence of diarrhea, but retching.

(3) When Huang Qin is added, this is called Ge Gen Jie Ji Tang, treats heat effusion, aversion to cold, headache, stiff nape, cold damage, and warm disease.

·Original Source：Zhong Jing

5. 葛根湯
·總結：發汗兼解肌
·組成：葛根, 麻黃, 桂枝, 白芍, 甘草, 大棗, 生薑
·主治：(1)治太陽病, 項背几几, 無汗惡風.

79

(2)亦治太陽陽明合病下利.

　·歸經：足太陽藥也.

　·方義：成氏曰：「輕可去實，葛根，麻黃之屬是也.」此以中風表實，故加二物于桂枝湯中.

　·變化方：(1)本方除麻黃，名桂枝加葛根湯，治前證汗出惡風者.

　　　　　　(2)本方加半夏，名葛根加半夏湯，治太陽陽明合病，不下利，但嘔.

　　　　　　(3)本方加黃芩，名葛根解肌湯，治發熱惡寒，頭痛項強，傷寒溫病.

　·來源：仲景

6. Ma Huang Fu Zi Xi Xin Tang. Ephedra, Asarum, and Prepared Aconite Decoction. 麻黃附子細辛湯

·**ACTIONS**：The foot lesser yin exterior pattern.

·**COMPOSITION**：Ma Huang, Fu Zi, Xi Xin, Gan Cao

·**INDICATIONS**：When lesser yin disease has just started, but there is heat effusion and the pulse is sunken.

·**CHANNELS ENTERED**：The lesser yin channel. [The kidney]

·**Analysis of Formula**：In greater yang pattern, there is heat effusion, and the pulse should be floating, but the pulse is sunken. In lesser yin pattern, the pulse is sunken, and there is absence of heat effusion, therefore it says that 'but the pulse is sunken'. Heat effusion indicates evil in the exterior, sweating should be promoted. The sunken pulse belongs to yin, warming should be used, therefore Fu Zi is used to warm lesser yin channel, Ma Huang is used to disperse the cold of greater yang and promote sweating, Xi Xin is kidney channel exterior herb.

·**Original Source**：Zhong Jing

6. 麻黃附子細辛湯

　·總結：少陰表證

　·組成：麻黃, 附子, 細辛, 甘草

　·主治：治傷寒少陰證, 始得之, 反發熱, 脈沉者.

　·歸經：足少陰藥也.

　·方義：太陽證發熱, 脈當浮, 今反沉；少陰證脈沉, 當無熱, 故曰反也. 熱爲邪在表, 當汗, 脈沉屬陰, 又當溫, 故以附子溫少陰之經, 以麻黃

散太陽之寒而發汗，以細辛腎經表藥，聯屬其間，是汗劑之重者.

·來源：仲景

7. Sheng Ma Ge Gen Tang. Cimicifuga and Kudzu Decoction. 升麻葛根湯

·ACTIONS： raises and disperses yang brightness

·COMPOSITION：Sheng Ma, Ge Gen, Gan Cao, Sheng Jiang, Bai Shao Yao

·INDICATIONS：(1) Yang brightness cold damage, headache in wind strike, generalized pain, heat effusion, aversion to cold, absence of sweating, thirst, eye pain, dry nose, and inability to lie down.

(2) Yang brightness macula which has a desire come out but fails, epidemic disease.

CHANNELS ENTERED：The foot yang brightness channel. [The stomach]

·MODIFICATIONS：(1) for headache, add Chuan Xiong and Bai Zhi.

(2) for generalized pain and stiff back, add Qiang Huo and Fang Feng.

(3) for heat which won't retreat, in spring add Chai Hu, Huang Qin, Fang Feng, In summer, add Huang Qin and Shi Gao.

(4) for face swelling, add Fang Feng, Jing Jie, Lian Qiao, Bai Zhi, Chuan Xiong, Niu Bang Zi, and Shi Gao.

(5) for sore throat, add Jie Geng.

(6) for macula which won't outthrust through the exterior, add Zi Cao Rong.

(7) If the pulse is weak, add Ren Shen.

(8) for decreased diet due to stomach vacuity, add Bai Zhu.

(9) for abdominal pain, double Shao Yao to harmonize.

·Analysis of Formula：(1) Yang brightness has much qi and much blood, if cold evil damages people, blood and qi will be congested.

(2) Pungent can reach exterior, something light can eliminate repletion, therefore the herbs which is light and pungent as Sheng Ma and Ge Gen, disperse the exterior evil of yang brightness. When yang evil is exuberant, yin qi is vacuous, therefore Shao Yao is used to restrain yin and harmonize blood. And Gan Cao regulates the defense qi.

(3) Sheng Ma and Gan Cao raise yang and resolve toxin, therefor

81

e treats seasonal epidemic.

·**Contraindication**：⑴ When macula has already come out, do not take this. It is afraid that this formula makes the exterior more vacuous.

⑵ When cold damage has not yet entered yang brightness, do not take this, it is afraid that this formula leads exterior evil to yang brightness.

·**Original Source**：**Quan Zhong Yang**

7. 升麻葛根湯
    ·總結：陽明升散
    ·組成：升麻，葛根，甘草，生薑，白芍
    ·主治：⑴治陽明傷寒，中風頭疼，身痛發熱惡寒，無汗口渴，目痛鼻乾，不得臥.

⑵及陽明發斑，欲出不出，寒暄不時，人多疾疫.

    ·加減：⑴如頭痛，加川芎，白芷.

⑵身痛背強，加羌活，防風.

⑶熱不退，春加柴胡，黃芩，防風；夏加黃芩，石膏.

⑷頭面腫，加防風，荊芥，連翹，白芷，川芎，牛蒡，石膏.

⑸咽痛加桔梗.

⑹斑出不透，加紫草茸.

⑺脈弱，加人參.

⑻胃虛食少，加白朮.

⑼腹痛，倍芍藥和之.

    ·歸經：足陽明藥也.
    ·方義：⑴陽明多氣多血，寒邪傷人，則血氣爲之壅滯.

⑵辛能達表，輕可去實，故以升，葛辛輕之品，發散陽明表邪. 陽邪盛則陰氣虛，故用芍藥斂陰和血. 又用甘草調其衛氣也.

⑶升麻，甘草升陽解毒，故又治時疫.

    ·禁　忌：⑴斑疹已出者勿服，恐反重虛其表也.

⑵傷寒未入陽明者勿服，恐反引表邪入陽明也.

    ·來源：錢仲陽

8. Chai Ge Jie Ji Tang. Bupleurum and Kudzu Decoction to Release the Muscle Layer. 柴葛解肌湯

·**ACTIONS**：The combination disease of greater yang yang brightness.

·**COMPOSITION**：Chai Hu, Ge Gen, Qiang Huo, Bai Zhi, Huang Qin, Shi Gao, Bai Shao Yao, Gan Cao, Jie Geng, Sheng Jiang, Da Zao

·**INDICATIONS**：In the combination disease of greater yang and yang brightness, pain in the head, eye, eye socket, dry nose, insomnia, aversion to cold, absence of sweating, the pulse which is slightly surging.

·**MODIFICATIONS**：(1) When there is absence of sweating and aversion to cold are severe, eliminate Huang Qin.

(2) In winter, add Ma Huang, in spring, add a little of it.

(3) In summer, add Su Ye.

·**CHANNELS ENTERED**：The foot greater yang and yang brightness channel. [The bladder and stomach]

·**Analysis of Formula**：(1) Cold evil in channel, Qiang Huo disperses the evil in greater yang, Bai Zhi and Ge Gen disperse the evil in yang brightness, and Chai Hu disperses evil in lesser yang.

(2) When cold is about to transform into heat, Huang Qin, Shi Gao, and Jie Geng clear heat. Shao Yao and Gan Cao restrain yin and harmonize the middle.

·**Original Source**：Jie An

8. 柴葛解肌湯

·總結：太陽陽明

·組成：柴胡，葛根，羌活，白芷，黃芩，石膏，白芍，甘草，桔梗，生薑，大棗

·主治：治太陽陽明合病，頭目眼眶痛，鼻乾不眠，惡寒無汗，脈微洪.

·加減：(1)無汗惡寒甚者，去黃芩.

(2)冬月加麻黃，春月少加.

(3)夏月加蘇葉.

·歸經：足太陽陽明藥也.

·方義：(1)寒邪在經，羌活散太陽之邪，芷，葛散陽明之邪，柴胡散少陽之邪.

(2)寒將爲熱，故以黃芩，石膏，桔梗清之；以芍藥，甘草和之也.

·來源：節庵

9. Chai Hu Sheng Ma Tang. Bupleurum and Cimicifuga Decoction. 柴胡升麻湯

·**ACTIONS**：The combination disease of lesser yang and yang brightness

·**COMPOSITION**：Chai Hu, Qian Hu, Huang Qin, Sheng Ma, Ge Gen, Sang Bai Pi, Jing Jie, Chi Shao, Shi Gao, Sheng Jiang, Dan Dou Chi

·**INDICATIONS**：(1) The combination disease of lesser yang and yang brightness, wind damage, invigorating heat effusion, aversion to wind, headache, generalized pain, nasal congestion, dry throat, exuberant phlegm, cough, and thick spittle.

(2) Depressed yang qi, sunken source qi, scourage epidemic.

·**CHANNELS ENTERED**： the foot lesser yang and yang brightness channel [The gall bladder and stomach]

·**Analysis of Formula**：(1) When there is yang brightness disease with lesser yang, it is impossible to attack both exterior and interior, one should harmonize and release the exterior and interior.

(2) Chai Hu pacifies the heat of lesser yang and Sheng Ma and Gen Gen disperse the evil of yang brightness. Qian Hu disperses phlegm, descends qi, and releases wind and cold, Sang Pi drains the lung, disinhibits damp, and stops phlegm cough, Jing Jie disperse wind and heat and clears the head and eyes, Chi Shao regulates construction and blood and disperses liver evil, Huang Qin clears fire in the upper and middle burner, Shi Gao drains heat in the lung and stomach.

(3) The pungent of Sheng Jiang, Dan Dou Chi raises yang and disperse the exterior.

·**Original Source**：Ju Fang

9. 柴胡升麻湯
　·總結：少陽陽明
　·組成：柴胡，前胡，黃芩，升麻，葛根，桑白皮，荊芥，赤芍，石膏，薑，豆鼓
　·主治：(1)治少陽陽明合病，傷風壯熱惡風，頭痛體痛，鼻塞咽乾，痰盛欬嗽，唾涕稠粘.
　　　　(2)及陽氣鬱遏，元氣下陷，時行瘟疫.
　·歸經：足少陽陽明藥也.
　·方義：(1)陽明而兼少陽，則表裏俱不可攻，祇宜和解.

84

(2)柴胡平少陽之熱，升葛散陽明之邪，前胡消痰下氣而解風寒，桑皮瀉肺利溲而止痰嗽，荊芥疏風熱而清頭目，赤芍調營血而散肝邪，黃芩清火于上中二焦，石膏瀉熱于肺胃之部.

(3)加薑，豉者，取其辛散而升發也.

·來源：局方

10. Jiu Wei Qiang Huo Tang. Nine-Herb Decoction with No topterygium. 九味羌活湯

·**ACTIONS**：releases the exterior

·**COMPOSITION**：Qiang Huo, Fang Feng, Xi Xin, Chuan Xiong, Bai Zhi, Sheng Jiang, Cong Bai, Sheng Di Huang, Huang Qin, Cang Zhu, Da Zao, Gan Cao

·**INDICATIONS**：(1) Cold damage and wind damage, aversion to cold and vigorous heat effusion, headache and generalized pain, nape pain and stiff back, vomiting and thirst, absence of sweating in greater yang pattern.

(2) Common cold due to untimely seasonal qi, warm disease and heat disease.

·**MODIFICATIONS**：(1) for spontaneous sweating as in wind strike, eliminate Cang Zhu and add Bai Zhu and Huang Qi.

(2) for thoracic fullness, eliminate Di Huang and add Zhi Ke and Jie Geng.

(3) for panting, add Xing Ren.

(4) in summer, add Shi Gao and Zhi Mu.

(5) when promotion of sweating and precipitation are needed to be used together, add **Da Huang**.

·**CHANNELS ENTERED**：This formula is commonly used to the pattern of the foot greater yang, and is applied instead of Gui Zhi Tang, Ma Huang Tang, Qing Long Tang, Gui Ma Ge Ban Tang, etc.

·**Analysis of Formula**：(1) The pungent belongs to metal and reinforces the healthy qi and eliminates the pathogenic factors. Qiang Huo, Fang Feng, Cang Zhu, Xi Xin, Chuan Xiong, and Bai Zhi, these are pungent.

Qiang Huo enters the foot greater yang, eliminates the pathogenic factors, and restores health.

Cang Zhu enters the foot greater yin, repels foul turbidity, and eliminates damp.

Bai Zhi enters the foot yang brightness and treats head

85

ache in the forehead.

Chuan Xiong enters the foot reverting yin and treats headache in the brain.

Xi Xin enters the foot lesser yin and treats headache in the foot lesser yin channel.

All of them can expel wind and disperse cold, and move qi and activate blood.

(2) If Huang Qin which enters the hand greater yin is added, this drains the heat in the qi. Sheng Di Huang enters the hand greater yin and drains the heat in the blood. Fang Feng is wind herb and there is no place where it can not reach, treats whole body pain, and acts as courier. Gan Cao is sweet and neutral, harmonizes every herbs.

(3) In this formula there is six channel herbs, this is commonly used to external contraction disease pattern in every season, doctors should modify this according to the pattern, must not adhere to one formula.

·**Original Source**：Zhang Yuan Su

10. 九味羌活湯

·總結：解表通劑

·組成：羌活，防風，細辛，川芎，白芷，生薑，蔥白，生地，黃芩，蒼朮，大棗，甘草

·主治：(1)治傷寒傷風，憎寒壯熱，頭痛身痛，項痛脊強，嘔吐口渴，太陽無汗.

(2)及感冒四時不正之氣，溫病熱病.

·加減：(1)如風證自汗者，去蒼朮，加白朮黃耆.

(2)胸滿，去地黃，加枳殼，桔梗.

(3)喘加杏仁.

(4)夏加石膏，知母.

(5)汗下兼行，加大黃.

·歸經：足太陽例藥，以代桂枝，麻黃，青龍名半等湯也.

·方義：(1)藥之辛者屬金，于人爲氣，故能匡正黜邪. 羌，防，蒼，細，芎，芷，皆辛藥也.

羌活入足太陽，爲撥亂反正之主藥.

蒼朮入足太陰，辟惡而去溼.

白芷入足陽明，治頭痛在額.

芎藭入足厥陰，治頭痛在腦.

細辛入足少陰，治本經頭痛.

86

皆能驅風散寒, 行氣活血.

(2)而又加黃芩入手太陰, 以泄氣中之熱；生地入手太陰, 以泄血中之熱；防風爲風藥卒徒, 隨所引而無不庄, 治一身盡痛爲使；甘草甘平, 用以協和諸藥也.

(3)藥備六經, 治通四時, 用者當隨證加或, 不可執一.

·來源：張元素

11. Shi Shen Tang. Ten-Immortal Decoction. 十神湯

·**ACTIONS**：common cold and seasonal qi

·**COMPOSITION**：Zi Su Ye Ge Gen Chuan Xiong Sheng Ma Bai Zhi Ma Huang Gan Cao Chen Pi Xiang Fu Chi Shao Yao Sheng Jiang Cong Bai

·**INDICATIONS**： contraction of wind and cold, seasonal qi and scourage epidemic, headache, heat effusion, aversion to cold, absence of sweating, cough, nasal congestion, deep voice.

·**CHANNELS ENTERED**：external contraction in three yang channel.

·**Analysis of Formula**：Wu He Gao says that when treating wind cold, ancient person always discriminates the pattern according to the six channel and then they use medicine, although there is heat effusion, headache, aversion to cold, and nasal congestion, but the pattern of the six channel is not remarkable, therefore herbs which courses and disinhibits qi are mainly used. Chuan Xiong, Ma Huang, Sheng Ma, Ge Gen (dry), Bai Zhi, Zi Su Ye, Chen Pi, and Xiang Fu are pungent and aromatic and disinhibit qi, therefore this formula can release qi blockage in common cold. Shao Yao is added to harmonize yin qi during promoting of sweating, and Gan Cao is added to harmonize yang qi during coursing and disinhibiting of qi.

·**Original Source**：Ju Fang

11. 十神湯

·總結：感冒時氣

·組成：紫蘇 葛根 川芎 升麻 白芷 麻黃 甘草 陳皮 香附 赤芍藥 生薑 葱白

·主治：治風寒兩感, 時氣瘟疫, 頭痛發熱, 惡寒無汗, 欬嗽, 鼻塞聲重.

·歸經：陽經外感之通劑也.

·方義：吳鶴皋曰：「古人治風寒, 必分六經見證用藥, 然亦有發熱頭

痛，惡寒鼻塞，而六經之證不甚顯者，亦總以疏利氣之藥主之．是方也，川芎，麻黃，升麻，乾葛，白芷，紫蘇，陳皮，香附，皆辛香利氣之品，故可以解感冒氣塞之證．而又加芍藥，和陰氣于發汗之中，加甘草，和陽氣于疏利之隊也．」

·來源：局方

12. Shen Zhu San. Wonderous Atractylodes Powder. 神术散

·**ACTIONS**：cold damage with absence of sweating

·**COMPOSITION**：Cang Zhu, Fang Feng, Gan Cao, Sheng Jiang Cong Bai

·**INDICATIONS**：(1) Internal damage due to cold drink, external contrac tion of cold evil with absence of sweating.

(2) Febrile convulsion with chills.

·**MODIFICATIONS**：(1) If there is greater yang pattern with heat effusio n, aversion to cold, and the pulse that is floating and tight, add Qiang Huo. If th e pulse is floating and tight with surging, and there is yang brightness pattern, a dd Huang Qin. If the pulse is floating and tight with string like and rapid and th ere is yang pattern, add Chai Hu.

(2) In case of women, add Dang Gui.

·**CHANNELS ENTERED**：The foot greater yang channel. [The bladder]

·**Analysis of Formula**：Fang Feng is pungent and warm, has the characte r of rising and floating, eliminates wind and prevails over damp, and is the mai n herb for controlling greater yang. Cang Zhu is sweet, warn, pungent, and hars h, disperses cold and promotes sweating, and repels foulness and raises yang. If Gan Cao is added, this makes formula get harmonious during dispersing.

·**RELATED FORMULA**：(1) If Cang Zhu is eliminated, Bai Zhu (two li ang), Sheng Jiang (Three Pian) are added, this is called Bai Zhu Tang (Wang H ai Zang), treats the pattern of Shen Zhu San with sweating, also treats febrile co nvulsion without chills.

(2) Tai Wu Shen Zhu San, ：Cang Zhu, Hou Po, Chen Pi, Gan Cao, Huo Xiang, Shi Chang Pu. This treats that when miasmic toxin contracts, t here is abhorrence of cold, invigorating heat effusion, generalized pain, swellin g of face, miasmic malaria, and seasonal toxin.

(3) Ju Fang Shen Zhu San, ：Cang Zhu, Chuan Xiong, Bai Zhi, Qiang Huo, Gao Ben, Xi Xin, Gan Cao (mix fried), Sheng Jiang, Cong Bai. Thi

s treats damage wind with headache, absence of sweating, nasal congestion, an
d deep voice, and cough due to wind and cold and seasonal diarrhea.

·**Original Source**：Wang Hai Zang

12. 神朮散
·總結：傷寒無汗
·組成：蒼朮，防風，甘草，薑，葱
·主治：(1)治內傷冷飲，外感寒邪而無汗者.
　　　(2)亦治剛痙.
·加減：(1)如太陽證發熱，惡寒，脈浮緊者，加羌活；浮緊帶洪者，是
兼陽明，加黃芩；浮緊帶弦數者，是兼少陽，加柴胡.
　　　(2)婦人加當歸.
·歸經：足太陽藥也.
·方義：防風辛溫升浮，除風勝溼，爲太陽主藥. 蒼朮甘溫辛烈，散寒
發汗，辟惡升陽. 加甘草者，發中有緩也.
·變化方：(1)本方除蒼朮，加白朮二兩，薑三片，不用葱，名白朮湯(海
藏)，治前證有汗者，亦治柔痙.
　　　(2)太無神朮散：蒼朮，厚朴，陳皮，甘草，藿香，石菖蒲. 治
感山嵐瘴氣，憎寒壯熱，一身盡痛，頭面腫大，瘴瘧時毒.
　　　(3)局方神朮散：蒼朮，川芎，白芷，羌活，藁本，細辛，炙甘
草，薑，葱. 治傷風頭痛無汗，鼻塞聲重，及風寒欬嗽，時行泄瀉.
·來源：海藏

13. Cong Chi Tang. Scallion and Prepared Soybean Decocti on. 葱豉湯

·**ACTIONS**：promotion of sweating in greater yang
·**COMPOSITION**：Cong Bai, Dan Dou Chi.
·**INDICATIONS**：in the initial stage of cold damage, there is headache, g
eneralized heat effusion, and the pulse is surging.
MODIFICATIONS：If there is absence of sweating, add Ge Gen.
·**CHANNELS ENTERED**：The foot greater yang channel. [The bladder]
·**Analysis of Formula**：(1) Cong Bai frees yang and promotes sweating,
Dan Dou Chi tends to rise, and disperses and promotes sweating.

　　　(2) At initial stage, evil is in the exterior, first of all take this Dec

89

oction to releases and disperses it, it can be used instead of Ma Huang Tang.

·**RELATED FORMULA**：If Dan Dou Chi is eliminated and Sheng Jiang is added, this is called Lian Zu Cong Bai Tang, treats same thing.

·**Original Source**：Zhou Hou Fang

13. 葱豉湯

    ·總結：太陽發汗

    ·組成：葱白，豉.

    ·主治：治傷寒初覺頭痛身熱，脈洪，便當服此.

    ·加減：如無汗，加葛根.

    ·歸經：足太陽藥也.

    ·方義：(1)葱通陽而發汗，豉升散而發汗.

        (2)邪初在表，宜先服此以解散之，免用麻黃湯者之多顧忌，用代麻黃者之多所紛更也.

    ·變化方：本方去淡豉，加生薑，名連鬚葱白湯，治同.

    ·來源：肘後

14. Ren Shen Bai Du San. Ginseng Powder to Overcome Pathogenic Influences Ren Shen. 人參敗毒散

·**ACTIONS**：influenza.

·**COMPOSITION**：Ren Shen, Qiang Huo, Du Huo, Chuan Xiong, Chai Hu, Qian Hu, Zhi Ke, Jie Geng, Fu Ling, Gan Cao, Sheng Jiang, Bo He.

·**INDICATIONS**：(1) Cold damage with headache, abhorrence of cold and invigorating heat effusion, stiff nape and dim vision, nasal congestion and deep voice, and wind phlegm with cough

    (2) Seasonal epidemic, miasmic toxin, and ghost malaria.

    (3) Voice as like frog, red eye (conjunctivitis), aphtha, deep multiple abscess due to damp toxin, leg swelling and mumps, throat impediment, toxin dysentery, every sore, and **macula**.

·**MODIFICATIONS**：(1) for dry mouth and tongue, add Huang Qin.

    (2) for leg qi, add Da Huang and Cang Zhu.

    (3) for itching in the skin, add Chan Tui.

·**CHANNELS ENTERED**：The foot greater yang and lesser yang and the hand greater yin channels. [The bladder, gall bladder, and lung]

·**Analysis of Formula**：(1) Qiang Huo enters greater yang and rectifies w andering wind. Du Huo enters lesser yin and rectifies hidden wind and also can eliminate damp and pain. Chai Hu disperses heat, raises clear yang, and with co operating with Chuan Xiong harmonizes blood and pacifies the liver to treat he adache and blurred vision. Qian Hu and Zhi Ke descend qi, move phlegm, and t hey cooperate with Jie Geng and Fu Ling to drain lung heat, eliminate damp, an d disperse swelling. Gan Cao harmonizes interior and disperses exterior. Ren S hen helps the right qi to repel evil.

⑵ This formula disperses and frees the channel and disperses ev il stagnation in the exterior, therefore it is called Bai Du (Overcome Pathogenic Influences).

·**RELATED FORMULA**：⑴ When Ren Shen is eliminated, this is calle d Bai Du San, treats same thing with Ren Shen Bai Du San. When there is wind heat, add Jing Jie and Fang Feng, this is called Jing Fang Bai Du San, also treat s intestinal wind bleeding with fresh blood.

⑵ When Ren Shen is eliminated and Lian Qiao and Jin Yin Hua are added, this is called Lian Qiao Bai Du San, treats sore toxin.

⑶ When Ren Shen is eliminated and Huang Qin is added, this is called Bai Du Jia Huang Qin Tang, treats warm disease without aversion to win d and cold but thirst.

⑷ When Ren Shen is eliminated and Da Huang and Mang Xiao are added, this is called Xiao Huang Bai Du San, disperses accumulation which is congested with heat toxin.

⑸ The combination of Bai Du San and Xiao Feng San is called Xiao Feng Bai Du San, treats urticarial due to wind toxin, wind edema and skin edema in the exterior, this should be released following promotion of sweating.

⑹ If Chen Cang Mi (old rice) is added, this is called Chen Cang San, treats food-denying dysentery.

·**Original Source**：Huo Ren

14. 人參敗毒散
·總結：感冒時行
·組成：人參, 羌活, 獨活, 川芎, 柴胡, 前胡, 枳殼, 桔梗, 茯苓, 甘草, 生薑, 薄荷.
·主治：⑴治傷寒頭痛, 憎寒壯熱, 項強睛暗, 鼻塞聲重, 風痰欬嗽
⑵及時氣疫癘, 嵐瘴鬼瘧.
⑶或聲如蛙鳴, 赤眼口瘡, 溼毒流注, 腳腫腮腫, 喉痺毒痢, 諸瘡斑疹.

·加減：(1)口乾舌燥加黃芩.

　　　　(2)腳氣加大黃, 蒼术.

　　　　(3)膚癢加蟬蛻.

·歸經：足太陽少陽手太陰藥也.

·方義：(1)羌活入太陽而理遊風. 獨活入少陰而理伏風, 兼能去溼除痛. 柴胡散熱升清, 協川芎和血平肝, 以治頭痛目昏. 前胡, 枳殼降氣行痰, 協桔梗, 茯苓以泄肺熱, 而除溼消腫. 甘草和裏而發表. 人參輔正以匡邪.

　　　　(2)疏導經絡, 表散邪滯, 故曰敗毒.

·變化方：(1)本方除人參名敗毒散, 治同. 有風熱, 加荊芥, 防風, 名荊防敗毒散, 亦治腸風下血清鮮.

　　　　(2)本方去人參, 加連翹, 金銀花, 名連翹敗毒散, 治瘡毒.

　　　　(3)除人參, 加黃芩, 名敗毒加黃芩湯, 治瘟病不惡風寒而渴.

　　　　(4)除人參, 加大黃, 芒硝, 名硝黃敗毒散, 消熱毒壅積.

　　　　(5)敗毒散合消風散, 名消風敗毒散, 治風毒癮疹, 及風水皮水在表, 宜從汗解者.

　　　　(6)本方加陳廩米, 名陳廩散, 治噤口痢.

·來源：活人

15. Chuan Xiong Cha Tiao San. Ligusticum Chuanxiong Powder to be Taken with Green Tea. 川芎茶調散

·**ACTIONS**：raising and dispersing of wind and heat

·**COMPOSITION**：Bo He, Chuan Xiong, Jing Jie, Qiang Huo, Bai Zhi, Fang Feng, Xi Xin, Gan Cao (mix fried), Xi Cha (powder)

·**INDICATIONS**：every wind attacking upward, unbiased and hemilateral headache, aversion to wind, sweating, abhorrence of cold, invigorating heat, nasal congestion exuberant phlegm, dizziness, and dizzy vision.

·**CHANNELS ENTERED**：The foot three yang channels.

·**Analysis of Formula**：(1) Qiang Huo treats greater yang headache, Bai Zhi treats yang brightness headache, Chuan Xiong treats lesser yang headache, Xi Xin treats lesser yin headache, Fang Feng is the top herb to treat wind, all of them can release exterior and disperse cold, because wind and heat are in the upper part, therefore the herb having an action of raising and dispersing should be used. In headache, wind herb should be used, because only wind herb can reach the top of the head.

　　　　(2) Bo He and Jing Jie can disperse wind and heat, clear inhibite

92

d head and eye, therefore they act as sovereign, with the other herbs ascend up ward to raise and clear yang, and disperse depressed fire. Add Gan Cao to mod erate the middle.

(3) Cha can clear the head and eyes.

·**RELATED FORMULA**：In another formula, Ju Hua and Jiang Can are added, this is called Ju Hua Cha Diao San, treats wind and heat in the head and eyes

·**Original Source**：Ju Fang

15. 川芎茶調散

·總結：升散風熱

·組成：薄荷, 川芎, 荊芥, 羌活, 白芷, 防風, 細辛, 炙甘草, 細茶末

·主治：治諸風上攻, 正偏頭痛, 惡風有汗, 憎寒壯熱, 鼻塞痰盛, 頭暈目眩.

·歸經：足三陽藥也.

·方義：(1)羌活治太陽頭痛, 白芷治陽明頭痛, 川芎治少陽頭痛, 細辛治少陰頭痛, 防風爲風藥卒徒, 皆能解表散寒, 以風熱在上, 宜于升散也. 頭痛必用風藥者, 以巔頂之上, 惟風可到也.

(2)薄荷, 荊芥並能消散風熱, 清利頭目, 故以爲君, 同諸藥上行, 以升清陽而散鬱火. 加甘草者, 以緩中也.

(3)用茶調者, 茶能上清頭目也.

·變化方：一方加菊花殭蠶, 名菊花茶調散, 治頭目風熱.

·來源：局方

16. Zai Zao San. Renewal Powder. 再造散

·**ACTIONS**：absence of sweating due to yang vacuity

·**COMPOSITION**：Ren Shen, Huang Qi, Gui Zhi, Gan Cao, Fu Zi, Xi Xi n, Qiang Huo, Fang Feng, Chuan Xiong, Wei Jiang (roasted ginger), Shao Yao, Da Zao.

·**INDICATIONS**：owing to yang vacuity, sweat cannot be issued.

·**MODIFICATIONS**：in summer, add Huang Qin and Shi Gao.

·**CHANNELS ENTERED**：The foot greater yang channel.

·**Analysis of Formula**：Nei Jing says that sweat which is transformed by the dispersing of yang qi is like the rain which falls from heaven. Absence of s weating in greater yang indicates exuberant evil and true yang vacuity. Therefo

re Ren Shen, Huang Qi, Gan Cao, Wei Jiang, Gui Zhi, and Fu Zi greatly supple
ment the yang. Qiang Huo, Fang Feng, Chuan Xiong, and Xi Xin disperse exter
ior evil. Shao Yao is added to restrain yin during supplementing yang and dispe
rsing evil.

·**Original Source**：Jie An

16. 再造散

　·總結：陽虛無汗

　·組成：人參，黃耆，桂枝，甘草，附子，細辛，羌活，防風，川芎，煨
薑，芍藥，棗.

　·主治：治陽虛不能作汗.

　·加減：夏加黃芩，石膏.

　·歸經：足太陽藥也.

　·方義：經曰：「陽之汗以天之雨名之.」太陽病汗之無汗，是邪盛而
眞陽虛也.

　　　　故以參，耆，甘草，薑，桂，附子，大補其陽

　　　　；而以羌，防，芎，細，發其表邪

　　　　加芍藥者，于陽中斂陰，散中有收也.

　·來源：節庵

17. Da Qiang Huo Tang. Major Notopterygium Decoction. 大羌活湯

·**ACTIONS**：double contraction of cold damage

·**COMPOSITION**：Qiang Huo, Du Huo, Fang Feng, Xi Xin, Fang Ji, Hu
ang Qin, Huang Lian, Cang Zhu, Bai Zhu, Gan Cao (mix fried), Zhi Mu, Chuan
Xiong, sheng Di Huang.

·**INDICATIONS**：double contraction of cold damage.

·**CHANNELS ENTERED**：yin and yang channels.

·**Analysis of Formula**：(1) When the qi and flavor of herb are bland and li
ght, this can disperse and diffuse, therefore Qiang Huo, Du Huo, Chang Zhu, F
ang Feng, Chuan Xiong, and Xi Xin are used to eliminate wind, disperse exteri
or, and raise and disperse the evil which tries to transport to another channel.

(2) Cold can prevail over heat, therefore Huang Qin, Huang Lian,
Zhi Mu, Sheng Di Huang, and Fang Ji are used to clear heat, disinhibit damp, a
nd enrich damaged yin.

(3) Bai Zhu and Gan Cao secure the middle and harmonize the qi of the exterior and interior.

·**Original Source**：Jie Gu

17. 大羌活湯

　·總結：兩感傷寒

　·組成：羌活，獨活，防風，細辛，防己，黃芩，黃連，蒼朮，白朮，炙甘草，知母，川芎，生地黃．

　·主治：治兩感傷寒．

　·歸經：陰陽兩解之藥也．

　·方義：(1)氣薄則發泄，故用羌活，獨，蒼，防，芎，細，袪風發表，升散傳經之邪．

　　　(2)寒能勝熱，故用芩，連，知母，生地，防己，清熱利溼，滋培受傷之陰．

　　　(3)又用白朮，甘草以固中州，而和表裏之氣，升不至峻，寒不至凝，間能回九死一生也．

　·來源：潔古

18. Gui Zhi Qiang Huo Tang. Cinnamon Twig and Notopterygium Decoction. 桂枝羌活湯

·**ACTIONS**：malaria in greater yang.

·**COMPOSITION**：Gui Zhi, Qiang Huo, Fang Feng, Gan Cao.

·**INDICATIONS**：　Malaria which occurs before Chu Shu (around July by the lunar calendar), headache and nape pain, the pulse that is floating, sweating, aversion to wind.

　·**MODIFICATIONS**：(1) for vomiting, add Ban Xia.

　　　(2) for absence of sweating, exchange Gui Zhi with Ma Huang, this is called Ma Huang Fang Feng Tang.

　·**CHANNELS ENTERED**：The foot greater yang channel.

·**Analysis of Formula**：　Malaria is treated according the six channel, therefore as like Zhong Jing's cold damage, Fang Feng and Qiang Huo disperse the evil of greater yang.

　·**Original Source**：Huo Fa Ji Yao

18. 桂枝羌活湯
　·總結：太陽瘧疾
　·組成：桂枝, 羌活, 防風, 甘草.
　·主治：治瘧疾發在處暑以前, 頭項痛, 脈浮, 有汗惡風.
　·加減：(1)或吐, 加半夏麴.
　　　　　(2)無汗, 桂枝易麻黃, 名麻黃防風湯.
　·歸經：足太陽藥也.
　·方義：瘧分六經, 故倣仲景傷寒例, 以防風, 羌活散太陽之邪.
　·來源：機要

Chapter 3. Ejection Formulas. 涌吐之劑

1. Gua Di San. Melon Pedicle Powder. 瓜蒂散

·**ACTIONS**：vomiting of replete evil.

·**COMPOSITION**：Gua Di (stir-bake to yellow), Chi Xiao Dou.

·**INDICATIONS**：(1) Wind stroke, confounding phlegm, drool congestion, mania and withdrawal, vexation and derangement, loss of consciousness, five epilepsy, phlegm congestion, surging upward of fire qi, difficulty of breathing due to throat problem, congested food in greater yin with desire to vomit but f ails to.

(2) In cold damage as Gui Zhi pattern, if there is absence of headache and s tiff nape, glomus and hardness in the chest, and qi surging upward with diffic ulty of taking breath, the pulse is faint and floating, this means that there is co ld in the chest, this should be treated with vomiting.

(3) Every acute jaundice.

·**CHANNELS ENTERED**：The foot greater yang and yang brightness ch annels. [The bladder and stomach]

·**Analysis of Formula**：(1) Phlegm and food in the chest is different with vacuity vexation, therefore the bitter of Gua Di is used to make them skip upwa rd and the sour of Chi Xiao Dou is to eject them, then if phlegm and food in the upper burner are removed through vomiting, water becomes soothed and uninhi bited, heaven and earth get to interact and all things also get to free.

(2) Even though there is a pattern which need vomiting, but stom ach is weak, change with Ren Shen Lu.

·**RELATED FORMULA**：(1) When Chi Xiao Dou is eliminated from thi s formula, this is called Du Sheng San, treats greater yang summerheat stroke, generalized heaviness and pain, and the pulse that is faint and weak.

(2) When Chi Xiao Dou is eliminated and Fang Feng and Li Lu a re added, this is called San Sheng San (Three-Sage Powder).

(3) When Chi Xiao Dou is eliminated and Yu Jin and Jiu Zhi are added, and then stimulating throat with a feather of goose to make one vomit, t his is also called San Sheng San (Three-Sage Powder), treats wind strike, wind epilepsy, and phlegm reversal headache.

(4) When Chi Xiao Dou is added and Quan Xie (five fen) is adde d, this is to make one vomit wind phlegm.

(5) When Dan Dou Chi is added, treats cold damage, and vexatio

n and oppression.

    ·**Original Source**：Zhong Jing

1. 瓜蒂散

    ·總結：吐實邪

    ·組成：甜瓜蒂(炒黃), 赤小豆.

    ·主治：(1)治卒中痰迷, 涎潮壅盛, 巔狂煩亂, 人事昏沉, 五癇痰壅, 及火氣上衝, 喉不得息, 食填太陰, 欲吐不出.

        (2)傷寒如桂枝證, 頭不痛, 項不强, 寸脈微浮, 胸中痞硬, 氣上衝喉不得息者, 胸有寒也, 當吐之.

        (3)亦治諸黃急黃.

    ·歸經：足太陽陽明藥也.

    ·方義：(1)胸中痰食與虛煩者不同, 越以瓜蒂之苦, 涌以赤小豆之酸, 吐去上焦有形之物, 則水得舒暢, 天地交而萬物通矣.

        (2)當吐而胃弱者, 改用參蘆.

    ·變化方：(1)本方除赤小豆, 名獨聖散, 治太陽中暍, 身重痛而脈微弱.

        (2)本方除赤豆, 加防風, 藜蘆, 名三聖散.

        (3)本方除赤豆, 加鬱金, 韭汁, 鵝翎探吐, 亦名三聖散, 治中風風癇, 痰厥頭痛.

        (4)本方除赤豆, 加全蠍五分, 吐風痰.

        (5)本方加淡豉, 治傷寒煩悶.

    ·來源：仲景

2. Shen Lu San. Ginseng Tops Powder. 參蘆散

    ·**ACTIONS**：vomiting of vacuity phlegm

    ·**COMPOSITION**：Ren Shen Lu

    ·**INDICATIONS**：weak constitution with congested phlegm.

  ·**CHANNELS ENTERED**：The hand greater yin and the foot greater yang channel. [The lung and bladder]

    ·**Analysis of Formula**：(1) Nei Jing says that when it is on high, trace [it] and disperse it. When phlegm and drool are congested in the upper part, this should be treated with making one vomit.

        (2) Because the patient is vacuous, therefore Len Lu is used instead of Li Lu and Gua Di to supplement and not to exhaust and damage source qi.

98

2. 參蘆散
·總結：吐虛痰
·組成：人參蘆
·主治：治虛弱人痰涎壅盛.
·歸經：此手太陰足太陽藥也.
·方義：(1)經曰：「在上者因而越之.」痰涎上壅, 法當涌之.
　　　　(2)病人虛羸, 故以參蘆代藜蘆, 瓜蒂, 宣猶代補, 不致耗傷
元氣也.

3. Zhi Zi Chi Tang. Gardenia and Soja Decoction. 梔子豉 湯

·**ACTIONS**：treating vacuity vexation through vomit.

·**COMPOSITION**：Zhi Zi and Dan Dou Chi

·**INDICATIONS**：(1) When in cold damage after promotion of sweating or v omiting or precipitation, there is vacuity vexation and inability to sleep, and if the condition is severe, with tossing and turning and anguish in the heart.

(2) and if after great precipitation, the generalized heat has not gone, and there is binding pain in the heart and phlegm in the diaphragm.

·**CHANNELS ENTERED**：The foot greater yang and yang brightness channel. [The bladder and stomach]

·**Analysis of Formula**：(1) Vexation is related with heat exuberance, Zhi Zi is bitter and cold, the red color enters the heart, therefore acts as sovereign.

The bitter of Dan Dou Chi can disperse evil heat, putridity qi prevails scorch qi (putridity qi enters the kidney, scorch qi enters the heart, kidney water prevails heart fire), assists Zhi Zi to vomit vacuity vexation, therefore acts as minister.

(2) ejection with sour and bitter belongs to yin, this formula makes vacuity vexation of formless to be ejected, if replete evil in the diaphragm, it is appropriate to treat with Gua Di San.

·**RELATED FORMULA**：(1) When Gan Cao is added, this is called Zhi Zi Gan Cao Chi Tang, treats the above pattern with shortage of qi.

(2) When Sheng Jiang is added, this is called Zhi Zi Sheng Jiang Chi Tang, treats the above pattern with retching.

(3) When Dan Dou Chi is eliminated and Gan Jiang is added, thi

99

s is called Zhi Zi Gan Jiang Tang, treats that when in cold damage great precipi
tation is performed, the generalized heat is not gone and there is mild vexation

(4) When Dan Dou Chi is eliminated and Hou Po and Zhi Shi are
added, this is called Zhi Zi Hou Po Tang, treats that in cold damage after precip
itation, there is heart vexation and abdominal fullness.

(5) When Da Huang and Zhi Shi are added, this is called Zhi Zi
Da Huang Tang, treats alcoholic jaundice with yellowing, the anguish in the he
art or heat pain in the chest and diaphragm, and also treats relapse due to dietar
y irregularity in the stage of cold damage.

(6) When Zhi Shi is added, this is called Zhi Shi Zhi Zi Tang, tre
ats cold damage taxation relapse.

(7) when Xie Bai is added, this is called Chi Xie Tang, treats that
when in cold damage after precipitation, there is stool as putrid flesh juice, red
vaginal discharge, latent qi, abdominal pain, and all of heat pattern.

(8) When Xi Jiao and Da Qing Ye are added, this is called Xi Jia
o Da Qing Tang, treats macula toxin and headache with heat exuberance.
·**Original Source**：Zhong Jing

3. 梔子豉湯
  ·總結：吐虛煩
  ·組成：梔子, 淡豉
  ·主治：(1)治傷寒汗吐下後, 虛煩不眠, 劇者反覆顛倒, 心下懊憹.
        (2)及大下後身熱不退, 心下結痛, 或痰在膈中.
  ·歸經：此足太陽陽明藥.
  ·方義：(1)煩爲熱盛, 梔子苦寒, 色赤人心, 故以爲君.
        淡豉苦能發熱, 腐能勝焦, 助梔子以吐虛煩, 故以
爲臣.
        (2)酸苦涌泄爲陰也, 此吐無形之虛煩, 若膈有實邪, 當用瓜
蒂散.
  ·變化方：(1)本方加甘草, 名梔子甘草豉湯治前證兼少氣者.
        (2)本方加生薑, 名梔子生薑豉湯, 治前證兼嘔者.
        (3)本方除淡豉, 加乾薑, 名梔子乾薑湯, 治傷寒誤下, 身熱
不去, 微煩者.
        (4)本方除淡豉, 加厚朴, 枳實, 名梔子厚朴湯, 治傷寒下後,
心煩腹滿.
        (5)本方加大黄, 枳實, 名梔子大黄湯, 治酒疸發黄, 心中懊

儂或熱痛；亦治傷寒食復.

(6)本方加枳實，名枳實梔子湯，治傷寒勞復.

(7)本方加薤白，名豉薤湯，治傷寒下利如爛肉汁，赤滯下，伏氣腹痛諸熱證.

(8)本方加犀角，大青，名犀角大青湯，治斑毒熱甚頭痛.

·來源：仲景

4. Xi Xian San. Drool Thinning Powder. 稀涎散

·**ACTIONS**：making one to vomit phlegm in wind stroke

·**COMPOSITION**：Zao Jiao, Bai Fan

·**INDICATIONS**：(1) hen in stroke, there is sudden collapse, phlegm-drool congestion, clenched jaw, and acute upper airway obstruction, first of all, clenched jaw is to be open, and make patient to mildly vomit thin drool, and then give medicine. (2) also treats throat impediment with inability to eat.

·**CHANNELS ENTERED**：The foot greater yin and reverting yin channel. [The spleen and liver]

·**Analysis of Formula**：(1) Wu He Gao says that clear yang is in the upper part and turbid yin in the lower part, this is like that the sky is above and land is below. If turbid evil counterflows upward, clear yang gets to lose the position and then locates the other way which is bottom, therefore sudden collapse occurs. Congested phlegm and wind exuberance with congested qi bring about this. Nei Jing says that when disease occurs in the condition of insufficiency, first treat the tip and then treat the root. This disease does not respond to the first applying of the root treatment which is to course wind and supplement vacuity, but responds to the first applying of vomiting phlegm-drool.

(2) The sour and bitter of Bai Fan can eject [phlegm-drool], the salty can soften stubborn phlegm, therefore acts as sovereign.

The pungent of Zao Jiao can free orifice, the salty can eliminate grime, and mainly treats wind wood, therefore acts as courier.

(3) teacher says that after vomiting of wind-phlegm when throat gets to course and free, then one must stop taking this decoction, if one keep draining or attacking the phlegm, there will be no humor for nourishing sinew, this can cause hemilateral withering.

·**RELATED FORMULA**：(1) Zhang Zi He adds Li Lu, Chang Shan, and Gan Cao to this formula, this is called Chang Shan San, makes one vomit malaria phlegm.

101

(2) When Xiong Huang and Li Lu are added, this is called Ru Sheng San, put this powder into nose, treats acute entwining throat wind and clenched jaw.

4. 稀涎散
·總結：中風吐痰
·組成：皂角，白礬
·主治：(1)治中風暴仆，痰涎壅盛，氣閉不通，先開其關，令微吐稀涎，續進他藥，

　　　　(2)亦治喉痹不能進食.
·歸經：此足太陰厥陰藥也.
·方義：(1)吳鶴皋曰：「清陽在上，濁陰在下，天冠地履，無暴仆也.

　　　　若濁邪逆上，則清陽失位而倒置矣，故令人暴仆.

　　　　所以痰涎壅塞者，風盛氣壅使然也.

　　　　經曰：『病發于不足，標而本之，先治其標，後治其本.』

　　　　治不與疏風補虛，而先吐其痰涎.」

　　　　(2)白礬酸苦，能湧泄，鹹能軟頑痰，故以爲君.

　　　　皂角辛能通竅，鹹能去垢，專治風木，故以爲使，故奪門之兵也.

　　　　(3)師曰：「反吐中風之痰，使咽喉疏通，能進湯藥便止，若盡攻其痰，則無液以養筋，令人攣急偏枯，此其禁也.」

·變化方：(1)張子和加藜蘆，常山，甘草，名常山散，吐瘧痰.

　　　　(2)本方加雄黃，藜蘆，名如聖散，爲末，搐鼻，治纏喉急痹，牙關緊閉.

5. Gan Huo Luan Tu Fang. Dry Cholera and Vomiting Decoction. 乾霍亂吐方

·**ACTIONS**：Cholera
·**COMPOSITION**：Salt (burned), heat Child's urine.
·**INDICATIONS**：dry cholera, a desire to vomit but inability to do, a desire to defecate but inability to do, and great pain in the abdomen.
·**CHANNELS ENTERED**：The foot greater yin and yang brightness. [The spleen and stomach]

·**Analysis of Formula**：(1) A desire to vomit but inability to do means evil binds in the middle burner, the salt can soften hardness and break stubborn phlegm and retained food. Stir-baked salt generates bitter, therefore this causes emetic actions.

(2) Child's urine originally descends qi of body, therefore this induces fire to descend and return fire to old way, and the flavor and character are salty and cold, therefore its action of descending fire is very rapid.

The salt makes one vomit in the upper part and urine drains fire in the lower part, then the middle gets free.

·**RELATED FORMULA**：Here, this formula uses only salt (burned) with hot water, and making one vomit with finger, this is called Shao Yan Zhi Tan Tu Fa, treats that when in food damage there is pain linked to chest and diaphragm, glomus and oppression, counterflow cold of the extremities, and the pulse in the cubit that does not feel. Qian Jin Fang uses this method of taking and vomiting three times, this generally treats cholera, parasitic toxin, retained food with abdominal pain, and cold qi and ghost qi.

·**Original Source**：San Yin Fang

5. 乾霍亂吐方

·總結：霍亂

·組成：燒鹽, 熱童便

·主治：治乾霍亂欲吐不得吐, 欲瀉不得瀉, 腹中大痛者.

·歸經：此足太陰陽明藥也.

·方義：(1)吐瀉不得, 邪結中焦, 鹹能軟堅, 可破頑痰宿食. 炒之則苦, 故能涌吐.

(2)童便本人身下降之氣, 引火下行, 乃歸舊路, 味又鹹寒, 故降火甚速.

鹽涌于上, 溺泄于下, 則中通矣.

·變化方：本方單用燒鹽, 熱水調飲, 以指探吐, 名燒鹽探吐法, 治傷食痛連胸膈, 痞悶不通, 手足逆冷, 尺脈全無. 千金用此法三飲三吐, 通治霍亂蠱毒, 宿食腹痛, 冷氣鬼氣.

·來源：三因

Chapter 4. Interior-Attacking Formulas. 攻裏之劑

1. Da Cheng Qi Tang. Major Order the Qi Decoction. 大承氣湯

·**ACTIONS**：great repletion and fullness in the stomach and intestines.

·**COMPOSITION**：Da Huang, Zhi Shi, Hou Po, Mang Xiao

·**INDICATIONS**：(1) treats cold damage yang brightness bowel pattern, yang evil which enters interior, stomach repletion with constipation, heat effusion, delirious speech, spontaneous sweating, absence of aversion to cold, glomus and oppression, distention and fullness, dry stool with hardness.

(2) In miscellaneous disease there is great heat in triple burner, and the pulse is sunken and replete.

(3) also treats yang brightness febrile convulsion with chills.

·**CHANNELS ENTERED**：this belongs to right yang yang brightness medicine.

·**Analysis of Formula**：(1) excessive heat in the interior should be treated with the salty and cold, something hard is softened by the salty, exuberant heat is dispersed by cold.

Therefore the salty and cold of Mang Xiao are used to moisten dryness and soften hardness. The bitter and cold of Da Huang drain heat and eliminate stasis by precipitating dry binds and draining strong stomach. The bitter and descending nature of Zhi Shi and Hou Po drain glomus, fullness, and repletion. Nei Jing says that depressed earth should be treated by despoliation.

(2) If the pattern does not belong to great repletion and fullness, it is not impossible to give without caution.

·**RELATED FORMULA**：(1) When Gan Cao is added, this is called San Yi Cheng Qi Tang, treats abdominal fullness and replete pain in Da Cheng Qi Tang pattern, delirious speech and diarrhea in the Tiao Wei Cheng Qi Tang pattern, interior heat with constipation in the Xiao Cheng Qi Tang pattern, heat amassment in the interior in the interior, distention and fullness, and dry stool with hardness in all kinds of cold damage miscellaneous disease pattern.

(2) When Chai Hu, Huang Qin, and Gan Cao are added, this is called Liu Yi Shun Qi Tang, treats tidal heat effusion, spontaneous sweating, thirst, delirious speech, mania and frenetic, yellow macule, abdominal fullness, replete stool, add right yang yang brightness bowel disease.

(3) When Ren Shen, Gan Cao, Dang Gui, Jie Geng, Sheng Jiang,

and Da Zao are added, this is called Huang Long Tang, treats heat evil which p
asses into the interior, dry stool in the stomach, hardness and pain below the he
art, generalized heat effusion, thirst, delirious speech, and diarrhea which is pur
e and clear water.

(4) When Mang Xiao is eliminated and Ma Zi Ren, Xing Ren, S
hao Yao are added (made into pill with Honey), this is called Ma Ren Wan, trea
ts that the anterior tibial pulse is floating and rough, the floating means that sto
mach qi is strong, and the rough indicates frequent urination. If the floating and
rough contend with each other, it will be hard to defecate and the spleen gets str
aitened.

·**Original Source**：Zhong Jing

1. 大承氣湯
  ·總結：胃腑大實滿
  ·組成：大黃, 枳實, 厚朴, 芒硝
  ·主治：(1)治傷寒陽明腑證, 陽邪入裡, 胃實不大便, 發熱譫語, 自汗
出, 不惡寒, 痞滿燥實堅全見.
  　　　 (2)雜病三焦大熱, 脈沈實者.
  　　　 (3)亦治陽明剛痙.
  ·歸經：此正陽陽明藥也.
  ·方義：(1)熱淫於內, 治以鹹寒, 氣堅者以鹹軟之, 熱盛者以寒消之.
  　　　 故用：芒硝之鹹寒, 以潤燥軟堅；大黃之苦寒, 以瀉熱去瘀,
下燥結, 泄胃強；枳實, 厚朴之苦降, 瀉痞滿實滿. 經所謂「土鬱奪之」
也.
  　　　 (2)然非大實大滿, 不可輕投, 恐有寒中結胸痞氣之變.
  ·變化方：(1)本方加甘草等分, 名三一承氣湯, 治大承氣證, 腹滿實痛,
調胃證, 譫語下利, 小承氣證, 內熱不便, 一切傷寒雜病, 畜熱內甚, 燥實
堅脹.
  　　　 (2)本方加柴胡, 黃芩, 甘草, 入鐵鏽水三匙, 墜熱開結, 名六
一順氣湯, 治潮熱自汗, 發渴, 譫語, 狂妄, 斑黃, 腹滿, 便實, 正陽明腑
病.
  　　　 (3)本方加人參, 甘草, 當歸, 桔梗, 薑, 棗煎, 名黃龍湯, 治
熱邪傳裡, 胃有燥屎, 心下硬痛, 身熱口渴, 譫語, 下利純清水.
  　　　 (4)本方去芒硝, 加麻仁, 杏仁, 芍藥, 蜜丸, 名麻仁丸, 治趺
陽脈浮而濇, 浮則胃氣強, 濇則小便數, 浮濇相搏, 大便則難, 其脾爲約.
  ·來源：仲景

2. Xiao Cheng Qi Tang. Minor Order the Qi Decoction. 小承氣湯

·**ACTIONS**：The repletion and fullness of the stomach and intestines.

·**COMPOSITION**：Da Huang, Hou Po, Zhi Shi

·**INDICATIONS**：(1) treats cold damage yang brightness pattern, delirious speech, hard stool, and tidal heat effusion with panting.

(2) and miscellaneous disease, glomus, fullness, and blockage in the upper burner.

·**CHANNELS ENTERED**： this is lesser yang yang brightness medicine.

·**Analysis of Formula**：(1) evil in the upper burner causes fullness and distention in the middle burner, stomach repletion brings about tidal heat effusion, yang evil overwhelming the heart causes mania, and stomach heat and dry lung give rise to panting.

Therefore Hou Po and Zhi Shi eliminate the glomus and fullness in the upper burner, and Da Huang eliminates replete heat in the stomach.

(2) here, glomus, fullness, dry stool, and hardness have not yet made, therefore Mang Xiao is eliminated in order not to damage other true yin in the lower burner.

·**RELATED FORMULA**：(1) Jin Gui Yao Lue uses this formula to treat propping rheum and thoracic fullness, this is called Hou Po Da Huang Tang.

(2) When Qiang Huo is added, this is called San Hua Tang, treats wind strike evil qi which causes replete pattern, and urinary and fecal stoppage.

·**Original Source**：Zhong Jing

2. 小承氣湯

·總結：胃腑實滿

·組成：大黃, 厚朴, 枳實

·主治：(1)治傷寒陽明證, 譫語便硬, 潮熱而喘.

(2)及雜病, 上焦痞滿不通.

·歸經：此少陽陽明藥也.

·方義：(1)邪在上焦則滿, 在中焦則脹, 胃實則潮熱, 陽邪乘心則狂, 胃熱干肺則喘.

故以枳, 朴去上焦之痞滿, 以大黃去胃中之實熱.

(2)此痞滿燥實堅未全者, 故除芒硝, 欲其無傷下焦真陰也.

·變化方：(1)金匱用本方治支飲胸滿, 更名厚朴大黃湯.

106

(2)本方加羌活，名三化湯，治中風邪氣作實，二便不通.
·來源：仲景

3. Tiao Wei Cheng Qi Tang. Regulate the Stomach and Order the Qi Decoction. 調胃承氣湯

·**ACTIONS**： mild attack to the stomach

·**COMPOSITION**：Da Huang, Mang Xiao, Gan Cao

·**INDICATIONS**：(1) treats cold damage yang brightness pattern, absence of aversion to cold, but aversion to heat, thirst, fecal block, delirious speech, abdominal fullness, and dryness and repletion in the middle burner.

(2) and when in cold damage after vomiting there is abdominal distention and fullness.

(3) When in yang brightness disease, neither vomiting nor precipitation was used and there is heart vexation.

(4) also treats thirst, middle wasting-thirst with thinness despite large food intake.

·**CHANNELS ENTERED**：The foot greater yang and yang brightness channel.

·**Analysis of Formula**：(1) Da Huang is bitter and cold, eliminates heat and flushes repletion. Mang Xiao is salty and cold, moistens dryness and softens hardness.

The moving downward of Da Huang and Mang Xiao is very fast, therefore the sweet and neutral of Gan Cao is used to moderate it and not to reach stomach damage, therefore this formula regulates the stomach and supports qi.

(2) Hou Po and Zhi Shi are eliminated in order not to attack the qi part in the upper burner.

·**RELATED FORMULA**：(1) When Dang Gui, Sheng Jiang, and Da Zao are added, this is called Dang Gui Cheng Qi Tang, treats interior heat and fire depression, or desiccated and dry skin, or dry throat and nose, or constipation and rough urination, or static blood with mania.

(2) When Mang Xiao is eliminated, this is called Da Huang Gan Cao Tang, Jin Gui Yao Lue uses this formula to treat vomiting after eating, Wai Tai Mi Yao uses this formula to treat vomiting of water.

(3) Da Huang (two liang), Mang Xiao, Gan Cao (respectively two liang), ; this is called Po Guan Dan, treats profuse sweating, great thirst, const

107

ipation, delirious speech, yang bind pattern, and every sore and swelling with h
eat.

·**Original Source**：Zhong Jing

3. 謂胃承氣湯
　·總結：胃實緩攻
　·組成：大黃, 芒硝, 甘草
　·主治：(1)治傷寒陽明證, 不惡寒, 反惡熱, 口渴便閉, 譫語腹滿, 中
焦燥實.
　　　　　(2)及傷寒吐後腹脹滿者.
　　　　　(3)陽明病不吐不下而心煩者.
　　　　　(4)亦治渴證, 中消善食而溲.
　·歸經：此足太陽陽明藥也.
　·方義：(1)大黃苦寒, 除熱蕩實. 芒硝鹹寒, 潤燥軟堅.
　　　　　二物下行甚速, 故用甘草甘平以緩之, 不致傷胃, 故謂調胃
承氣.
　　　　　(2)去枳, 朴者, 不欲其犯上焦氣分也.
　·變化方：(1)本方加當歸, 薑, 棗煎, 名當歸承氣湯, 治裡熱火鬱, 或
皮膚枯燥, 或咽燥鼻乾, 或便溺祕結, 或瘀血發狂.
　　　　　(2)方本方除芒硝, 名大黃甘草湯, 金匱用治食已即吐, 外臺
用治吐水.
　　　　　(3)本方用大黃二兩半, 芒硝甘草名二兩, 又名破棺丹, 治多
汗, 大渴, 便祕, 譫語, 陽結之證及諸瘡腫熱.
　·來源：仲景

4. Tao Ren Cheng Qi Tang. Peach Pit Decoction to Order t he Qi. 桃仁承氣湯

·see number 13 in the chapter 8. Blood-Rectifying Formulas.

5. Da Xian Xiong Tang. Major Sinking into the Chest Deco ction. 大陷胸湯

·**ACTIONS**：chest binds

·**COMPOSITION**：Da Huang, Mang Xiao, Gan Sui

·**INDICATIONS**：(1) treats that when in cold damage, precipitation was used too early, exterior evil enters the interior, there is fullness, hardness, and pain below the heart.

(2) or if sweating is promoted repeatedly, yet precipitation is also used and there is inability to defecate for five or six days, a dry tongue and thirst, tidal heat effusion in the late afternoon, and hardness, fullness, and pain, extending from below the heart to the lesser abdomen and which the person will not allow anyone even to get near.

(3) or there is absence of great heat effusion, slight sweat issuing only from the head, and the pulse is sunken, this is water chest bind.

·**CHANNELS ENTERED**：The foot greater yang channel. [The bladder]

·**Analysis of Formula**：Exterior evil enters the interior, binds in the high location, and this gets to reach the repletion of triple burner, the pain is so severe that anyone cannot get to near, this is emergency sign, this cannot be treated with common usual medicine, therefore the bitter and cold of Gan Sui moves water, acts as sovereign, Mang Xiao is salty and cold, softens hardness, acts as minister. Da Huang is bitter and cold, flushes the repletion, and acts as courier.

·**Original Source**：Zhong Jing

5. 大陷胸湯
　·總結：結胸
　·組成：大黃, 芒硝, 甘遂
　·主治：(1)治傷寒下之早, 表邪入裡, 心下滿而鞭痛.
　　　　　(2)或重汗而復下之, 不大便五, 六日, 舌上燥渴, 日晡潮熱, 從心至小腹鞭滿, 痛不可近；
　　　　　(3)或無大熱, 但頭微汗出, 脈沈, 爲水結胸.
　·歸經：此足太陽藥也.
　·方義：表邪入裡, 結于高位, 以致三焦俱實, 手不可近, 證爲危急, 非常藥所能平, 故以甘遂苦寒行水直達爲君, 芒硝鹹寒軟堅爲臣, 大黃苦寒蕩滌爲使.
　·來源：仲景

6. Xiao Xian Xiong Tang. Minor Sinking into the Chest Dec oction. 小陷胸湯

·**ACTIONS**：minor chest bind

·**COMPOSITION**：Huang Lian, Ban Xia, Gua Lou

·**INDICATIONS**：(1) treats when in cold damage after precipitation erron eously, minor chest bind is directly below the heart and painful when pressure i s applied, and the pulse is floating and slippery.

(2) phlegm heat obstructing chest.

·**CHANNELS ENTERED**：The foot lesser yang channel. [The gall blad der]

·**Analysis of Formula**：(1) the bitter and cold of Huang Lian drains heat, t he cold of Gua Lou flushes grime, the pungent and warm of Ban Xia disperses binds.

(2) Chest bind occurs mainly due to the binding of phlegm and h eat, the three herbs eliminate phlegm and heat.

·**Original Source**：Zhong Jing

6. 小陷胸湯

·總結：小結胸

·組成：黃連，半夏，栝蔞

·主治：(1)治傷寒誤下，小結胸正在心下，按之則痛，脈浮滑者.
　　　(2)及痰熱塞胸.

·歸經：此足少陽藥也.

·方義：(1)黃連性苦寒以泄熱，栝蔞性寒以滌垢，半夏性辛溫以散結.
　　　(2)結胸多由痰熱結聚，故用三物以除痰去熱也.

·來源：仲景

7. Da Xian Xiong Wan, Major Sinking into the Chest Pill, 大陷胸丸

·**ACTIONS**：chest bind

·**COMPOSITION**：Da Huang, Mang Xiao, Ting Li, Xing Ren

·**INDICATIONS**：treats that when in cold damage chest bind, there is sti ff nape as the form of soft tetany.

·**CHANNELS ENTERED** ： The foot greater yang and yang brightness ch annels. [The bladder and stomach]

·**Analysis of Formula** ： The bitter and cold of Da Huang drains heat, the salty and cold of Mang Xiao softens hardness, the bitter and sweet of Xing Ren descends qi, Ting Li and Gan Sui move water, Honey moistens and lubricates the action of the other herbs and the sweet moderates.

·Original Source ： Zhong Jing

7. 大陷胸丸

    ·總結：結胸

    ·組成：大黄，芒硝，葶藶，杏仁

    ·主治：治傷寒結胸項强，如柔痙狀.

    ·歸經：此足太陽陽明藥也.

    ·方義：大黄性苦寒以泄熱，芒硝性鹹寒以軟堅，杏仁性苦甘以降氣，葶藶，甘遂取其行水而直達，白蜜取其潤滑而甘緩.

    ·炮製：葶藶炒，杏仁去皮尖.

    ·來源：仲景

8. Shi Zao Tang. Ten-Jujube Decoction. 十棗湯

·**ACTIONS** ： deep-lying rheum and accumulated phlegm

·**COMPOSITION** ： Yuan Hua, Gan Sui, Da Ji, Da Zao

·**INDICATIONS** ： (1) treats that when in greater yang wind strike with diarrhea, retching counterflow, the exterior has resolved, one can attack..

    (2) When the person has drizzly sweating, hard glomus and fullness below the heart and pain extending under rib-side, dry retching, short of breath, sweating, and absence of aversion to cold, this means that the exterior has resolved and the interior is not yet harmonized.

    (3) evil heat which is amassed in the interior and deep-lying rheum.

·**CHANNELS ENTERED** ： The foot greater yang channel. [The bladder]

·**Analysis of Formula** ： (1) Yuan Hua and Da Ji are pungent and bitter, and expel water rheum. Gan Sui is bitter and cold, can reach directly where water qi binds and attacks water rheum.

    (2) the three herbs are too drastic, therefore Da Zao is used to moderate them with the sweet and to overcome water through boosting earth, thi

s formula makes water rheum come out through defecation and urination.

·Original Source：Zhong Jing

8. 十棗湯

　·總結：伏飲積痰

　·組成：芫花，甘遂，大戟，大棗

　·主治：⑴治太陽中風，下利嘔逆，表解者乃可攻之.

　　　　　⑵其人漐漐汗出，頭痛，心下痞硬，引脅下痛，乾嘔短氣，汗
出不惡寒，此表解而裏未和.

　　　　　⑶邪熱內蓄，有伏飲者.

　·歸經：此足太陽藥也.

　·方義：⑴芫花，大戟性辛苦以逐水飲. 甘遂苦寒，能直達水氣所結之
處，以攻決爲用.

　　　　　⑵三藥過峻，故用大棗之甘以緩之，益土所以勝水，使邪從
二便而出也.

　·來源：仲景

9. San Wu Bei Ji Wan Three-Substance Pill for Emergencie s 三物備急丸

·**ACTIONS**：food damage with acute pain.

·**COMPOSITION**：Ba Dou Shuang, Da Huang, Gan Jiang

·**INDICATIONS**：⑴ treats food retention in the intestines and stomach, irregularities of cold and heat, abdominal distention with rapid breathing, pain and fullness as if the person is about to die.

　　　　　⑵ malignity stroke and visiting hostility, all kinds of sudden and acute disease.

·**CHANNELS ENTERED**：The hand and foot yang brightness channels. [The large intestine and stomach]

·**Analysis of Formula**：⑴ Da Huang is bitter and cold and precipitates heat binds. Ba Dou Shuang is pungent and heat and precipitates cold binds. Gan Jiang is pungent and is added to disperse and free.

　　　　　⑵ those three herbs are drastic and harsh, if the condition is not in emergency, do not use, therefore this is called Bei Ji.

·Original Source：Tian Jin Yao Fang

112

9. 三物備急丸

　·總結：傷食急痛

　·組成：巴豆霜, 大黃, 乾薑

　·主治：(1)治食停腸胃, 冷熱不調, 腹脹氣急, 痛滿欲死.

　　　　　(2)及中惡客忤, 卒暴諸病.

　·歸經：此手足陽明藥也.

　·方義：(1)大黃苦寒以下熱結. 巴霜辛熱以下寒結. 加乾薑辛散以宣通
之.

　　　　　(2)三藥峻屬, 非急莫施, 故曰備急.

　·來源：千金

10. Nao Sha Wan. Sal Ammomiac Pill. 硇砂丸

·**ACTIONS**：all kinds of aggregation-accumulation

·**COMPOSITION**：Nao Sha, Ba Dou, San Leng, Gan Jiang, Bai Zhi, Mu Xiang, Qing Pi, Hu Jiao, Da Huang, Gan Qi, Bing Lang, Rou Dou Kou

·**INDICATIONS**：treats all kinds of aggregation-accumulation and phlegm, pulling pain in the heart and rib-side.

·**Analysis of Formula**：(1) treats flesh accumulation, qi accumulation, and blood accumulation.

　　　　(2) Nao Sha digests meat, Gan Qi disperses static blood, Mu Xiang and Qing Pi move qi stagnation, San Leng breaks blood and moves qi, Rou Dou Kou warms the stomach and harmonizes the middle, Bai Zhi disperses wind and eliminates damp, Gan Jiang and Hu Jiao eliminate deep and intractable cold, Da Huang and Ba Dou can precipitate accumulated phlegm.

　　　　(3) there is lots of herbs with pungent and heat in this formula, these are used to break cold and attack hardness. Only Da Huang is bitter and cold, this flushes heat and eliminates repletion.

　　　　Generally when aggregation-accumulation has already been severe, the attacking treatment cannot be drastic.

　　　　(4) Vinegar is used to promote contraction by sour flavor.

·**Original Source**：Ben Shi Fang

10. 硇砂丸

　·總結：一切積聚

　·組成：硇砂, 巴豆, 三稜, 乾薑, 白芷, 木香, 青皮, 胡椒, 大黃, 乾

漆，檳榔，肉豆蔻

　·主治：治一切積聚痰飲，心脅引痛.

　·方義：(1)此治肉積氣積血積通劑也.

　　　　　(2)硇砂化肉食，乾漆散瘀血，木香，青皮行氣滯，三稜破血而行氣，肉蔻暖胃而和中，白芷散風而除溼，乾薑，胡椒除沈寒錮冷，大黃，巴豆能斬關奪門.

　　　　　(3)方內多辛熱有毒之品，用之以破冷攻堅，惟大黃苦寒，假之以蕩熱去實.

　　　　　　　蓋積聚既深，攻治不得不峻.

　　　　　(4)用醋者酸以收之也.

　·來源：本事

11. Mu Xiang Bing Lang Wan. Aucklandia and Betel Nut Pills. 木香檳榔丸

·**ACTIONS**：accumulation and diarrhea.

·**COMPOSITION**：Mu Xiang, Xiang Fu, Qing Pi, Chen Pi, Huang Lian, Huang Bai, Bing Lang, Hei Chou, Da Huang, Zhi Ke, Mang Xiao, E Zhu, San Leng

·**INDICATIONS**：(1) treats accumulation in the chest and abdomen, glomus, fullness, and binding pain, urinary and fecal stoppage.

　　　　　(2) or diarrhea, tenesmus, food malaria, and replete accumulation.

·**CHANNELS ENTERED**：The hand and foot yang brightness channel. [The large intestine and stomach]

·**Analysis of Formula**：(1) damp-heat in the qi part of triple burner. Mu Xiang and Xiang Fu are the herbs to move qi, they can free triple burner and resolve six depressions.

　　　　　Chen Pi rectifies the upper burner and lung qi.
　　　　　Qing Pi pacifies the lower burner and liver qi.
　　　　　Zhi Ke soothe intestines and disinhibits qi.
　　　　　Hei Chou and Bing Lang are most fast in descending qi. When qi moves, glomus, fullness, and tenesmus will disappear.

　　　　　(2) Malaria with diarrhea is originated from the depression of damp-heat and irregularities of qi and blood.
　　　　　Huang Bai and Huang Lian dry damp and clear heat,
　　　　　San Leng can break qi stagnation in blood.
　　　　　E Zhu can break blood stagnation in qi.

114

Da Huang and Mang Xiao are the herbs which belong to blood part, they can eliminate latent heat in blood, free and move accumulation, and also are drastic herbs for smashing hardness and transforming glomus. When the accumulation of damp-heat is eliminated, then defecation and urination get regulated and triple burner calm.

Generally owing to retained grime and some unclear, clear yang is unable to rise, therefore this formula is used to push and flush out them. If the accumulation pattern does not belong to repletion, it is impossible to use.

(4) Dang Gui is added to moisten dryness and harmonize blood.

·Original Source：Zhang Zi He

11. 木香檳榔丸
　·總結：積滯瀉痢
　·組成：木香，香附，青皮，陳皮，黃連，黃柏，檳榔，黑丑，大黃，枳殼，芒硝，莪朮，三稜
　·主治：(1)治胸腹積滯，痞滿結痛，二便不通.
　　　　　(2)或瀉泄下痢，裏急後重，食瘧實積.
　·歸經：此手足陽明藥也.
　·方義：(1)濕熱三焦氣分. 木香，香附行氣之藥，能通三焦，解六鬱；
　　　　　　　陳皮理上焦肺氣；
　　　　　　　青皮平下焦肝氣；
　　　　　　　枳殼寬腸而利氣；
　　　　　　　而黑丑，檳榔又下氣之最速者也. 氣行則無痞滿後重之患矣.
　　　　　(2)瘧痢由于濕熱鬱積，氣血不和.
　　　　　　　黃柏黃連燥濕清熱之藥；
　　　　　　　三稜能破血中氣滯；
　　　　　　　莪朮能破氣中血滯；
　　　　　　　大黃芒硝血分之藥，能除血中伏熱，通行積滯，並為摧堅化痞之峻品. 濕熱積滯去，則二便調而三焦泰矣.
　　　　　　　蓋宿垢不淨，清陽終不得升，故必假此以推蕩之，亦通因通用之意.
　　　　　　　然非實積，不可輕投.
　　　　　(4)加當歸者，潤燥和其血也.
　·來源：子和

115

12. Zhi Shi Dao Zhi Wan. Immature Bitter Orange Pill to Guide Out Stagnation. 枳實導滯丸

·**ACTIONS**：food damage

·**COMPOSITION**：Da Huang, Zhi Shi, Huang Qin, Huang Lian, Shen Qu, Bai Zhu, Fu Ling, Ze Xie

·**INDICATIONS**：treats food damage that has the nature of damp-heat, inability to digest, glomus, oppression, and disquiet, hardness and pain in the abdomen, accumulation, and diarrhea.

·**CHANNELS ENTERED**：The foot greater yin and yang brightness channel. [The spleen and stomach]

·**Analysis of Formula**：(1) in case of stagnation due to food damage which causing pain and accumulation, without pushing and flushing of food stagnation, it is impossible to move it. When accumulation has not yet eliminated the disease never recover, therefore Da Huang and Zhi Shi attack to precipitate, then rather, pain and diarrhea allay. Nei Jing says that the stopped is treated by stopping.

(2) for damage to damp-heat, Huang Qin and Huang Lian are used as assistant to clear heat. Fu Ling and Ze Xie act assistant to disinhibit damp.

(3) in case of accumulation due to wine, something steamed or fumed such as Shen Qu transforms food and resolves wine, because this is a similar kind with wine, this disperses wine with the warm.

(4) Huang Qin, Huang Lian, and Da Huang are very bitter and cold, there is worry of damaging the stomach by them, therefore the sweet and warm of Bai Zhu are used to supplement earth and secure the middle.

·**Original Source**：Li Dong Yuan

12. 枳實導滯丸

·總結：傷食

·組成：大黃, 枳實, 黃芩, 黃連, 神麴, 白朮, 茯苓, 澤瀉

·主治：治傷溼熱之物, 不得施化, 痞悶不安, 腹內硬痛, 積滯泄瀉.

·歸經：此足太陰陽明藥也.

·方義：(1)飲食傷滯, 作痛成積, 非有以推蕩之, 則不行. 積滯不盡, 病終不除. 故以大黃, 枳實攻而下之, 而痛瀉反止, 經所謂「通因通用」也.

(2)傷由溼熱, 黃芩, 黃連佐之以清熱. 茯苓, 澤瀉佐之以利溼.

(3)積由酒食，神麴蒸窨之物，化食解酒，因其同類，溫而消之.

(4)芩連大黃，苦寒太甚，恐其傷胃，故又以白朮之甘溫，補土而固中也.

·來源：東垣

13. Mi Jian Dao Fa. Honey Enema. 蜜煎導法

·**ACTIONS**：frees the stool

·**COMPOSITION**：Honey

·**INDICATIONS**：treats yang brightness patter, spontaneous sweating, uninhibited urination, constipation.

·**CHANNELS ENTERED**：The hand yang brightness.

·**Analysis of Formula**：(1) Honey can moisten intestines, the heat can move qi, Zao Jiao can free orifice.

(2) Shang Han Lun says that if exterior has resolved and there is the other pattern, even though the stomach is replete, attacking method [precipitation] is contraindicated. Therefore freeing the stool with enema externally is used in order not to damage the stomach with bitter and cold.

·**Taking Method**：Place the above ingredient in a copper pot. Cook it with a mild flame. It must congeal to a form like malt sugar, stir to prevent it from burning and sticking to the pot. Wait until the consistency is correct to form a pill, and then roll it into a cun long, it is urgent to use it while hot, as it will harden when cold. Insert into the grain tract and hold the buttocks closed with the hand, releasing the buttocks when the person is about to defecate. It is doubted that this is Zhang Zhong Jing's formula, but it proves to be very effective.

·**Original Source**：Zhong Jing

13. 蜜煎導法

·總結：通大便

·組成：蜂蜜

·主治：治陽明證，自汗，小便利，大便秘者.

·歸經：此手陽明藥也.

·方義：(1)蜜能潤腸，熱能行氣，皂能通竅.

(2)經曰：「表解無證者，胃雖實，忌攻.」故外導而通之，不欲以苦寒傷胃也.

117

·煎服法：用調器微火熬，頻攪，勿令焦，候凝如飴，捻作挺子，頭銳如指.

糝皂角末少許，乘熱納殼道中，用手抱住，欲大便時去之.

·來源：仲景

14. Pig's Bile Enema. Zhu Dan Dao Fa. 豬膽導法

·**ACTIONS**：frees the stool

·**COMPOSITION**：gall bladder from one large pig.

·**INDICATIONS**：treats yang brightness pattern, spontaneous sweating, uninhibited urination, constipation.

·**CHANNELS ENTERED**：the hand yang brightness channel. [The large intestine]

·**Analysis of Formula**：(1) When constipation belongs to dryness and heat, spontaneous sweating means humor collapse, then at this condition urination is inhibited, but now, it is uninhibited, this indicates that heat has not yet got replete, therefore it is impossible to attack.

(2) the cold of gall bladder overcomes heat, the clear moistens dryness, the bitter can descend, the sour of vinegar tends to enter well, therefore this can induce honey to enter the large intestine and free the stool.

·**Taking Method**：Take the gallbladder from one large pig and drain the juice. Mix with a small amount of cooking vinegar and pour into the grain tract, leaving in for about the time it takes to eat meal. The stool should issue forth with the abiding food and bad substances. It is very effective.

·**Original Source**：Zhong Jing

14. 豬膽導法

·總結：通大便

·組成：豬膽一枚

·主治：治陽明證，自汗，小便利，大便秘者.

·歸經：此手陽明藥也.

·方義：(1)便祕者屬燥屬熱，自汗者爲亡津液，當小便不利，今反利，是熱猶未實，故不可攻.

(2)豬膽汁寒勝熱，清潤燥，苦能降；醋酸善入，故能引入大腸而通之也.

·煎服法：取汁入醋少許，以灌殼道中，如一食頃，當大便出宿食惡物，

118

甚效.
　·來源：仲景

Chapter 5. Exterior-Interior Formulas. 表裏之劑

1. Da Chai Hu Tang. Major Bupleurum Decoction. 大柴胡湯

·**ACTIONS**：lesser yang yang brightness pattern. resolves exterior and attacks interior.

·**COMPOSITION**：Chai Hu, Huang Qin, Ban Xia, Sheng Jiang, Da Zao, Zhi Shi , Da Huang, Bai Shao Yao

·**INDICATIONS**：(1) treats cold damage, heat effusion, sweating without resolving, yang evil which entered interior, heat binding in the interior, glomus and hardness below the heart, retching and diarrhea.

(2) or alternating aversion to cold and heat effusion, vexation, thirst, delirious speech, abdominal fullness, and constipation.

(3) when exterior pattern has not yet eliminated, interior pattern also is urgent, the pulse is surging or sunken, replete, string-like, and rapid.

·**CHANNELS ENTERED**：The foot lesser yang and yang brightness channels. [The gall bladder and stomach]

·**Analysis of Formula**：(1) Because exterior pattern has not yet eliminated, therefore Chai Hu is used to resolve exterior. The interior pattern is dry and replete, therefore Da Huang and Zhi Shi are used to attack the interior.

Shao Yao quiets the spleen and restrains yin. Huang Qin abates heat and allays thirst, Ban Xia harmonizes the stomach and checks retching. Sheng jiang disperses with the pungent, Da Zao moderates with the sweet, they used to regulate Construction and Defense and move liquid and humor.

(2) This treats exterior and interior, and is gentle formula of precipitating.

·**Original Source**：Zhong Jing

1. 大柴胡湯
  ·總結：少陽陽明，解表攻裏
  ·組成：柴胡，黃芩，半夏，生薑，大棗，枳實，大黃，白芍
  ·主治：(1)治傷寒發熱，汗出不解，陽邪入裡，熱結在裏，心下痞硬，嘔而下利.
       (2)或往來寒熱，煩渴譫語，腹滿便秘.
       (3)表證未除，裏證又急，脈洪或沈實弦數者.

·歸經：此足少陽陽明藥也.
　·方義：(1)表證未除，故用柴胡以解表. 裡證燥實，故用大黃，枳實以
攻裡.

　　　　　　　芍藥安脾斂陰. 黃芩退熱解渴，半夏和胃止嘔，薑
辛散而棗甘緩，以調營衛而行津液.
　　　　　　(2)此表裡交治，下劑之緩者也.
　·來源：仲景

2. Chai Hu Jia Mang Xiao Tang. Bupleurum Decoction Plu s Mirabilite Decoction. 柴胡加芒硝湯

·**ACTIONS**：lesser yang yang brightness. resolves exterior and attacks in terior.

·**COMPOSITION**：Xiao Chai Hu Tang with Mang Xiao

·**INDICATIONS**：(1) treats that when in cold damage the disease has not resolved in thirteen days, and there is fullness in the chest and rib-side, retching, late afternoon tidal heat effusion, and shortly afterward mild diarrhea.

　　　　　(2) this is originally Chai Hu pattern, one knows the physician pr ecipitate with a pill medicine and this is not the correct treatment.

　　　　　(3) tidal heat effusion means repletion. It is appropriate to first ta ke Xiao Chai Hu Tang in order to resolve the exterior aspect. Afterward, Chai Hu Jia Mang Xiao Tang governs.

·**CHANNELS ENTERED**：　The lesser yang and yang brightness chann els. [The gall bladder and stomach]

·**Analysis of Formula**：(1) erroneous treatment of precipitation is applied to exterior pattern, evil heat enters the stomach by exploiting vacuity, and then diarrhea, thoracic and abdominal fullness, retching, tidal heat effusion occur.

　　　　　Therefore Chai Hu Tang is given to resolve lesser yan g and Mang Xiao is added to flush stomach heat.

　　　　　(2) This also treats both exterior and interior as Da Chai Hu Tan g.

·**Original Source**：Zhong Jing

2. 柴胡加芒硝湯
　·總結：少陽陽明解表攻裏
　·組成：小柴胡湯加芒硝

·主治：⑴治傷寒十三日不解，胸脅滿而嘔，日晡潮熱，已而微利.

⑵此本柴胡證，知醫以圓藥下之，非其治也.

⑶潮熱者，實也. 先以小柴胡湯以解外，後以加芒硝湯主之.

·歸經：此少陽陽明藥也.

·方義：⑴表證誤下，邪熱乘虛入胃，以致下利而滿嘔，潮熱之證猶在.
故仍與柴胡湯以解少陽. 加芒硝以蕩胃熱.

⑵亦與大柴胡兩解同意.

·來源：仲景

3. Gui Zhi Jia Da Huang Tang. Cinnamon Twig Decoction Plus Rhubarb. 桂枝加大黄湯

·**ACTIONS**：greater yang and greater yin, resolves exterior and attacks interior.

·**COMPOSITION**：Gui Zhi Tang with Da Huang and Shao Yao

·**INDICATIONS**：treats that when in greater yang disease, precipitation is used erroneously, this passed into greater yin, and there is abdominal fullness with repletion.

·**CHANNELS ENTERED**：The foot greater yang and greater yin channels. [The bladder and spleen]

·**Analysis of Formula**：⑴ When wrong precipitation causes chest bind, evil locates in the upper part, this belongs to greater yang. Now the abdominal fullness with replete pain means that evil has already entered greater yin.

⑵ In Shang Han Lun, most of pain belong to replete pattern. Pain relieves through precipitation, therefore Gui Zhi Tang is used to resolve exterior evil which has not yet resolved, and Da Huang is added to precipitate evil heat which has fallen inward.

·**Original Source**：Zhong Jing

3. 桂枝加大黄湯

·總結：太陽太陰解表攻裏

·組成：桂枝湯加大黄，芍藥

·主治：治太陽誤下，轉屬太陰，腹滿大實痛者.

·歸經：此足太陽太陰藥也.

·方義：⑴誤下而作結胸，則邪在上，仍屬太陽. 今腹滿而大實痛，則邪以已入太陰.

122

(2)經曰：「諸痛爲實．」痛隨利減，故用桂枝以解未盡之表邪，加大黃以下內陷之邪熱.

·來源：仲景

4. Shui Jie San. Release Water Powder. 水解散

·**ACTIONS**：warm epidemic, resolves both exterior and interior.

·**COMPOSITION**：Ma Huang, Gui Xin, Gan Cao, Da Huang, Huang Qin, Bai Shao Yao.

·**INDICATIONS**：treats that when heaven current epidemic lasts for one or two days, there is headache and invigorating heat.

·**CHANNELS ENTERED**：The foot greater yang and yang brightness channels. [The bladder and stomach]

·**Analysis of Formula**：(1) Ma Huang can open the flesh and promote sweating, Gui Xin can induce blood to transform into sweat, Huang Qin clears the heat in the supper and middle part, Da Huang drains the heat in the middle and lower part, Gan Cao and Bai Shao Yao can regulate the stomach and harmonize the middle.

(2) Generally in heaven current warm epidemic, depressed heat reaches exterior from interior, this is different of cold damage in which heat passes from exterior to interior, therefore though the disease has last only one or two day, but promotion of sweating and precipitation can be used together, there is no need to be same with the treatment of cold damage.

·**Original Source**：Zhou Hou Fang

4. 水解散

·總結：溫疫表裏兩解

·組成：麻黃，桂心，甘草，大黃，黃芩，白芍

·主治：治天行一，二日，頭痛壯熱.

·歸經：此足太陽陽明藥也.

·方義：(1)麻黃能開腠發汗，桂心能引血化汗，黃芩以清上中之熱，大黃以瀉中下之熱，甘草，白芍能調胃而和中.

(2)蓋天行溫疫，鬱熱自內達外，與傷寒由表傳裡者不同. 故雖一，二日之淺，可以汗下兼行，不必同于傷寒之治法也.

·炮製：甘草炙.

·來源：肘後

123

5. Fang Feng Tong Sheng San. Saposhnikovia Powder that Sagely Unblocks. 防風通聖散

·**ACTIONS**︰repletion of both the exterior and interior.

·**COMPOSITION**︰Fang Feng, Jing Jie, Bo He, Ma Huang, Da Huang, Mang Xiao, Shan Zhi Zi , Hua Shi, Jie Geng, Shi Gao, Huang Qin, Lian Qiao, Dang Gui, Chuan Xiong, Bai Shao Yao, Bai Zhu, Gan Cao, Sheng Jiang, Cong Bai

·**INDICATIONS**︰(1) treats all kinds of wind, cold, summerheat, and damp, excessive hunger and bellyful, taxation, both interior and exterior damage by evil.

(2) depression of qi and blood, repletion of exterior, interior, and triple burner, abhorrence of cold and invigorating heat.

(3) dizzy head and blurred vision, painful redness of the eyes, tinnitus, nasal congestion, bitter taste in the mouth dry tongue, discomfort in the throat, spitting of spittle which is thick and sticky, cough with dyspnea. .

(4) constipation, inhibited voiding of reddish urine.

(5) swelling and toxin of sore and ulcer swelling, knocks and falls, static blood and hematochezia, intestinal wind, and hemorrhoids and fistulas.

(6) the spasm and relaxation of the limbs, fright mania and delirium, cinnabar macule and urticaria.

·**MODIFICATIONS**︰(1) for white diarrhea, eliminate Mang Xiao.

(2) for spontaneous sweating, eliminate Ma Huang and add Gui Zhi.

(3) for drool with cough, add Sheng Jiang (processed with Ban Xia).

·**CHANNELS ENTERED**︰The exterior, interior, blood, and qi of the foot greater yang and yang brightness.

·**Analysis of Formula**︰(1) Fang Feng, Jing Jie, Bo He, and Ma Huang are light, tend to float, raise, and disperse, and resolve exterior and disperse cold, they make wind-heat to disperse in the upper part through promotion of sweating.

Da Huang, Mang Xiao break binds and frees dark-gate, Zhi Zi and Hua Shi descend fire and disinhibit water, they make wind heat to come out through defecation and drain them in the lower part.

When excessive wind in the interior enters the lung and stomach, Jie Geng and Shi Gao clear the lung and drain the stomach.

When wind causes disease, the liver is supplied with it, Chuan Xiong, Dang Gui, and Shao Yao harmonize blood and supplement the li

124

ver.

        Huang Qin clears the fire in the upper and middle part.

        Lian Qiao disperses accumulated qi and congealing bl

ood.

        Gan Cao moderates drastic formula and harmonize the

middle.

        Bai Zhu fortifies the spleen and dries damp.

(2) this formula disperse the upper and lower part separately, treats both exterior and interior, and can warm and nourish during dispersing and draining the middle, therefore promotion of sweating does not damage the exterior and precipitation does not damage the interior.

·**RELATED FORMULA**：(1) Ren Shen is added to supplement qi, Shu Di Huang is added to boost blood, Huang Bai and Huang Lian eliminate heat, Qiang Huo, Du Huo, Tian Ma, Xi Xin, Quan Xie eliminates wind, make this into pill with Honey. This is called Qu Feng Zhi Bao Dan.

(2) When Da Huang and Mang Xiao are added, this is called Shu ang Jie San.

·**Original Source**：Liu He Jian's formula

5. 防風通聖散
 ·總結：表裏俱實
 ·組成：防風, 荊芥, 薄荷, 麻黃, 大黃, 芒硝, 山梔子, 滑石, 桔梗, 石膏, 黃芩, 連翹, 當歸, 川芎, 白芍, 白术, 甘草, 生薑, 葱白
 ·主治：(1)治一切風寒暑溼, 飢飽勞役, 內外諸邪所傷.
        (2)氣血怫鬱, 表裡三焦俱實, 憎寒壯熱.
        (3)頭目昏運, 目赤睛痛, 耳鳴鼻塞, 口苦舌乾, 咽喉不利, 唾涕稠黏, 咳嗽上氣.
        (4)大便秘結, 小便赤澀.
        (5)瘡瘍腫毒, 折跌損傷, 瘀血便血, 腸風痔漏.
        (6)手足瘈瘲, 驚狂譫妄, 丹斑癮疹.
 ·加減：(1)自利去硝黃.
        (2)自汗去麻黃, 加桂枝.
        (3)涎嗽加薑製半夏.
 ·歸經：此足太陽陽明表裡血氣藥也.
 ·方義：(1)防風, 荊介, 薄荷, 麻黃, 輕浮升散, 解表散寒, 使風熱從汗出而散之于上.
        大黃, 芒硝, 破結通幽；梔子, 滑石降火利水；使

風熱從便出而泄之于下.

> 風淫于內, 肺胃受邪, 桔梗, 石膏清肺瀉胃.
> 風爲之患, 肝木受之, 川芎, 歸, 芍, 和血補肝.
> 黃芩清中上之火.
> 連翹散氣聚血凝.
> 甘草緩峻而和中.
> 白术健脾而燥溼.

(2)上下分消, 表裡交治, 而能散瀉之中, 猶寓溫養之意, 所以汗不傷表, 不下傷裡也.

·變化方：(1)本方再加人參補氣, 熟地益血, 黃柏, 黃連除熱, 羌活, 獨活, 天麻, 細辛, 全蝎祛風, 蜜丸彈子大, 每服一丸, 茶酒任下, 名祛風至寶丹.

(2)本方除大黃, 芒硝, 名雙解散.

·來源：河間

6. Ge Gen Huang Qin Huang Lian Tang. Kudzu, Coptis, and Scutellaria Decoction. 葛根黃連黃芩湯

·ACTIONS：greater yang yang brightness, resolves exterior and clears interior

·COMPOSITION：Ge Gen, Gan Cao, Huang Qin, Huang Lian

·INDICATIONS：treats that when in a greater yang disease the condition is Gui Zhi Tang pattern, but the physician precipitates, causing incessant diarrhea and a pulse that is skipping, it means that the exterior has not resolved, when there is panting and sweating, this formula governs.

·CHANNELS ENTERED：The foot greater yang and yang brightness channels.

·Analysis of Formula：(1) exterior pattern still exists, but the physician precipitates erroneously, evil enters the bowel of yang brightness. Qi surging upward causes panting and Qi falling downward brings about diarrhea. Therefore Gui Zhi is abandoned and Ge Gen is used to treat only the exterior of yang brightness. Huang Qin and huang lian clear interior heat, Gan Cao regulates the stomach qi.

(2) this does not treat diarrhea, but diarrhea gets to stop spontaneously. And this does not treats panting, but panting gets to relieve spontaneously. Also this is modified method to resolve both the exterior and interior of the g

126

reater yang.

    ·**Original Source**：Zhong Jing

6. 葛根黄連黄芩湯

    ·總結：太陽陽明解表清裏

    ·組成：葛根，甘草，黃芩，黃連

    ·主治：治太陽病桂枝證，醫反下之，利遂不止，脈促者，表未解也，喘而汗出者，此湯主之.

    ·歸經：此足太陽陽明藥也.

    ·方義：(1)表證尚在，醫反誤下，邪入陽明之腑，其汗外越，氣上奔則喘，下陷則利. 故舍桂枝而用葛根，專治陽明之表；加芩，連以清裡熱，甘草調胃氣.

        (2)不治利而利自止，不治喘而喘自止矣. 又太陽表裡兩解之變法.

    ·來源：仲景

7. San Huang Shi Gao Tang. Three-Yellow and Gypsum Decoction. 三黃石膏湯

·**ACTIONS**：effuses the exterior and clears the interior

·**COMPOSITION**：Huang Lian, Huang Qin, Huang Bai, Zhi Zi, Ma Huang, Dan Dou Chi, Shi Gao

·**INDICATIONS**：(1) treats cold damage warm toxin, heat in both the exterior and interior, shouting frenetically with a desire to run, vexation and agitation with great thirst, reddish complexion and dry nose, reddish eyes like fire, generalized contracture, inability to sweat.

    (2) or promotion of sweating or precipitation are already used, the disease passed the channel without resolving, there is great heat in triple burner, delirious mania and nosebleed, yellowish eyes and whole body, six pulses that are surging and rapid, and yang toxin with macule.

·**CHANNELS ENTERED**：The foot greater yang and the hand lesser yang channels.

·**Analysis of Formula**：(1) the evil of the exterior and interior are exuberant, one desires to treat interior but the exterior pattern still remains, and one desires to effuse the exterior but the interior is also urgent, therefore Huang Qin drains the fire of the upper burner, Huang Lian drains the fire of the middle burne

127

r, Huang Bai drains the fire of the lower burner, Zhi Zi frees and drains the fire of triple burner, Ma Huang and Dan Dou Chi disperse exterior evil, Shi Gao is heavy and drains stomach fire and can resolve the flesh.

(2) this formula also disperses the exterior and interior separately.

·**Original Source**：Tao Yao

7. 三黃石膏湯
    ·總結：發表清裏
    ·組成：黃連, 黃芩, 黃柏, 梔子, 麻黃, 淡豆豉, 石膏
    ·主治：(1)治傷寒溫毒, 表裏俱熱, 狂叫欲走, 煩燥大渴, 面赤鼻乾,
兩目如火, 身形拘急, 而不得汗.
          (2)或已經汗下, 過經不解, 三焦大熱, 譫狂鼻衄, 身目俱黃,
六脈洪數, 及陽毒發斑.
    ·歸經：此足太陽手少陽之藥也.
    ·方義：(1)表裏之邪俱盛, 欲治內則表未除, 欲發表則裏又急. 故以黃
芩瀉上焦之火, 黃連瀉中焦之火, 黃柏瀉下焦之火, 梔子通瀉三焦之火,
而以麻黃, 淡豆豉發散表邪, 石膏體重, 瀉胃火, 能解肌.
          (2)亦表裏分消之藥也.

8. Wu Ji San. Five-Accumulation Powder. 五積散

·**ACTIONS**：effuses the exterior and warms the interior

·**COMPOSITION**：Ma Huang, Bai Zhi, Gan Jiang, Rou Gui, Cang Zhu, Hou Po, Ban Xia, Chen Pi, Fu Ling, Dang Gui, Chuan Xiong, Bai Shao Yao, Gan Cao, Jie Geng, Zhi Ke, Sheng Jiang, Cong Bai

·**INDICATIONS**：(1) treats lesser yin cold damage.

(2) and external contraction of wind cold, coldness engendered by internal damage, generalized heat effusion without sweating, headache and generalized pain, contracture of nape and back.

(3) thoracic fullness, aversion to eat, retching and vomiting, abdominal pain, alternating aversion to cold and heat effusion.

(4) leg qi with swelling and pain, cold constipation and cold abdominal colic, cold malaria, aversion to cold and absence of sweating.

(5) irregularities of menstruation.

·**MODIFICATIONS**：(1) for sweating, eliminate Cang Zhu and Ma Huang.

128

　　　　　　　(2) for qi vacuity, eliminate Zhi Ke and Jie Geng and add Ren Sh en and Bai Zhu.

　　　　　　　(3) for abdominal pain with qi stagnation, add Wu Zhu Yu.

　　　　　　　(4) for stomach cold, add Sheng Jiang (roast).

　　　　　　　(5) for yin pattern in cold damage, cold limbs and vacuous sweat ing, add Fu Zi.

　　　　　　　(6) for irregularities of menstruation, add Ai Ye (stir-bake with v inegar).

　　　·**CHANNELS ENTERED**：yin yang exterior interior

·**Analysis of Formula**：(1) this is commonly used to yin, yang, exterior, and interi or.

　　　　　　　(2) Ma Huang and Gui Zhi resolve exterior and disperse cold.

　　　　　　　　　Gan Cao and Shao Yao harmonize the middle and reli eve pain.

　　　　　　　　　Cang Zhu and Hou Po pacify stomach earth and elimi nate dampness.

　　　　　　　　　Chen Pi and Ban Xia move counterflow qi and elimina te phlegm.

　　　　　　　　　Chuan Xiong, Dang Gui, Sheng Jiang, and Bai Zhi ent er blood part and eliminate cold damp.

　　　　　　　　　Zhi Ke and Jie Geng disinhibit chest and diaphragm a nd clear cold and heat.

　　　　　　　　　Fu Ling drains heat, disinhibits water, quiets the heart, and boosts the spleen.

　　　　　　　(3) Therefore this formula resolve the exterior, warm the middle, eliminates damp, removes phlegm, disperses glomus, and regulates menstruatio n.

　　　　　　　　　This formula treats lots of disease, only wise doctor ca n apply this formula to various diseases.

·**RELATED FORMULA**：　combining with Ren Shen Bai Du San, this is called Wu Ji Jiao Jia San, treats cold-damp, generalized heaviness and pain, and aching lu mbus and leg.

　　　·**Original Source**：Ju Fang

8. 五積散
　·總結：發表溫裏
　·組成：麻黃，白芷，乾薑，肉桂，蒼朮，厚朴，半夏，陳皮，茯苓，當

129

歸, 川芎, 白芍, 甘草, 桔梗, 枳殼, 生薑, 葱白

　　·主治：⑴治少陰傷寒.

　　　　　　⑵及外感風寒, 內傷生冷, 身熱無汗, 頭痛身痛, 項背拘急.

　　　　　　⑶胸滿惡食, 嘔吐腹痛, 寒熱往來.

　　　　　　⑷腳氣腫痛, 冷秘寒疝, 寒癧, 惡寒無汗.

　　　　　　⑸婦人經水不調.

　　·加減：⑴ 有汗去蒼朮, 麻黃.

　　　　　　⑵ 氣虛去枳, 桔, 加人參, 白朮.

　　　　　　⑶ 腹痛挾氣加吳茱萸.

　　　　　　⑷ 胃寒加煨薑.

　　　　　　⑸ 陰證傷寒, 肢冷虛汗, 加附子.

　　　　　　⑹ 婦人調經, 加醋艾.

　　·歸經：陰陽表裏通用之劑也.

　　·方義：⑴此陰陽表裡通用之劑也.

　　　　　　⑵麻黃, 桂枝所以解表散寒.

　　　　　　　　甘草, 芍藥, 所以和中止痛.

　　　　　　　　蒼朮, 厚朴平胃土而祛溼.

　　　　　　　　陳皮, 半夏, 行逆氣而除痰.

　　　　　　　　芎, 歸, 薑, 芷, 入血分而祛寒溼.

　　　　　　　　枳殼, 桔梗, 利胸膈而清寒熱.

　　　　　　　　茯苓瀉熱利水, 寧心益脾.

　　　　　　⑶所以爲解表溫中除溼之劑, 祛痰消痞調經之方也.

　　　　　　　　一方統治多病, 惟活法者變而通之.

　　·變化方：本方合人參敗毒散, 名五積交加散, 治寒溼身體重痛, 腰腳酸疼.

　　·來源：局方

9. Ma Huang Bai Zhu Tang. Ephedra and Atractylodes Ma crocephala Decociton. 麻黃白朮湯

·**ACTIONS**：resolves the exterior, clears the interior, and supplements the middle.

·**COMPOSITION**：Qing Pi, Chen Pi, Huang Lian, Huang Bai, Gan Cao, Sheng Ma, Chai Hu, Gui Zhi, Ren Shen, Huang Qi, Hou Po, Zhu Ling, Fu Ling, Ze Xie, Wu Zhu Yu, Bai Dou Kou, Shen Qu (stir-bake), Ma Huang, Xing Ren

·**INDICATIONS**：(1) treats constipation, inhibited voiding of reddish uri
ne, swelling of eyes and whole body, yellowish skin, and numbness [of skin].

(2) generalized heaviness as mountain, panting with forceless, vo
miting of phlegm and spitting of spittle.

(3) heat effusion and periodic vexation, chilling after vexation, coldness in
the nape and forehead, heat pain in the eyes as flowing fire.

(4) loss of smell, stirring qi in the umbilicus, acute pain in the les
ser abdomen.

·**CHANNELS ENTERED**：The foot three yang and three yin.

·**Analysis of Formula**：(1) the above pattern is due to damage of both ext
erior and interior, yang qi is oppressed so that this is unable to raise, therefore
wind, fire, damp, and heat are depressed and disease occurs.

(2) Gui Zhi and Ma Huang resolve exterior and eliminate wind.

Sheng Ma and Chai Hu raise yang and disperse fire.

Huang Lian and Huang Bai dry damp and clear heat.
Huang Bai also can supplement the kidney and nourish yin.

Qing Pi, Chen Pi, Bai Dou Kou, and Hou Po disinhibit
qi and disperse fullness. Qing Pi and Chai Hu also can pacify the liver. Bai Dou
Kou and Hou Po also can warm the stomach.

Xing Ren disinhibits the lung and descends qi. Shen Q
u transforms stagnation and regulates the middle. Wu Zhu Yu warms the kidne
y and liver.

Ren Shen, Huang Qi, Gan Cao, Chang Zhu, and Bai Z
hu supplement the spleen and boost qi.

Zhu Ling, Fu Ling, and Ze Xie free and disinhibit urin
ation, if damp is eliminated, and then heat also removes.

(4) although there is absence of herbs to free stool, generally wh
en clear yang raises, turbid yin spontaneously descends.

·**Original Source**：Li Dong Yuan

9. 麻黃白朮湯

·總結：解表清裏補中

·組成：青皮, 陳皮, 黃連, 黃柏, 甘草, 升麻, 柴胡, 桂枝, 人參, 黃
耆, 厚朴, 豬苓, 茯苓, 澤瀉, 吳茱萸, 白豆蔻, 炒麴, 麻黃, 杏仁

·主治：(1)治大便不通, 小便赤澀, 身面俱腫, 色黃麻木.

(2)身重如山, 喘促無力, 吐痰唾沫.

(3)發熱時躁, 躁已振寒, 項額如冰, 目中溜火.

(4)鼻不聞香，臍有動氣，小腹急痛．

・歸經：此足三陽三陰通治之劑也．

・方義：(1)前證蓋因表裡俱傷，陽氣抑不得升，故風火溼熱鬱而爲病也．

(2)桂枝，麻黃解表袪風．

升麻，柴胡，升陽散火．

黃連，黃柏，燥溼清熱；而黃柏又能補腎滋陰．

青，陳，蔻，朴利氣散滿；而青，柴又能平肝；蔻，朴又能溫胃．

杏仁利肺下氣；神麴化滯調中；吳萸暖腎溫肝；

參，耆，甘草，蒼白二朮補脾益氣；

二苓，澤瀉通利小便，使溼去而熱亦行．

(4)方內未嘗有通大便之葯，蓋清陽升則濁陰自降矣．

・來源：東垣

10. Shen Su Yin. Ginseng and Perilla Leaf Decoction. 參蘇飲

・**ACTIONS**：external contraction and internal damage

・**COMPOSITION**：Ren Shen, Ban Xia, Fu Ling, Chen Pi, Gan Cao, Zhi Ke, Ge Gen (dry), Zi Su Ye, Qian Hu, Mu Xiang, Jie Geng, Sheng Jiang, Da Zao

・**INDICATIONS**：(1) treats external contraction and internal damage, heat effusion and headache, retching and cough, phlegm blocking the middle burner, dizziness, gastric upset, vexation, wind damage with diarrhea.

(2) and when in cold damage, promotion of sweating has used, but there is incessant heat effusion

・**MODIFICATIONS**：(1) if external contraction is more severe, eliminate Da Zao and add Cong Bai.

(2) for fire in the lung, eliminate Ren Shen and add Xing Ren and Sang Bai Pi.

(3) for diarrhea, add Bai Zhu, Bian Dou, and Lian Rou.

・**CHANNELS ENTERED**：The hand and foot greater yin channels.

・**Analysis of Formula**：Wind and cold should be treated with resolving exterior, therefore Zi Su Ye, Ge Gen, and Qian Hu are used.

Taxation damage should be treated with supplementing the middle, therefore Ren Shen, Fu Ling, and Gan Cao are used.

132

Chen Pi and Ban Xia eliminate phlegm and check retching.

Zhi Ke and Jie Geng disinhibit diaphragm and soothe intestines.

Mu Xiang moves qi and breaks stagnation.

This formula makes both interior and exterior harmonious, and then evil disperses.

·**RELATED FORMULA**：When Ren Shen and Qian Hua are eliminated and Chuan Xiong, Chai Hu, Sheng Jiang, Da Zao are added, this is called Xiong Su Yin, treats damage to wind and cold, heat effusion, headache, and aversion to cold in the exterior, cough, vomiting of phlegm, counterflow qi in the interior.

·**Original Source**：Yi Lei Yuan Rong

10. 參蘇飲

·總結：外感內傷

·組成：人參, 半夏, 茯苓, 陳皮, 甘草, 枳殼, 乾葛, 紫蘇, 前胡, 木香, 桔梗, 生

薑, 大棗

·主治：(1)治外感內傷, 發熱頭痛, 嘔逆咳嗽, 痰塞中焦, 眩運嘈煩, 傷風泄瀉.

　　　　(2)及傷寒汗已, 發熱不止.

·加減：(1)外感多者去棗, 加葱白.

　　　　(2)肺中有火, 去人參, 加杏仁, 桑白皮.

　　　　(3)泄瀉加白朮, 扁豆, 蓮肉.

·歸經：此手足太陰藥也.

·方義：風寒宜解表, 故用蘇, 葛, 前胡；

　　　　勞傷宜補中, 故用參, 苓, 甘草；

　　　　橘, 半除痰止嘔；

　　　　枳, 桔利膈寬腸；

　　　　木香行氣破滯.

　　　　使內外俱和, 則邪散矣.

·變化方：本方去人參, 前胡加川芎, 柴胡, 薑, 棗煎, 名芎蘇飲, 治傷風寒, 外有發熱頭痛惡寒, 內有咳嗽吐痰氣湧.

·來源：元戎

11. Xiang Su San. Cyperus and Perilla Leaf Powder. 香蘇

飲

·**ACTIONS**：external contraction and internal damage

·**COMPOSITION**：Xiang Fu, Zi Su Ye, Chen Pi(eliminate white), Gan Cao, Sheng Jiang, Da Zao

·**INDICATIONS**：(1) treats seasonal common cold, headache, and heat effusion.

(2) or with internal damage, there is fullness and oppression in the chest and diaphragm, belching, and aversion to food.

·**MODIFICATIONS**：(1) for food damage, add digestant medicinal.

(2) for cough, add Xing Ren and Sang Pi.

(3) for phlegm, add Ban Xia.

(4) for headache, add Chuan Xiong and Bai Zhi.

(5) for wind damage with spontaneous sweating, add Gui Zhi.

(6) for cold damage with absence of sweating, add Ma Huang, Gan Jiang.

(7) for wind damage with nasal congestion and dizziness, add Qiang Huo and Jing Jie.

(8) for sudden pain in the heart, add Yan Hu Suo with one cup of wine.

·**CHANNELS ENTERED**：The hand greater yin channel.

·**Analysis of Formula**：Zi Su Ye courses exterior qi and disperses external cold. Xiang Fu moves interior qi and disperses internal congestion. Ju Hong also can move the exterior and interior as an assistant. Gan Cao harmonizes the middle, and also can resolve the exterior acting as courier.

·**Original Source**：Ju Fang

11. 香蘇飲
·總結：外感內傷
·組成：香附, 紫蘇, 陳皮(去白), 甘草, 生薑, 大棗
·主治：(1)治四時感冒, 頭痛發熱.
(2)或兼內傷, 胸膈滿悶, 噯氣惡食.
·加減：(1)傷食加消導藥.
(2)咳嗽加杏仁, 桑皮.
(3)有痰加半夏.
(4)頭痛加川芎, 白芷.

(5)傷風自汗加桂枝.

(6)傷寒無汗加麻黃, 乾薑.

(7)傷風鼻塞頭昏, 加羌活, 荊芥.

(8)心中卒痛加延胡索酒一杯.

·歸經：此手太陰藥也.

·方義：紫蘇疏表氣而散外寒；香附行裡氣而消內壅；橘紅能兼行表裡以佐之；

甘草和中, 亦能解表, 爲使也.

·來源：局方

12. Yin Chen Wan. Artemisia Scoparia Pills. 茵陳丸

·**ACTIONS**：promotion of sweating, vomiting, and precipitation.

·**COMPOSITION**：Yin Chen, Zhi Zi, Bie Jia, Mang Xiao, Da Huang, Chang Shan, Xing Ren, Ba Dou, Dan Dou Chi

·**INDICATIONS**：treats seasonal qi, miasmic toxin, jaundice, all kinds of malaria, red or white dysentery, and so on.

·**CHANNELS ENTERED**：The foot greater yang, greater yin, yang brightness, and reverting yin channels. [The bladder, spleen, stomach, and liver]

·**Analysis of Formula**：(1) the composition of Zhi Zi and Dan Dou Chi is Zhi Chi Tang. Combining with Chang Shan can make one vomit, Xing Ren can resolve the flesh.

(2) the composition of Da Huang and Mang Xiao is Cheng Qi Tang, this can flush heat and eliminate repletion. Yin Chen can disinhibit damp and abate jaundice.

(3) Ba Dou is great heat, eliminates accumulated cold in the viscera and bowels. Bie Jia nourishes yin and abates cold and heat in the blood part.

(4) there is all treatments of promotion of sweating, vomiting, and precipitation in this formula, therefore this can treat all kinds of disease.

·**Original Source**：Wai Tai Mi Yao

12. 茵陳丸

·總結：汗吐下兼行

·組成：茵陳, 梔子, 鱉甲, 芒硝, 大黃, 常山, 杏仁, 巴豆, 豉

135

·主治：治時氣瘴氣，黃病痎瘧，赤白痢等證．

·歸經：此足太陽太陰陽明厥陰葯也．

·方義：(1)梔子淡豉，梔豉湯也．合常山可以涌吐，合杏仁可以解肌．

　　　　(2)大黃芒硝承氣湯也，可以蕩熱去實．合茵陳可以利溼退黃．

　　　　(3)加巴豆大熱，以袪臟腑積寒．加鱉甲滋陰，以退血分寒熱．

　　　　(4)此方備汗吐下三法，故能統治諸病．

·來源：外臺

136

Chapter 6. Harmonizing Formulas. 和解之劑

1. Xiao Chai Hu Tang. Minor Bupleurum Decoction. 小柴胡湯

·**ACTIONS** : half-exterior half-interior pattern.

·**COMPOSITION** : Chai Hu, Huang Qin, Ban Xia, Sheng Jiang, Ren Shen, Gan Cao, Da Zao

·**INDICATIONS** : (1) When in cold damage wind strike the evil is in lesser yang, there is alternating aversion to cold and heat effusion, fullness in the chest and rib-side, and taciturnity with no desire for food or drink, heart vexation and frequent retching

(2) or possibly there is pain in the abdomen, or pain below rib-side, or thirst, or cough, or diarrhea, or palpitations with inhibited urination, or absence of thirst with bitter taste in the mouth, deafness, the pulse that is string like, or unresolved residual heat after sweating.

(3) or there is seasonal malaria in spring, or malaria with alternating aversion to cold and heat effusion. When in cold damage of women, heat entered blood chamber.

(4) also treats that when cold damage has lasted for five or six days, there is sweating from the head, mild aversion to cold, cold extremities, fullness below the heart, absence of desire to eat, hard stool, and a pulse that is fine, this means mild yang bind

·**MODIFICATIONS** : (1) for counterflow retching, add Sheng Jiang and Chen Pi.

(2) for vexation without retching, eliminate Ban Xia and Ren Shen, add Gua Lou.

(3) for thirst, eliminate Ban Xia, add Tian Hua Fen.

(4) if there is absence of thirst, and mild heat effusion, eliminate Ren Shen, add Gui Zhi, and then take mild sweating.

(5) for cough, eliminate Ren Shen, Da Zao, and Sheng Jiang, add Wu Wei Zi and Gan Jiang.

(6) for vacuity vexation, add Zhu Ye and Geng Mi.

(7) for dry teeth without fluids, add Shi Gao.

(8) for copious phlegm, add Gua Lou and Bei Mu.

⑼ for abdominal pain, eliminate Huang Qin, add Shao Yao.

⑽ for glomus and hardness below the heart, eliminate Da Zao, add Mu Li.

⑾ for pain below the heart, add Qing Pi and Shao Yao.

⑿ for palpitation below the heart and inhibited urination, eliminate Huang Qin, add Fu Ling.

⒀ for headache in the lesser yang channel, add Chuan Xiong.

⒁ for yellowing, adds Yin Chen.

·**CHANNELS ENTERED** : The foot lesser yang channel.

·**Analysis of Formula** : (1) The gall bladder is the organ of clear and pure, in which nothing comes out and enter, the channel of it is in half-exterior half-interior, it is impossible to use promotion of sweating, vomiting, and precipitation, it should be harmonized. When evil enters the lesser yang channel, this is going to enter interior from exterior, this should be treated with dispersing heat and releasing exterior, so as not to transport evil to greater yin.

(2) Chai Hu is bitter and slightly cold. This is the main herb of lesser yang, raises yang to reach exterior, and acts as sovereign.

Huang Qin is bitter and cold. This nourishes yin and abates heat, and acts as minister.

Ban Xia is pungent and warm. This can fortify the spleen and harmonize the stomach, and disperses counterflow qi to stop retching.

Ren Shen and Gan Cao supplement right qi and harmonize the middle to make evil not to enter interior, and act as assistant.

When evil is in half interior half exterior, Construction and Defense contend with each other, therefore the pungent and sweet of sheng jiang and Da Zao are used to harmonize Construction and Defense and act as courier.

·**RELATED FORMULA** : (1) When Qian Hu is used instead of Chai Hu, this is called Xiao Qian Hu Tang, treats same thing with above.

(2) When Chen Pi and Shao Yao are added, this is called Chai Hu Shuang Jie San, treats same thing with the above.

(3) When Mang Xiao is added, this is called Chai Hu Jia Mang Xiao Tang.

(4) When Gui Zhi is added, this is called Chai Hu Jia Gui Zhi Tang, treats that when cold damage has lasted for six and seven days, there is heat effusion, mild aversion to cold, vexation pain in the limb and joint, mild retching, and tightness below the heart. This means that the exterior pattern has not yet resolved.

138

(5) When Huang Qin and Gan Cao are eliminated and Gui Zhi, Fu Ling, Long Gu, Mu Li, Qian Dan, and Da Huang are added, this is called Chai Hu Jia Long Gu Mu Li Tang, treats that when cold damage has lasted for eight or nine days precipitation is used, there is thoracic fullness, vexation and fright, inhibited urination, delirious speech, heaviness of the entire body, and inability to turn sides.

(6) when Ban Xia, Ren Shen, Shen Jiang, and Da Zao are eliminated and Gui Zhi, Gan Jiang, Tian Hua Fen, and Mu Li are added, this is called Chai Hu Gui Zhi Gan Jiang Tang, treats when cold damage has lasted five or six days, and sweating has been promoted and then precipitation has been used and there is fullness in the chest and rib-side and mild bind, inhibited urination, thirst without retching, sweating only from the head, alternating aversion to cold and heat effusion, and heart vexation. And also treats malaria with heat effusion and aversion to cold (with the aversion to cold more pronounced than the heat effusion), or only aversion to cold without heat effusion.

(7) When Ban Xia is eliminated and Tian Hua Fen is added, this is called Chai Hu Qu Ban Xia Jia Gua Lou Gen Tang, treats alternating aversion to cold and heat effusion with thirst, and taxation malaria.

(8) When Chai Hu and Huang Qin are eliminated, and Hou Po is added, this is called Hou Po Sheng Jiang Ban Xia Gan Cao Ren Shen Tang, treats abdominal distention and fullness after promotion of sweating.

(9) When Ban Xia is eliminated and Dang Gui, Bai Shao Yao, and Da Huang are added, this is called Chai Hu Yin Zi, treats flesh heat, steaming heat, accumulated heat, residual heat after promotion of sweating, a pulse that is surging, replete, string like, and rapid. Also treats malaria.

(10) When Qiang Huo and Fang Feng are added, this is called Chai Hu Qiang Huo Tang, treats scourage epidemic which belongs to lesser yang pattern.

(11) When Jie Geng is added, this is called Chai Hu Jie Geng Tang, treats spring cough.

(12) When Ping Wei San is combined with this formula, this is called Chai Ping Tang, treats damp malaria with generalized pain and heaviness.

(13) When Qing Dai and the juice of Sheng Jiang are added and made into pills with rice, this is called Qing Zhen Wan, treats vomiting, a pulse which is string like, headache, and heat cough.

(14) The combination of this formula (one fen) and Si Wu Tang (two fen) is called Chai Hu Si Wu Tang, treats enduring vacuity taxation of women with mild aversion to cold and heat effusion.

⒂ The combination of this formula (half) and Si Wu Tang (half) is called Tiao Jiang Tang.

·**Original Source**：Zhong Jing

1. 小柴胡湯
　·總結：半表半裏
　·組成：柴胡，黃芩，半夏，生薑，人參，甘草，大棗
　·主治：⑴治傷寒中風少陽證，往來寒熱，胸脅痞滿，黙黙不欲食，心煩喜嘔.

　　　　⑵或腹中痛，或脅下痛，或渴，或欬，或利，或悸，小便不利，或不渴，口苦耳聾，脈弦，或汗後餘熱不解.

　　　　⑶及春月時嗽，瘧發寒熱. 婦人傷寒，熱入血室.

　　　　⑷亦治傷寒五、六日，頭出汗，微惡寒，手足冷，心下滿，不欲食，大便硬，脈細者，爲陽微結.

　·加減：⑴嘔逆加生薑，陳皮.

　　　　⑵煩而不嘔，去半夏，人參，加栝蔞.

　　　　⑶渴者去半夏，加花粉.

　　　　⑷若不渴，外有微熱，去人參，加桂枝，覆取微汗.

　　　　⑸欬嗽去參，棗，生薑，加五味子，乾薑.

　　　　⑹虛煩加竹葉，粳米.

　　　　⑺齒燥無津加石膏.

　　　　⑻痰多加栝蔞，貝母.

　　　　⑼腹痛去黃芩，加芍藥.

　　　　⑽脅下痞硬，去大棗，加牡蠣.

　　　　⑾脅下痛，加青皮，芍藥.

　　　　⑿心下悸，小便不利，去黃芩，加茯苓.

　　　　⒀本經頭痛加川芎.

　　　　⒁發黃加茵陳.

　·歸經：足少陽藥
　·方義：⑴膽爲清淨之府，無出無入，其經在半表半裡，不可汗吐下，法宜和解. 邪入本經，乃由表而將至裡，當微熱發表，迎而奪之，勿令傳太陰.

　　　　⑵柴胡味苦微寒，少陽主藥，以升陽達表爲君.

　　　　　　黃芩苦寒. 以養陰退熱爲臣.

　　　　　　半夏辛溫，能健脾和胃，以散逆氣而止嘔.

140

人參，甘草，以補正氣而和中，使邪不得復傳入裡爲佐.

邪在半裡半表，則營衛爭. 故用薑，棗之辛甘，以和營衛爲使也.

·變化方：(1)本方以前胡代柴胡，名小前胡湯（崔氏），治同.

(2)本方加陳皮，芍藥，名柴胡雙解散，治同.

(3)本方加芒硝，名柴胡加芒硝湯.

(4)本方加桂枝，名柴胡加桂枝湯，治傷寒六、七日，發熱，微惡寒，支節煩痛，微嘔，心下支結. 外證未去者.

(5)本方除黃芩，甘草，加桂枝，茯苓，龍骨，牡蠣，鉛丹，大黃，名柴胡加龍骨牡蠣湯，治傷寒八、九日下之，胸滿煩驚，小便不利，譫語，身重不可轉側.

(6)本方去半夏，人參，薑，棗，加桂枝，乾薑，花粉，牡蠣，名柴胡桂枝乾薑湯，治傷寒汗下後，胸脇滿，微結，小便不利，渴而不嘔，但頭汗出，往來寒熱，心煩者. 亦治瘧發寒多熱少，或但寒不熱.

(7)本方去半夏，加花粉，名柴胡去半夏加栝蔞根湯，治往來寒熱而渴，及勞瘧.

(8)本方去柴胡，黃芩，加厚朴，名厚朴生薑半夏甘草人參湯，治發汗後腹脹滿者.

(9)本方除半夏，加當歸，白芍，大黃，名柴胡飲子，治肌熱蒸熱積熱，汗後餘熱，脈洪實弦數. 亦治瘧疾.

(10)本方加羌活，防風，名柴胡羌活湯，治瘟疫少陽證.

(11)本方加桔梗，名柴胡桔梗湯，治春嗽.

(12)本方合平胃散，名柴平湯，治溼瘧身痛，身重.

(13)本方加青黛，薑汁糊丸，名清鎮丸，治嘔吐脈弦頭痛及熱嗽.

(14)本方一分，加四物二分，名柴胡四物湯，治婦人日久虛勞，微有寒熱.

(15)本方與四物各半，名調經湯.

·來源：仲景

2. Huang Lian Tang. Coptis Decoction. 黃連湯

·**ACTIONS**：raises and descends yin and yang

·**COMPOSITION**：Huang Lian, Gan Jiang, Gui Zhi, Ban Xia, Ren Shen,

141

Gan Cao, Da Zao

·**INDICATIONS**：in cold damage, there is heat in the chest, a desire to re
tch, cold in the stomach, and abdominal pain.

·**CHANNELS ENTERED**：The foot yang brightness channel.

·**Analysis of Formula**：(1) Huang Lian is bitter cold, drains heat and desc
ends yang.

(2) Sheng Jiang and Gui Zhi are pungent and warm. They elimin
ate cold and raise yin.

(3) Ren Shen assists the right qi and eliminates evil.

(4) Ban Xia harmonizes the stomach and stops retching.

(5) Gan Cao and Da Zao regulate the middle and relieve pain.

When in the upper and middle burners cold and heat contend wi
th each other, this harmonizes and resolves those conditions.

·**Original Source**：Zhong Jing

2. 黃連湯
　·總結：升降陰陽
　·組成：黃連, 乾薑, 桂枝, 半夏, 人參, 甘草, 大棗
　·主治：治傷寒胸中有熱而欲嘔, 胃中有寒而腹痛.
　·歸經：足陽明藥
　·方義：(1)黃連苦寒泄熱以降陽.
　　　　　(2)薑, 桂辛溫除寒以升陰.
　　　　　(3)人參助正祛邪.
　　　　　(4)半夏和胃止嘔.
　　　　　(5)甘草, 大棗調中止痛.
　　　　　　上中二焦寒熱交戰, 以此和解之.
　·來源：仲景

3. Huang Qin Tang. Scutellaria Decoction. 黃芩湯

·**ACTIONS**：resolves both greater yang and lesser yang.

·**COMPOSITION**：Huang Qin, Bai Shao Yao, Gan Cao, Da Zao.

·**INDICATIONS**：The combination disease of greater yang and lesser ya
ng, spontaneous diarrhea.

·**CHANNELS ENTERED**：The foot greater yang and lesser yang chann
els

142

·**Analysis of Formula**：Cheng Wu Ji says that one who is vacuous and is not replete, is consolidated with bitter and restrained with sour. Huang Qin and Shao Yao are bitter and sour, they consolidate and restrain the qi of the intestines and stomach. One who is weak and insufficient, is supplemented with sweet. Da Zao and Gan Cao are sweet, supplement the weakness of the intestines and stomach.

·**RELATED FORMULA**：(1) When Ban Xia and Sheng Jiang are added, this is called Huang Qin Jia Ban Xia Sheng Jiang Tang, treats the above pattern with retching. And also treats cough due to gall bladder, vomiting of bitter water as like bile.

(2) When Da Zao is eliminated, this is called Huang Qin Shao Yao Tang, treats nosebleed due to fire raising, and heat diarrhea.

·another formula of Huang Qin Tang of Wai Tai Mi Yao Fang, ：Huang Qin, Ren Shen, Gan Jiang, Gui Zhi, Ban Xia, Da Zao, this treats dry retching and diarrhea.

·**Original Source**：Zhong Jing

3. 黃芩湯
    ·總結：太陽少陽兩解
    ·組成：黃芩 白芍 甘草 大棗
    ·主治：治太陽少陽合病，自下利者.
    ·歸經：足太陽少陽藥也
    ·方義：成氏曰「虛而不實者，苦以堅之，酸以收之；黃芩，芍藥之苦酸，以堅斂腸胃之氣. 弱而不足者力甘以補之；大棗，甘草味甘，以補腸胃之弱.」
    ·變化方：(1)本方加半夏，生薑，名黃芩加半夏生薑湯，治前證兼嘔者. 亦治膽腑發欬，嘔苦水如膽汁.
        (2)本方除大棗，名黃芩芍藥湯，治火升鼻衄，及熱痢.
    ·又附方：外臺黃芩湯：黃芩，人參，乾薑，桂枝，半夏，大棗，治乾嘔下痢.
    ·來源：仲景

4. Shao Yao Gan Cao Tang. Peony and Licorice Decoction. 芍藥甘草湯

·**ACTIONS** : abdominal pain

·**COMPOSITION** : Bai Shao Yao, Gan Cao

·**INDICATIONS** : (1) disharmony and pain in the abdomen.

(2) Zhong Jing uses this formula to treat the reversal cold of the l imbs after erroneous treatment of dispersing of exterior, there is reversal, tense d leg, and vomiting, first give Gan Jiang Gan Cao Tang to restore yang, If a cou nterflow patient recovers, and the feet become warm, one can use Shao Yao Ga n Cao Tang to harmonize yin, and then the feet will then be able to stretch.

·**MODIFICATIONS** : (1) If the pulse is moderate, this means water dama ge, add Gui Zhi and Sheng Jiang.

(2) If the pulse is surging, this means metal damage, add Huang Qin and Da Zao.

(3) If the pulse is rough, this means blood damage, add Dang Gu i.

(4) If the pulse is string-like, this means qi damage, add Shao Ya o.

(5) if the pulse is slow, this means cold damage, add Gan Jiang.

·**CHANNELS ENTERED** : The foot greater yin and yang brightness cha nnels.

·**Analysis of Formula** : (1) Because qi and blood are not in harmony, ther efore abdominal pain occurs. The sour of Bai Shao Yao promotes astriction and the bitter drains, and this can move Construction qi. The warm of Gan Cao disp erses and the sweet moderates, this can harmonize conterflow qi.

(2) The pain is related with exuberant wood overwhelming earth, Bai Shao Yao can drain the liver, Gan Cao can moderate the liver and harmoniz e the spleen.

·**RELATED FORMULA** : (1) When Shao Yao is eliminated and Gan Jia ng is added, this is called Gan Cao Gan Jiang Tang, in Jin Gui Yao Lue, this for mula is used to treat lung wilting and cold lung, vomiting of drool, and frequent urination.

(2) When Fu Zi is added, this is called Shao Yao Gan Cao Fu Zi Tang.

(3) When Huang Qin is added, this is called Huang Qin Shao Ya o Tang, treats heat diarrhea, abdominal pain, tenesmus, generalized heat effusio

144

n, pus and blood which are sticky, incessant nose bleed, and the pulse which is surging and rapid.

(4) When Bai Zhu is added, this is called Bai Zhu Shao Yao Tang, treats water diarrhea due to spleen damp, generalized heaviness, and fatigue and weakness.

4. 芍藥甘草湯
　·總結：腹痛
　·組成：白芍藥, 甘草
　·主治：(1)治腹中不和而痛.
　　　　　(2)仲景用治誤表發厥, 脚攣吐逆, 與乾薑甘草湯以復其陽, 厥愈足溫者, 更作此湯以和其陰, 其脚卽伸.
　·加減：(1)脈緩傷水, 加桂枝, 生薑.
　　　　　(2)脈洪傷金, 加黃芩, 大棗.
　　　　　(3)脈濇傷血, 加當歸.
　　　　　(4)脈弦傷氣, 加芍藥.
　　　　　(5)脈遲傷寒, 加乾薑.
　·歸經：足太陰陽明藥也
　·方義：(1)氣血不和, 故腹痛；白芍酸收而苦泄, 能行營氣；炙草溫散而甘緩, 能和逆氣.
　　　　　(2)又痛爲木盛剋土, 白芍能瀉肝, 甘草能緩肝和脾也.
　·變化方：(1)本方去芍藥, 加乾薑, 名甘草乾薑湯, 金匱用此治肺痿肺冷, 吐涎沫, 小便數.
　　　　　(2)本方加附子, 名芍藥甘草附子湯.
　　　　　(3)本方加黃芩, 名黃芩芍藥湯, 治熱痢, 腹痛, 後重, 身熱, 濃血稠黏. 及鼻衂不止. 脈洪數.
　　　　　(4)本方加白朮, 名白朮芍藥湯, 治脾溼水瀉, 身重困弱.

5. Gua Lou Xie Bai Bai Jiu Tang. Trichosanthes Fruit, Chinese Chive, and Wine Decoction. 栝蔞薤白白酒湯

　·**ACTIONS**：chest impediment
　·**COMPOSITION**：Gua Lou, Xie Bai, Wine
·**INDICATIONS**：chest impediment, panting, cough and spittle, chest pain stretching through to the back, shortness of breath.

·**CHANNELS ENTERED**：The upper burner and chest center

·**Analysis of Formula**： Zhong Jing, when this disease is slight, uses Xie Bai and Wine to boost yang, and when this is severe, uses Fu Zi and Gan Jiang to disperse yin. But the other doctors do not know what chest impediment is, th erefore they habitually use Bai Dou Kou, Mu Xiang, He Zi, San Leng, Shen Qu, Mai Ya, and so on, without any reason, they exhaust yang in the chest.

·**RELATED FORMULA**：⑴ When Ban Xia is added, this is called Gua Lou Xie Bai Ban Xia Tang, treats chest impediment with inability to sleep, hear t pain stretching through to the back.

⑵ When wine is eliminated and Zhi Shi, Hou Po, and Gui Zhi a re added, this is called Zhi Shi Xie Bai Gui Zhi Tang, treats chest impediment, qi binding in the chest, thoracic fullness, qi which counterflows from below the heart to the heart.

·**Original Source**：Jin Gui Yao Lue

5. 栝蔞薤白白酒湯

·總結：胸痺

·組成：栝蔞　薤白　白酒

·主治：治胸痺喘息，欬唾，胸背痛，短氣．

·歸經：上焦膻中藥

·方義：仲景微則用薤白，白酒以益其陽，甚則用附子，乾薑以消其陰．世醫不知胸痺爲何病，習用豆蔻，木香，訶子，三稜，神麴，麥芽等藥，坐耗其胸中之陽，亦相懸矣．

·變化方：⑴本方加半夏，名栝蔞薤白半夏湯，治胸痺不得臥，心痛徹背．

⑵本方除白酒，加枳實，厚朴，桂枝，名枳實薤白桂枝湯，治胸痺氣結在胸，胸滿脇下逆搶心．

·來源：金匱

6. Wen Dan Tang. Warm the Gallbladder Decoction. 溫膽湯

·**ACTIONS**：insomnia

·**COMPOSITION**：Ban Xia, Chen Pi, Fu Ling, Gan Cao, Zhi Shi, Zhu R u, Sheng Jiang, Da Zao, Huang Lian

·**INDICATIONS**：gall bladder vacuity, phlegm heat, insomnia, vacuity v exation, fright palpitations, bitter taste in the mouth, and vomiting of drool.

·**MODIFICATIONS**：(1) for heart vacuity, add Ren Shen and Zao Ren.

(2) for vexation heat in the heart, add Huang Lian and Mai Men Dong.

(3) for dry mouth and dry tongue, eliminate Ban Xia, add Mai M en Dong, Wu Wei Zi, and Tian Hua Fen.

(4) for exterior heat which has not been cleared, add Chai Hu.

(5) for heart vexation due to interior repletion, add Zhi Zi.

(6) for spontaneous diarrhea due to interior vacuity, eliminate Zh i Shi, add Bai Zhu.

·**CHANNELS ENTERED**： the foot lesser yang and yang brightness ch annels

·**Analysis of Formula**：(1) ① the pungent and warm of Ban Xia, Chen Pi, and Sheng Jiang abduct phlegm and stop retching, through this function, this fo rmula warms gall bladder.

② Zhi Shi breaks stagnation.

③ Gan Cao harmonizes the middle.

④ Fu Ling drains damp.

⑤ Zhu Ru opens the stagnation of stomach earth, clea rs the dry of lung metal, and cools lung metal. This calms Jia Wood.

(2) Nei Jing says that when the stomach is not in harmonious, fidgetiness o ccurs when lying. And also says that when yang qi is exuberant, this is unable t o enter yin, then yin qi gets vacuity, therefore vision is not clear. Ban Xia can h armonize the stomach and make yin and yang interact, therefore in Nei Jing it i s used to treat insomnia.

Er Chen Tang not only warms gall bladder but also ha rmonizes the stomach.

·**RELATED FORMULA**：When Ren Shen, Yuan Zhi, Zao Ren, and Shu Di Huang are added, this is called Shi Wei Wen Dan Tang, treats dream emissi on, and fright and anxiety.

·**Original Source**：Ji Yan Fang

6. 溫膽湯
　·總結：不眠
　·組成：半夏, 陳皮, 茯苓, 甘草, 枳實, 竹茹, 生薑, 大棗, 黃連
　·主治：治膽虛痰熱不眠, 虛煩驚悸, 口苦嘔涎.

147

·加減：(1)如心虛，加人參，棗仁.

   (2)心內煩熱，加黃連，麥冬.

   (3)口燥舌乾，去半夏，加麥冬，五味，花粉.

   (4)表熱未清，加柴胡.

   (5)內實心煩，加黑梔子.

   (6)內虛大便自利，去枳實，加白朮.

·歸經：足系陽陽明藥也

·方義：(1)①半，橘，生薑之辛溫，以之導痰止嘔，即以之溫膽.

    ②枳實破滯.

    ③甘草和中.

    ④茯苓滲溼.

    ⑤竹茹開胃土之鬱，清肺金之燥，涼肺金即所以甲木也.

   (2)經又曰：「胃不和則臥不安.」又曰：「陽氣滿不得入于陰，陰氣虛故目不得瞑」半夏能和胃而通陰陽，故內經用治不眠.

    二陳非特溫膽，亦以和胃也.

·變化方：本方加人參，遠志，棗仁，熟地，名十味溫膽湯，治夢遺驚惕.

·來源：集驗

7. Xiao Yao San. Rambling Powder. 消遙散

·**ACTIONS**：abates heat and regulates menstruation

·**COMPOSITION**：Fu Ling, Bai Zhu, Gan Cao (mix fried), Bai Shao Yao, Dang Gui, Chai Hu

·**INDICATIONS**：treats blood vacuity and dry liver, steaming bone and taxation heat, cough and tidal heat effusion, alternation aversion to cold and heat effusion, dry mouth and constipation, menstrual irregularities.

·**CHANNELS ENTERED**：The foot lesser yang and reverting yin channels. [The gall bladder and liver]

·**Analysis of Formula**：(1) When wood is exuberant, earth gets debilitated. Gan Cao and Bai Zhu harmonize the middle and supplement earth.

   (2) Liver vacuity causes blood disease. Dang Gui and Shao Yao nourish blood and restrain yin.

   (3)Chai Hu raises yang and disperses heat, with Shao Yao pacifi

148

es the liver and makes wood to reach orderly.

　　　　(4) Fu Ling clears heat and disinhibits damp, and assists Gan Cao and Bai Zhi to boost earth, and makes heart qi quiet.

　　　　(5) Sheng Jiang warms the stomach and eliminates phlegm, and regulates the middle and resolves depression.

　　　　(6) Bo He tracks the liver and drains the lung, and rectifies blood and disperses wind.

　　·**RELATED FORMULA**：When Mu Dan Pi and Zhi Zi are added, this is called Ba Wei Xiao Yao San, treats anger qi damaging the liver and scant blood with dim vision.

　　·**Original Source**：Ju Fang

7. 消遙散

　·總結：退熱調經

　·組成：茯苓，白朮，炙甘草，白芍，當歸，柴胡

　·主治：治血虛肝燥，骨蒸勞熱，欬嗽潮熱，往來寒熱，口乾便澀，月經不調.

　·歸經：足少陽厥陰藥也

　·方義：(1)木盛則土衰，甘草，白朮和中而補土.

　　　　(2)且肝虛則血病，當歸，芍藥養血而斂陰.

　　　　(3)柴胡升陽散熱，合芍藥以平肝，而使木得條達.

　　　　(4)茯苓清熱利溼，助甘朮以益土，而令心氣安寧.

　　　　(5)生薑暖胃祛痰，調中解鬱.

　　　　(6)薄荷搜肝瀉肺，理血消風.

　·變化方：本方加丹皮，栀子，名八味逍遙散，治怒氣傷肝，血少目暗.

　·來源：局方

8. Liu He Tang. Harmonize the Six Decoction. 六和湯

　·**ACTIONS**：regulates and harmonizes Six Qi.

　·**COMPOSITION**：Ren Shen, Bai Bian Dou, Bai Zhu, Gan Cao, Xiang Ru, Hou Po, Sha Ren, Xing Ren, Huo Xiang, Ban Xia, Chi Fu Ling, Mu Gua, Sheng Jiang, Da Zao

　·**INDICATIONS**：(1) treats irregularities of food in summer, internal damage engendering coldness, external damage to summerheat qi, alternation occurring of aversion to cold and heat effusion, sudden turmoil, vomiting, and diar

149

rhea.

(2) and latent summerheat with vexation and oppression, fatigue and a tendency to lie down, thirst with reddish urine, damage to wine, and so on.

·**MODIFICATIONS**：(1) for summerheat damage, add Xiang Ru.

(2) for cold damage, add Zi Su Ye.

·**CHANNELS ENTERED**：The foot greater yin and yang brightness channels.

·**Analysis of Formula**：(1) The bland of Bian Dou and Chi Fu Ling can drain damp and clear heat. Bian Dou also can disperse summerheat and harmonize the spleen.

(2) Ban Xia is pungent and warm, disperses counterflow qi and checks retching.

(3) Bai Zhu and Ren Shen are sweet and warm, supplement the right qi by eliminating of evil.

(4) The aroma of Xing Ren, Huo Xiang, Hou Po, and Sha Ren can soothe the spleen, the pungent can move qi. And Sha Ren and Hou Po also can transform food.

(5) The sour of Mu Gua can pacify the liver and soothe sinews.

(6) Gan Cao supplements the middle and harmonizes every herbs.

(7) Sheng Jiang and Da Zao disperse and regulate Construction and Defense.

(8) Xiang Ru is used to eliminate summerheat. Zi Su Ye is added to effuse the exterior and disperse cold.

·**Original Source**：Ju Fang

8. 六和湯

·總結：調和六氣

·組成：人參，白扁豆，甘草，香薷，厚朴，砂仁，杏仁，藿香，半夏，赤茯苓，木瓜，生薑，大棗

·主治：(1)治夏月飲食不調，內傷生冷，外傷暑氣，寒熱交作，霍亂吐瀉.

(2)及伏暑煩悶，倦怠嗜臥，口渴便赤，中酒等證.

·加減：(1)傷暑加香薷.

(2)傷冷加紫蘇.

·歸經：足太陰陽明藥也

·方義：(1)扁豆，赤苓，淡能滲溼清熱；而扁豆又能散暑和脾.

(2)半夏辛溫，散逆而止嘔.

(3)朮，參甘溫，補正以匡邪.

(4)杏仁，藿香，厚朴，砂仁，香能舒脾，辛能行氣； 而砂仁，厚朴，兼能化食.

(5)木瓜酸能平肝舒筋.

(6)甘草補中，協和諸藥.

(7)薑，棗發散而調營衛.

(8)或加香薷者，用以祛暑. 加紫蘇者，用以發表散寒也.

·來源：局方

9. Huo Xiang Zheng Qi San. Agastache Powder to Rectify the Qi. 藿香正氣散

·**ACTIONS**：external contraction with internal damage

·**COMPOSITION**：Huo Xiang, Zi Su Ye, Jie Geng, Bai Zhi, Hou Po, Da Fu Pi, Chen Pi, Ban Xia, Fu Ling, Bai Zhu, Gan Cao, Sheng Jiang, Da Zao

·**INDICATIONS**：(1) treats external contraction of wind cold, internal damage to food and drink, abhorrence of cold and invigorating heat, headache, retching, fullness and oppression in the chest and diaphragm, and cough with qi panting.

(2) also cold damage, damp damage, malaria, summerheat damage, sudden turmoil, vomiting, and diarrhea.

Generally when miasmic toxin contracts, the dose should be modified.

·**MODIFICATIONS**： for severe food damage, add digestant medicinal

·**CHANNELS ENTERED**：The hand greater yin and foot yang brightness channels.

·**Analysis of Formula**：(1) Huo Xiang is pungent and warm, rectifies qi and harmonizes the middle, repels something malign, checks retching, and also treats both the exterior and interior, acts as sovereign.

(2) Zi Su Ye, Bai Zhi, and Jie Geng disperse cold and disinhibit diaphragm, and assist the other herbs to effuse exterior evil.

(3) Hou Po and Da Fu Pi move water and disperse fullness.

(4) Ban Xia and Ju Pi disperse counterfolw qi and eliminate phlegm, assist the other herbs to course interior stagnation.

151

(5) Gan Cao, Bai Zhi, Fu Ling boosts the spleen and eliminate damp, and supplement the right qi, acts as minister and courier.

(6) When the right qi frees, counterflow evil gets to pause spontaneously.

·**RELATED FORMULA**：When this herb is combined with San Wei Xiang Rou Yin, this is called Huo Ru Tang, treats latent summerheat with vomiting, diarrhea, and cramp.

·Another Side Formula：in another formula of Huo Xiang Zheng Qi San, Mu Gua is added.

·**Original Source**：Ju Fang

9. 藿香正氣散

·總結：外感內傷

·組成：藿香，紫蘇，桔梗，白芷，厚朴，大腹皮，陳皮，半夏，茯苓，白朮，甘草，生薑，大棗

·主治：(1)治外感風寒，內傷飲食，憎寒壯熱，頭痛嘔逆，胸膈滿悶，欬嗽氣喘.

(2)及傷冷傷溼，瘧疾中暑，霍亂吐瀉.

凡感嵐瘴不正之氣者，宜增減用之.

·加減：傷食重者，加消食藥.

·歸經：手太陰足陽明藥也

·方義：(1)藿香辛溫，理氣和中，辟惡止嘔，兼治表裡爲君.

(2)蘇，芷，桔梗散寒利膈，佐之以發表邪.

(3)厚朴，大腹，行水消滿.

(4)半夏，橘皮，散逆除痰，佐之以疏裡滯.

(5)甘，朮，苓，益脾去溼，以輔正氣爲臣，使也.

(6)正氣通暢，則邪逆自除矣.

·變化方：本方合三味香薷飲，名藿薷湯，治伏暑吐瀉轉筋.

·又附方：一方加木瓜.

·煎服法：每服五錢，加薑，棗煎.

·來源：局方

10. San Jie Tang. Three Resolving Tang. 三解湯

·**ACTIONS**：epidemic yang malaria

·**COMPOSITION**：Ma Huang, Chai Hu, Ze Xie

·**INDICATIONS**：this is common formula to treat epidemic malaria.

·**CHANNELS ENTERED**：The foot lesser yang channel.

·**Analysis of Formula**：Wu He Gao says that disease can exist in the three part, in the exterior, in the interior, and in half exterior half interior. Malaria evil hides in fl esh, evil qi and right qi contend with each other, if they are combined in the exterio r, the disease is in the exterior, if in the interior, the disease is in the interior, if they have not yet been combined, the disease is in half exterior and half interior.

⑴ Ma Huang is pungent, can disperse exterior evil by sweating and effusing.

⑵ Chai Hu raises yang and effuses heat, harmonizes and resolve s between the interior and exterior.

⑶ Ze Xie is salty, can induce interior evil to come out through u rination.   ⑷ This only can treat replete malaria, in case of vacui ty pattern, first identify the qi and blood and then add tonifying medicinal.

10. 三解湯

　·總結：時行陽瘧

　·組成：麻黃，柴胡，澤瀉

　·主治：治時行瘧之通劑.

　·歸經：足少陽藥也

　·方義： 吳鶴皋曰：「病有三在， 在表在裡及在半表半裡也. 瘧邪藏 于分內之間， 邪正分爭， 併于表則在表， 併于裡則在裡， 未有所併則在半 表半裡.

　　　⑴麻黃之辛, 能散表邪由汗而泄.

　　　⑵柴胡升陽發熱, 居表裡之間而和解之.

　　　⑶澤瀉味鹹, 能引裡邪由溺而泄.

　　　⑷此但可以治實瘧, 虛者當辨其氣血而加補劑. 」

11. Qing Pi Yin. Clear the Splee Decoction. 清脾飲

·**COMPOSITION**：Qing Pi, Chai Hu, Hou Po, Ban Xia, Huang Qin, Cao Guo, Fu Ling, Gan Cao (mix fried), Bai Zhu

·**INDICATIONS**：treats malaria with the heat effusion more pronounced than the aversion to cold, bitter taste in the mouth, dry throat, inhibited voiding of reddish urine, and a pause when it comes, which is string-like.

·**MODIFICATIONS**：(1) for great thirst, add Mai Men Dong and Zhi Mu.

(2) for incessant malaria, add Chang Shan (stir-bake with wine), Wu Mei.

·**CHANNELS ENTERED**：The foot lesser yang and greater yin channels.

·**Analysis of Formula**：(1) Malaria is related with the evil of the liver and gall bladder, but this often occurs due to the damage of the spleen and stomach. The spleen belongs to damp earth, if it contracts to damp again, damp generates heat, and heat generates phlegm, therefore the above pattern shows.

(2) ① When the spleen contracts disease, wood also restrains it, therefore Qing Pi and Chai Hu are used to break stagnation and quell the liver.

② Hou Po and Ban Xia move phlegm and pacify the stomach.

③ Huang Qin is used to clear heat.

④ Cao Guo is pungent and heat, can disperse accumulated cold of greater yin, eliminate phlegm, and interrupt malaria.

⑤ Fu Ling is used to drain damp.

⑥ This formula first eliminates the evil which damages the spleen, and then Bai Zhu and Gan Cao is used to regulate and supplement the spleen.

·**Original Source**：Yan Yong He

11. 清脾飲
　·組成：青皮, 柴胡, 厚朴, 半夏, 黃芩, 草果, 茯苓, 炙甘草, 白朮
　·主治：治瘧疾熱多寒少, 口苦嗌乾, 小便赤澀, 脈來弦數.
　·加減：(1)大渴, 加麥冬, 知母.

(2)瘧不止, 加酒紗常山, 烏梅.
　·歸經：足少陽太陰藥也
　·方義：(1)瘧爲肝膽之邪, 然多因脾胃受傷而起. 脾屬溼土, 重感于溼, 溼生熱, 熱生痰, 故見前證也.

(2)①脾旣受病, 木又剋之, 故用青皮, 柴胡, 以破滯而伐肝.
②厚朴, 半夏, 以行痰而平胃.
③黃芩用以清熱.
④草果辛熱, 能散太陰之積寒, 除痰而截瘧.
⑤茯苓用以滲溼.
⑥蓋先去其害脾者, 而以白朮, 甘草調而補之也.

·來源：嚴用和

12. Tong Xie Yao Fang. Important Formula for Painful Dia rrhea. 痛瀉要方.

·**ACTIONS**：abdominal pain and diarrhea.
·**COMPOSITION**：Bai Shao Yao, Bai Zhu, Chen Pi, Fang Feng
·**INDICATIONS**：treats abdominal pain and incessant diarrhea.
·**MODIFICATIONS**：for enduring diarrhea, add Sheng Ma.
·**CHANNELS ENTERED**：The foot greater yin and reverting yin chann els

·**Analysis of Formula**：(1) Shao Yao drains liver fire, the sour restrains c ounterfolw qi, moderates the middle, and relieves pain.

(2) The bitter of Bai Zhu dries damp, the sweet supplements the spleen, and the warm harmonizes the middle.

(3) The pungent of Chen Pi can disinhibit qi, the aroma of stir ba ke can dry damp and enliven the spleen, and makes qi move to relieve the pain,

(4) The pungent of Fang Feng can disperse the liver, the aroma c an soothe the spleen, the wind can overcome damp. This is a key herb of rectify ing the spleen and channel conductor.

·**Original Source**：Liu Cao Chuang

12. 痛瀉要方
　·總結：痛瀉
　·組成：白芍, 白朮, 陳皮, 防風
　·主治：治痛瀉不止.
　·加減：久瀉加升麻.
　·歸經：足太陰厥陰藥也
　·方義：(1)芍藥瀉肝火, 酸斂逆氣, 緩中止痛.
　　　　　(2)白朮苦燥溼, 甘脯脾, 溫和中.
　　　　　(3)陳皮辛能利氣, 少香丸能燥溼醒脾, 使氣行則痛止.
　　　　　(4)防風辛能散肝, 香能舒脾, 風能勝溼, 爲理脾引經要藥.
　·來源：劉草窻

13. Huang Lian E Jiao Wan. Coptis and Ass Hide Glue Pill

155

s. 黃連阿膠丸

·**ACTIONS**：cold and heat dysentery

·**COMPOSITION**：Huang Lian, E Jiao, Fu Ling

·**INDICATIONS**：treats irregularities of cold and heat, red or white diarrhea, tenesmus, static pain in the umbilicus and abdomen, dry mouth, vexation with thirst, inhibited urination.

·**CHANNELS ENTERED**：The hand and foot yang brightness channels

·**Analysis of Formula**：(1) Huang Lian drains fire and dries damp, opens depression and disperses stasis, and pacifies the pain and heat.

(2) E Jiao supplements yin, boosts blood, moistens dryness, inhibits intestines, and harmonizes internal tense.

(3) Fu Ling can make lung qi descend with linking to the bladder, clears heat, disinhibits water, allays thirst, and eliminates vexation. This is common herb to clear heat and resolve.

·**Another Side Formula**：(1) Zhong Jing's Huang Lian E JiaoTang：Huang Lian, Huang Qin, Shao Yao, E Jiao, and Ji Zi huang; treats that when in lesser yin disease that has lasted more than two or three days, there is vexation in the heart and inability to sleep.

(2) Wang Hai Zang's Huang Lian E JiaoTang：Huang Lian, Huang Bai, E Jiao, Zhi Zi.

·**Original Source**：Ju Fang

13. 黃連阿膠丸

·總結：冷熱痢

·組成：黃連, 阿膠, 茯苓

·主治：治冷熱不調, 下痢赤白, 裡急後重, 臍腹瘀痛, 口燥煩渴, 小便不利.

·歸經：手足陽明藥也

·方義：(1)黃連瀉火燥溼, 開鬱消瘀, 以平其痛熱.

(2)阿膠補陰益血, 潤燥利腸, 以和其裡急.

(3)茯苓能令肺氣下降, 通于膀胱, 清熱利水, 止渴除煩, 爲清熱解之平劑.

·又附方：(1)仲景黃連阿膠湯：黃連, 黃芩, 芍藥, 阿膠, 雞子黃治傷寒少陰病得之二, 三日以上, 心煩不得臥.

(2)海藏黃連阿膠湯：黃連, 黃柏, 阿膠, 山±

·來源：局方

156

14. Lu Gen Tang. Rhizoma Phragmitis Decoction. 蘆根湯

·**ACTIONS**：vomiting and hiccup.

·**COMPOSITION**：Lu Gen, Zhu Ru, Geng Mi, Sheng Jiang

·**INDICATIONS**：treats that after cold damage, there is vomiting, hiccup, and inability to descend food.

·**CHANNELS ENTERED**：The foot greater yin and yang brightness channels

·**Analysis of Formula**：(1) Lu Gen is sweet and cold, descends latent fire, and disinhibits urine.

(2) Zhu Ru is sweet and cold, eliminates stomach heat, and clears dry metal.

(3) Sheng Jiang is pungent and warm, eliminates cold rheum, and disperses counterfolw qi. The three can harmonize the stomach. When the stomach is in harmony, vomiting gets to be checked.

(4) Geng Mi is added to regulate the stomach and spleen.

·**Original Source**：Tian Jin Yao Fang

14. 蘆根湯

·總結：嘔穢

·組成：蘆根，竹茹，粳米，生薑

·主治：治傷寒病後，嘔噦不下食.

·歸經：足太陰陽明藥也

·方義：(1)蘆根甘寒，降伏火，利小水.

(2)竹茹甘寒，除胃熱，清燥金.

(3)生薑辛溫，祛寒飲，散逆氣. 三者皆能和胃，胃和則嘔止.

(4)加粳米者，亦藉以調中州也.

·來源：千金

15. Yin Yang Shui. yin yang water. 陰陽水

·**ACTIONS**：sudden turmoil

·**COMPOSITION**：hot water, well water

·**INDICATIONS**：treats sudden turmoil with vomiting and diarrhea.

·**CHANNELS ENTERED**：This formula divides and manages yin and yang in the middle burner.

157

·**Analysis of Formula**：(1) Yin and yang are not harmonious and contend with each other, therefore vomiting on the upper part, diarrhea in the lower part, and sudden turmoil occur.

(2) Taking of this makes vomiting and diarrhea stop, and dividing and managing of yin and yang harmonizes and pacifies the stomach and spleen.

15. 陰陽水
　·總結：霍亂
　·組成：沸湯, 井水
　·主治：治霍亂吐瀉有神功.
　·歸經：中焦分理陰陽之藥也
　·方義：(1)陰陽不和而交爭, 故上吐下瀉而霍亂.
　　　　　(2)飲此輒定者, 分其陰陽使和平也.
　·煎服法：各半鍾和服

16. Gan Cao Hei Dou Tang. Licorice and Black Soybean Decociton. 甘草黑豆湯

·**ACTIONS**：resolves toxin
·**COMPOSITION**：Gan Cao, Hei Dou
·**INDICATIONS**：resolves toxin of every medicinal, treats sinews mounting (shan).
·**CHANNELS ENTERED**：The foot yang brightness channel.
·**Analysis of Formula**：(1) Gan Cao harmonizes the middle to resolve toxin, Hei Dou disperses heat to resolve toxin.

(2) When treating sinews mounting, one should use the twig of Gan Cao.
·**RELATED FORMULA**：When Da Huang is added, this is called Da Huang Gan Cao Tang, treats wasting-thirst in triple burner.

16. 甘草黑豆湯
　·總結：解毒
　·組成：甘草, 黑豆
　·主治：解百藥毒, 兼治筋疝.
　·歸經：足陽明藥也

·方義：⑴甘草和中以解毒，黑豆散熱以解毒.
　　　　⑵若治筋疝，當用甘草梢.
·變化方：本方加大黃，名大黃甘草湯. 治上中下三焦消渴.

Chapter 7. Qi-Rectifying Formulas. 理氣之劑

1. Bu Zhong Yi Qi Tang. Tonify the Middle and Augment the Qi Decoction. 補中益氣湯

·**ACTIONS**：raises yang and supplements the middle

·**COMPOSITION**：Bai Zhu, Huang Qi, Sheng Ma, Chai Hu, Ren Shen, Gan Cao (mix fried), Dang Gui, Chen Pi

·**INDICATIONS**：(1) treats vexed taxation, internal damage, generalized heat effusion, heart vexation, headache, aversion to cold, laziness to speak, aversion to eat, a pulse that is surging, large, and vacuous.

(2) or panting, or thirst, or spontaneous sweating due to yang vacuity, or qi vacuity failing to control blood.

(3) or malaria and dysentery with spleen vacuity, have not recovered for long time.

(4) all kinds of clear yang that falls downward, insufficient pattern of the middle qi.

·**MODIFICATIONS**：(1) for blood insufficiency, add Dang Gui.

(2) for lassitude of essence-spirit, add Ren Shen and Wu Wei Zi.

(3) for lung heat with cough, eliminate Ren Shen.

(4) for dry throat, add Ge Gen.

(5) for headache, add Man Jing Zi, for severe pain, add Chuan Xiong.

(6) for brain pain, add Gao Ben and Xi Xin.

(7) for contention of wind and damp with generalized pain, add Qiang Huo and Fang Feng.

(8) for phlegm, add Ban Xia and Sheng Jiang.

(9) for stomach cold with qi stagnation, add Qing Pi, Kou Ren, Mu Xiang, and Yi Zhi Ren.

(10) for abdominal distention, add Zhi Shi, Hou Po, Mu Xiang, and Sha Ren.

(11) for abdominal pain, add Bai Shao Yao and Gan Cao.

(12) for heat pain, add Huang Lian.

(13) for ability to eat with glomus below the heart, add Huang Lian.

160

(14) for sore throat, add Jie Geng.

(15) for cold, add Rou Gui.

(16) for excessive damp, add Cang Zhu.

(17) for yin fire, add Huang Bai and Zhi Mu.

(18) for yin vacuity, eliminate Sheng Ma and Chai Hu, add Shu D
i Huang, Shan Zhu Yu, Shan Yao.

(19) for constipation, add Da Huang (roast with wine).

(20) for cough, in spring add Xuan Fu Hua and Kuan Dong Hua, i
n summer add Mai Men Dong and Wu Wei Zi, in fall add Ma Huang and Huan
g Qin, in winter add Ma Huang, when whether is cold, add Gan Jiang.

(21) For diarrhea, eliminate Dang Gui and add Fu Ling, Cang Z
hu, and Yi Zhi Ren.

·**CHANNELS ENTERED** ： The foot greater yin and yang brightness cha
nnels

·**Analysis of Formula** ： (1) The lung is the root of qi, Huang Qi suppleme
nts the lung and secures the exterior, acting as sovereign.

(2) The spleen is the root of the lung. Ren Shen and Gan Cao sup
plement the spleen, boost qi, harmonize the middle, and drain fire, acting as mi
nister.

(3) Bai Zhu dries damp and strengthens the spleen, and Dang Gu
i harmonizes blood and nourishes yin, acting as assistant.

(4) Sheng Ma raises the clear qi of yang brightness, Chai Hu rais
es the clear qi of lesser yang. When yang rises, all things engender. When clear
qi raises, yin turbidity descends.

(5) Chen Pi is added to free and disinhibit qi.

(6) Sheng Jiang is pungent and warm, Da Zao is sweet and cold, they are u
sed to harmonize Construction and Defense, free and open the flesh, and transform
liquid and humor.

(7) When treating all kinds of insufficient pattern, first one shoul
d supplement the middle, what is the middle? It is the spleen and stomach.

·**RELATED FORMULA** ： (1) When Dang Gui and Bai Zhu is eliminated,
and Mu Xiang and Cang Zhu are added, this is called Tiao Zhong Bu Qi Tang,
treats the irregularities of the spleen and stomach, thoracic fullness, fatigued cu
mbersome limbs, scant food, shortness of breath, inability to taste food, and im
mediate vomting of ingest food.

(2) When Bai Shao Yao and Wu Wei Zi are added, this is also ca
lled Tiao Zhong Yi Qi Tang, treats qi vacuity with profuse sweating, and the ot

161

her signs which are same with the above.

(3) Double of Chang Zhu, Ban Xia, and Huang Qin (respectively three fen) are added, this is called Shen Zhu Yi Wei Tang, treats internal damage with taxation and fatigue, dry heat with shortness of breath, thirst with no desire to eat, sloppy stool with yellow color.

(4) When Bai Zhu is eliminated and Cao Dou Kou, Shen Qu, Ban Xia, and Huang Bai are added, this is called Sheng Yang Shun Qi Tang, treats damage to food and drink, taxation and fatigue, fullness and oppression, shortness of breath, no desire to eat, inability to taste food, periodic aversion to cold.

(5) When Huang Qin and Shen Qu are added, this is called Yi Wey Sheng Yang Tang, treats irregularities of menstruation, or reduced eating and water diarrhea after blood collapse.

(6) When Huang Bai and Sheng Di Huang are added, this is called Bu Zhong Yi Qi Jia Huang Bai Sheng Di Huang Tang, treats yin fire overwhelming yang, heat effusion which is severe at day, spontaneous sweating, shortness of breath, thirst with inability to taste. .

(7) When Bai Shao Yao, Xi Xin, Chuan Xiong, and Man Jing Zi are added, this is called Shun Qi He Zhong Tang, treats clears yang failing to raise, headache, aversion to wind, a pulse that is string-like, weak, and fine.

(8) When Qiang Huo, Fang Feng, Xi Xin, and Chuan Xiong are added, this is called Tiao Ying Yang Wei Tang, treats cold damage of overexerted and fatigue person, generalized pain and heat effusion, aversion to cold, mild thirst, sweating, a pulse that is floating with forceless.

·Original Source：Li Dong Yuan

1. 補中益氣湯
   ·總結：升陽補中
   ·組成：白朮, 黃耆, 升麻, 柴胡, 人參, 炙甘草, 當歸, 陳皮
   ·主治：(1)治煩勞內傷, 身熱心煩, 頭痛惡寒, 懶言惡食, 脈洪大而虛.
   　　　　(2)或喘或渴, 或陽虛自汗, 或氣虛不能攝血.
   　　　　(3)或瘧痢脾虛, 久不能愈.
   　　　　(4)一切清陽下陷, 中氣不足之證.
   ·加減：(1)如血不足, 加當歸.
   　　　　(2)精神短少, 加人參, 五味.
   　　　　(3)肺熱欬嗽, 去人參.
   　　　　(4)嗌乾, 加葛根.
   　　　　(5)頭痛, 加蔓荊子；痛甚加川芎.

162

(6)腦痛加藁本, 細辛.

(7)風溼相搏, 一身盡痛, 加羌活, 防風.

(8)有痰, 加半夏, 生薑.

(9)胃寒氣滯, 加青皮, 蔻仁, 木香, 益智.

(10)腹脹, 加枳實, 厚朴, 木香, 砂仁.

(11)腹痛, 加白芍, 甘草.

(12)熱痛, 加黃連.

(13)能食而心下痞, 加黃連.

(14)咽痛, 加桔梗.

(15)有寒, 加肉桂.

(16)溼勝, 加蒼朮.

(17)陰火, 加黃柏, 知母.

(18)陰虛, 去升柴, 加熟地, 山茱, 山藥.

(19)大便祕, 加酒煨大黃.

(20)欬嗽, 春加旋覆, 款冬; 夏加麥冬, 五味; 秋加麻黃, 黃芩; 冬加不去根節麻黃; 天寒加乾薑.

(21)泄瀉, 去當歸, 加茯苓, 蒼朮, 益智.

·歸經：足太陰陽明藥也

·方義：(1)肺者氣之本, 黃耆補肺固表爲君.

(2)脾者肺之本, 人參, 甘草, 補脾益氣, 和中瀉火爲臣.

(3)白朮燥溼強脾, 當歸和血養陰爲佐.

(4)升麻以升陽明清氣, 柴胡以升少陽清氣, 陽升則萬物生, 清升則陰濁降.

(5)加陳皮者, 以通利其氣.

(6)生薑辛溫, 大棗甘寒, 用以和營衛, 開腠理, 致津液諸虛不足.

(7)先建其中, 中者何？脾胃是也.

·變化方：(1)本方除當歸, 白朮, 加木香, 蒼朮, 名調中益氣湯, 治脾胃不調, 胸滿肢倦, 食少短氣, 口不知味, 及食入反出.

(2)本方加白芍, 五味子, 亦名調中益氣湯, 治氣虛多汗, 餘治同前.

(3)本方加蒼倍分, 半夏, 黃芩各三分, 名參朮益胃湯, 治內傷勞倦, 燥熱短氣, 口渴無味, 大便溏黃.

(4)本方去白朮, 加草蔻, 神麴, 半夏, 黃柏, 名升陽順氣湯, 治飲食勞倦所傷, 滿悶短氣, 不思食, 不知味, 時惡寒.

163

(5)本方加紗芩，神麴，名益胃升陽湯，治婦人經水不調，或脫血後食少水瀉.

(6)本方加黃柏，生地，名補中益氣加黃柏生地湯，治陰火乘陽，發熱晝甚，自汗短氣，口渴無味.

(7)本方加白芍，細辛，川芎，蔓荊，名順氣和中湯，治清陽不升，頭痛惡風，脈弦微細.

(8)本方加羌活，防風，細辛，川芎，名調榮養衛湯，治勞倦傷寒，身痛，體熱，惡寒，微渴，汗出，身痛，脈浮無力.

·來源：東垣

2. Wu Yao Shun Qi San. Lindera Powder to Smooth the Flow of Qi. 烏藥順氣散

·**ACTIONS**：soothes qi and eliminates wind

·**COMPOSITION**：Wu Yao, Ju Hong, Ma Huang, Chuan Xiong, Bai Zhi, Jie Geng Zhi Ke, Bai Jiang Can, Gan Jiang, Gan Cao, Sheng Jiang, Cong Bai

·**INDICATIONS**：treats stroke with generalized numbness, pain in the bone and joints, difficulty to walk, sluggish speech, deviated eye and mouth, rapid breathing with phlegm in the throat.

·**MODIFICATIONS**：(1) for vacuity sweating, eliminate Ma Huang and add Huang Qi.

(2) for inability to raise and move the hand and foot, add Fang Feng, Xu Duan, and Wei Ling Xian.

(3) for stiffness and tension in the limbs, add Mu Gua.

(4) for leg qi, add Niu Xi, Wu Jia Pi, Du Huo.

·**CHANNELS ENTERED**：The hand greater yin and foot reverting yin channels.

·**Analysis of Formula**：(1) When wind is exuberant, fire is intense, therefore phlegm fire surges and counterfolw upward, this is the counterflow of interior qi of the viscera and bowels. But wind strike occurs owing to external contraction to wind cold, when the interior is vacuous, exterior evil exploits this, this is the counterflow of exterior qi.

(2)① Wu Yao can free and move all kinds of stagnated evil.

② Jiang Can clears, transforms, and disperses binds.

③ Chuan Xiong and Bai Zhi are the medicinal for head and face, disperses wind and activates blood. Zhi Ke and Jie Geng disinhibit qi and move

164

phlegm.

④ Hei Jiang (blast fried ginger) warms channels and f rees yang. Gan Cao harmonizes the middle and drains fire.

⑤ Ma Huang and Jie Geng belong to the medicinal fo r the lung, promote sweating and eliminate cold.

(3) This formula first resolves exterior qi and then soothes interi or qi. When qi soothes, wind gets to disperse.

(4) Stroke owing to wind evil should first treat the tip, but if the qi is vacuous and the disease has lasted for long time, this treating of tip first is not appropriate.

·**Original Source**：Yan Yong He

2. 烏藥順氣散

·總結：順氣祛風

·組成：麻黃，陳皮，烏藥，川芎，白芷，白僵蠶，枳殼，桔梗，乾薑，甘草

·主治：治中風遍身頑麻，骨節疼痛，步履艱難，語言謇澀，口眼喎邪，喉中氣急有痰.

·加減：(1)虛汗者，去麻黃，加黃耆.

(2)手足不能舉動，加防風，續斷，威靈仙.

(3)拘攣，加木瓜.

(4)腳氣，加牛膝，五加皮，獨活.

·歸經：手太陰足厥陰藥也

·方義：(1)風盛則火熾，故有痰火衝逆而上，此裡氣逆也. 然中風必由外感風寒而發，內虛而外邪乘之，此表氣逆也.

(2)①烏藥能通行邪滯諸氣.

②殭蠶清化散結.

③川芎，白芷，頭面之藥，散風而活血. 枳，桔利氣行痰.

④黑薑溫經通陽. 甘草和中瀉火.

⑤麻黃，桔梗，肺家之藥，發汗而祛寒.

(3)此乃先解表氣而兼順裡氣者，氣順則風散.

(4)風邪卒中，當先治標，若氣虛病久者，非所宜也.

·來源：嚴用和

3. Su Zi Jiang Qi Tang. Perilla Fruit Decoction for Directing Qi Downward. 蘇子降氣湯

·**ACTIONS**：descends qi

·**COMPOSITION**： Su Zi, Ban Xia, Qian Hu, Hou Po, Chen Pi, Dang Gui, Sheng Jiang, Zhen Xiang, Gan Cao, Da Zao, Rou Gui.

·**INDICATIONS**：treats vacuity yang attacking the upper part, qi failing to ascend and descend, exuberance in the upper part and vacuity in the lower part, phlegm-drool congestion with panting and cough, vomiting of blood, or constipation. .

·**CHANNELS ENTERED**：The hand greater yang channel.

·**Analysis of Formula**：(1) Su Zi, Qian Hu, Hou Po, Ju Hong, and Ban Xia, ; they can descend counterfolw qi, and also eliminate phlegm. When qi moves, phlegm moves.

A few herbs in this formula also can effuse exterior, this formula courses internal congestion and disperses external cold.

(2) Dang Gui moistens and harmonizes blood.

(3) Gan Cao moderates the middle with the sweet.

(4) The lower part is vacuous and the upper part is exuberant, therefore Rou Gui is used to return fire to the origin.

·**Another Side Formula**：in another formula there is Chen Xiang without Rou Gui.

·**Original Source**：Ju Fang

3. 蘇子降氣湯

·總結：降氣

·組成：紫蘇子, 前胡, 半夏, 厚朴, 陳皮, 生薑, 枕香, 當歸, 甘草, 大棗

·主治：治虛陽上攻, 氣不升降, 上盛下虛, 痰涎壅盛, 喘嗽嘔血, 或大便不利.

·歸經：手太陽藥也

·方義：(1)蘇子, 前胡, 厚朴, 橘紅, 半夏, 皆能降逆下之氣, 兼能除痰, 氣行則痰行也. 數藥亦能發表, 既以疏內壅, 兼以散外寒也.

(2)當歸潤以和血.

(3)甘草甘以緩中.

(4)下虛上盛, 故又用桂引火歸元也.

·又附方：一方無桂, 有沈香.

·煎服法：加薑煎.

·來源：局方

4. Mu Xiang Shun Qi Tang. Aucklandia Decoction to Smooth the Flow of Qi. 木香順氣湯

·**ACTIONS**：regulates the middle and soothes qi

·**COMPOSITION**：Mu Xiang, Qing Pi, Chen Pi, Hou Po, Dang Gui, Cao Dou Kou, Yi Zhi Ren, Cang Zhu, Ban Xia, Wu Zhu Yu, Gan Jiang, Fu Ling, Ze Xie, Sheng Ma, Chai Hu

·**INDICATIONS**：treats abdominal and thoracic congestion and stagnation, qi failing to diffuse and free, glomus and oppression in the chest and diaphragm, distention and fullness in the abdomen and rib-side, and constipation.

·**CHANNELS ENTERED**：The foot greater yang and yang brightness channels

·**Analysis of Formula**：(1) ① Mu Xiang, Hou Po, Qing Pi, and Chen Pi are pungent, they can move qi and pacify the liver.

② The aroma of Cao Dou Kou and Yi Zhi Ren can soothe the spleen.

③ The dry of Cang Zhu and Ban Xia overcome damp.

④ The warm of Gan Jiang and Wu Zhu Yu can disperse cold.

⑤ The bland of Fu Ling and Ze Xie drain the yin.

⑥ The lightness of Sheng Ma and Chai Hu raise yang.

(2) Generally the spleen is central pivot, when the central pivot moves, clear qi raises and turbid qi descends, the upper and lower diffuse and free, yin and yang can take right position. When using Qi Medicinal, it is worry for them to cause dryness too much, therefore Dang Gui is used to moisten blood, and there is the effect of boosting the spleen and dispersing distention.

·**Original Source**：Li Dong Yuan

4. 木香順氣湯

·總結：調中順氣

·組成：木香, 青皮, 陳皮, 厚朴, 當歸, 草蔻仁, 益智, 蒼朮, 半夏, 吳茱萸, 乾薑, 茯苓, 澤瀉, 升麻, 柴胡

167

·主治：治陰陽壅滯，氣不宣通，胸膈痞悶，腹脇脹滿，大便不利．
·歸經：足太陽陽明藥也
·方義：(1)①木香，厚朴，青皮，陳皮，辛能行氣，兼能平肝．
　　　　②草蔻，益智，香能舒脾．
　　　　③蒼朮，半夏，燥能勝溼．
　　　　④乾薑，吳茱，溫能散寒．
　　　　⑤苓，瀉之淡，以泄其陰．
　　　　⑥升，柴之輕，以升其陽．

　　　(2)蓋脾爲中樞，使中樞運轉，則清升濁降，上下宣通，而陰陽得位矣．然皆氣藥，恐其過燥，故重用當歸以濡其血，共成益脾消脹之功也．
·來源：東垣

5. Si Mo Tang. Four Milled-Herbs Decoction. 四磨湯

·**ACTIONS**：seven emotions with qi counterfolw.

·**COMPOSITION**：Wu Yao, Ren Shen, Chen Xiang, Bing Lang

·**INDICATIONS**：treats seven emotions with qi counterfolw, dyspnea, panting, fullness and oppression in the chest with interrupting to eat.

·**CHANNELS ENTERED**：The hand greater yin channel.

·**Analysis of Formula**：(1) Qi in the upper part abnormally should descend, therefore Bing Lang and Chen Xiang are used.

　　　　(2) Counterfolw qi should soothe, therefore Wu Yao is used.

　　　　(3) Ren Shen is added to raise during descending, supplement during draining, and in order not to damage qi.

　　　　(4) for one with great replete pattern, Zhi Ke is used.

·Another Side Formula：(1) in another formula, Ren Shen is exchanged to Zhi Ke.

　　　　(2) in another formula, Ren Shen is eliminated and Zhi Shi and Mu Xiang are added, this is called Wu Ma Yin Zi, treats sudden stroke with sudden angry, this is called 'qi reverting'.

·**Original Source**：Yan Shi

5. 四磨湯
·總結：七情氣逆

·組成：烏藥, 人參, 沈香, 檳榔

·主治：治七情氣逆, 上氣喘急, 妨悶不食.

·歸經：手太陰藥也

·方義：(1)氣上宜降之, 故用檳榔, 沈香.

(2)氣逆宜順之, 故用烏藥.

(3)加人參者, 降中有升, 瀉中帶補, 恐傷其氣也.

(4)大實者, 仍宜枳殼.

·又附方：(1)一方人參易枳殼.

(2)一方去人參, 加枳實, 木香, 白酒磨服, 名五磨飲子. 治暴
怒卒死, 名曰氣厥.

·來源：嚴氏

6. Yue Ju Wan. Escape Restraint Pill. 越鞠丸

·**ACTIONS**：six depressions

·**COMPOSITION**：Xiang Fu, Cang Zhu, Chuan Xiong, Shan Zhi Zi, Shen Qu

·**INDICATIONS**：treats six depressions, glomus and oppression in the chest and diaphragm, acid regurgitation, vomiting, and indigestion of food.

·**MODIFICATIONS**：(1) for damp depression, add Fu Ling and Bai Zhi.

(2) for fire depression, add Qing Dai.

(3) for phlegm depression, add Nan Xing, Ban Xia, Gua Lou, Hai Shi.

(4) for blood depression, add Tao Ren, Hong Hua.

(5) for qi depression, add Mu Xiang, Bing Lang.

(6) for food depression, add Mai Ya, Shan Zha, Sha Ren.

(7) for being complicated with cold, add Wu Zhu Yu.

(8) in spring, add Fang Feng.

(9) in summer, add Ku Shen.

(10) in winter, add Wu Zhu Yu.

·**CHANNELS ENTERED**：The hand and foot greater yin and the hand lesser yang channels.

·**Analysis of Formula**：(1) Chuan Xiong regulates blood depression, Xiang Fu opens qi depression, Cang Zhu dries damp depression, Zhi Zi resolves fire depression, and Shen Qu disperses food depression.

169

(2) Chen Lai Zhang says that this rectifies qi. When qi is uninhib ited, depression gets to soothe.

·**Original Source**：Dan Xi

6. 越鞠丸
·總結：六鬱
·組成：香附, 蒼朮, 川芎, 山梔子, 神麴
·主治：統治六鬱胸膈痞悶, 吞酸嘔吐, 飲食不消.
·加減：(1)如溼鬱加茯苓, 白芷.
　　　　(2)火鬱加青黛.
　　　　(3)痰鬱加南星, 半夏, 栝蔞, 海石.
　　　　(4)血鬱加桃仁, 紅花.
　　　　(5)氣鬱加木香, 檳榔.
　　　　(6)食鬱加麥芽, 山查, 砂仁.
　　　　(7)挾寒加吳茱萸.
　　　　(8)又或春加防風.
　　　　(9)夏加苦參.
　　　　(10)冬加吳茱萸.
·歸經：手足太陰手少陽藥也
·方義：(1) 撫芎調血鬱, 香附開氣鬱, 蒼朮燥溼鬱, 梔子解火鬱, 神麴消食鬱.」
　　　　(2)陳來章曰：「皆理氣也, 氣暢而鬱舒矣.」
·來源：丹溪

7. Qi Qi Tang. Seven-Qi Decoction. 七氣湯

·**ACTIONS**：moves qi and disperses phlegm

·**COMPOSITION**：Fu Ling, Zi Su Ye, Hou Po, Ban Xia

·**INDICATIONS**：(1) treats qi depression of seven emotions, binding of p hlegm with difficulty to spit and swallow, thoracic fullness, and panting.

(2) or cough, or retching, or surging pain.

·**CHANNELS ENTERED**：The hand and foot greater yin channels

·**Analysis of Formula**：(1) When qi is depressed, phlegm is accumulated, first one should move qi and transform phlegm.

(2)① Fu Ling is sweet and bland, drains damp, boosts the spleen,

170

and makes the heart and kidney interact.

       ② Zi Su Ye is pungent and warm, soothes the middle, disinhibits the lung, calms panting, and disperses phlegm.

       ③ Hou Po is bitter and warm, descends qi and disperses fullness.

       ④ Ban Xia is pungent and warm, eliminates phlegm and opens depression.

       (3) When phlegm is eliminated and qi moves, binds get to disperse and depression gets to resolve, and then all kinds of pattern gets calm.

·**RELATED FORMULA**：When Bai Shao Yao, Chen Pi, Ren Shen, and Gui Xin are added, this is also called Qi Qi Tang, treats depression and binds of seven emotions, irregularities of yin and yang, alternation vomiting and diarrhea, aversion to cold, heat effusion, dizziness, glomus and fullness in the chest and diaphragm, and inhibited digestion.

7. 七氣湯
  ·總結：行氣消痰
  ·組成：茯苓, 紫蘇, 厚朴, 半夏
  ·主治：(1)治七清氣鬱, 痰涎結聚, 咯不出, 嚥不下, 胸滿喘急.
       (2)或欬或嘔, 或攻衝作痛.
  ·歸經：手足太陰藥也
  ·方義：(1)氣鬱則痰聚, 故散鬱必以行氣化痰爲先.
       (2)①茯苓甘淡滲溼, 益脾通心交腎.
         ②紫蘇辛溫, 寬中暢肺, 定喘消痰.
         ③厚朴苦溫, 降氣散滿.
         ④半夏辛溫, 除痰開鬱.
       (3)痰去氣行, 則結散鬱解, 而諸證平矣.
  ·變化方：本方加白芍, 陳皮, 人參, 桂心, 亦名七氣湯, 治七情鬱結, 陰陽反戾, 吐利交作, 寒熱眩運, 痞滿噎塞.

8. Si Qi Tang. Four-Seven Decoction. 四七湯

·**ACTIONS**：warms the middle and resolves depression
·**COMPOSITION**：Rou Gui, Ren Shen, Ban Xia, Gan Cao
·**INDICATIONS**：treats Seven emotions with qi depression, accumulated phlegm, vacuous cold, dyspnea, or gripping pain in the heart and abdomen, ext

ension and distention in the chest and epigastric region, and panting.

·**CHANNELS ENTERED**：The hand greater yin channel

·**Analysis of Formula**：Li Shi Cai says that excessive seven emotions gen erally damage the qi. Dan Xi controls this disease with Yue Yue Ju Wan, but th is formula is different with Dan Xi's. Generally enduring depression gets to blo ck turbid qi and clear qi becomes weak, therefore even though there is pain and distension, Mu Xiang and Zhi Ke are not used but Ren Shen is used to invigora te the organ [lung] which governs qi. Rou Gui is used to restrain the depression of strategies [liver]. Enduring depression generates phlegm, Ban Xia expels it. Depression causes disharmony of the organs, therefore Gan Cao is used to regu late them. Rou Gui is pungent and warm, courses qi quickly. Therefore depressi on is eliminated and recover occurs. In the name of this formula, Si Qi means t hat seven emotions are treated with four flavors.

8. 四七湯

·總結：溫中解鬱

·組成：官桂, 人參, 半夏, 甘草

·主治：治七清氣鬱, 痰涎結聚, 虛冷上氣, 或心腹絞痛, 或膨脹喘急.

·歸經：手太陰藥也

·方義： 李士材曰：「夫七情過極, 皆傷其氣. 丹溪以越鞠丸主之, 而此獨異者, 蓋鬱久則濁氣閉塞, 而清氣日薄矣. 故雖痛雖膨, 而不用木 香, 枳殼, 用人參以壯主氣之臟. 官桂以制謀慮之鬱. 鬱久生痰, 半夏爲之 驅逐. 鬱故不和, 國老爲之調停. 況桂性辛溫, 疏氣甚捷, 鬱結者還爲和暢 矣. 湯名四七者, 以四味治七情也.」

9. Xuan Fu Dai Zhe Shi Tang. Inula and Hematite Decoctio n. 旋覆代赭石湯

·**ACTIONS**：hard glomus below the heart, belching

·**COMPOSITION**：Xuan Fu Hua, Dai Zhe Shi, Ren Shen, Gan Cao, Da Zao, Ban Xia, Sheng Jiang

·**INDICATIONS**：treats that when in cold damage, sweating is promoted or vomiting or precipitation is used and after resolution of the exterior disease, t here is a hard glomus below the heart and belching that is not eliminated,

·**CHANNELS ENTERED**：The foot yang brightness channel.

·**Analysis of Formula**：Cheng Wu Ji says that ：(1) timidity causes qi to float. The heaviness of Dai Zhe Shi settles vacuous counterfolw.

172

(2) Hard glomus makes qi hard, the salty of Xuan Fu Hua softens hard glomus.

(3) Pungent flavor can disperse. The pungent of Sheng Jiang disperses vacuous glomus.

(4) Sweet flavor can moderate. The sweet of Ren Shen, Gan Cao, and Da Zao supplements weak stomach.

·**Original Source**：Zhong Jing

9. 旋覆代赭石湯
　·總結：痞鞕噫氣
　·組成：旋覆花, 代赭石, 人參, 甘草, 大棗, 半夏, 生薑
　·主治：治傷寒發汗, 若吐若下, 解後心下痞硬, 噫氣不除.
　·歸經：足陽明藥也
　·方義：成氏曰：(1)怯則氣浮, 代赭之重以鎮虛逆.
　　　　　(2)硬則氣堅, 施覆之鹹以輭痞硬.
　　　　　(3)辛者散也, 生薑之辛以散虛痞.
　　　　　(4)甘者緩也, 人參, 甘草, 大棗之甘, 以補胃弱.
　·來源：仲景

10. Ding Xiang Shi Di Tang. Clove and Persimmon Calyx Decoction. 丁香柿蒂湯

·**ACTIONS**：hiccup

·**COMPOSITION**：Ding Xiang, Shi Di, Ren Shen, Sheng Jiang

·**INDICATIONS**：treats enduring hiccup which occurs due to cold.

·**CHANNELS ENTERED**：The foot yang brightness and lesser yin channels

·**Analysis of Formula**：(1) Ding Xiang drains the lung and warms the stomach and kidney.

(2) The bitter and astringent of Shi Di descends qi.

(3) Ren Shen supplements the true qi.

(4) Sheng Jiang eliminates phlegm, opens depression, and disperses cold.

(5) This is also used to hiccup due to fire.

·**RELATED FORMULA**：(1) When Ren Shen and Sheng Jiang are elimi

173

nated, this is also called Ding Xiang Shi Di Tang, treats same things with above.

(2) When Ren Shen and Sheng Jiang are eliminated and Zhu Ru and Ju Hong are added, this is called Ding Xiang Shi Di Zhu Ru Tang and also called Ju Hong Zhu Ru Tang.

(3) In Wei Sheng Bao Jian, Ren Shen is eliminated and Qing Pi and Chen Pi are added.；In San Yin Fang, Ren Shen is eliminated and Liang Jiang and Gan Cao are added, this is called Ding Xiang San, treats same thing.

·**Original Source**：Yan Shi

10. 丁香柿蒂湯
　　·總結：呃逆
　　·組成：丁香，柿蒂，人參，生薑
　　·主治：治久病呃逆，因于寒者.
　　·歸經：足陽明少陰藥也
　　·方義：⑴丁香泄肺溫胃而暖腎.
　　　　　　⑵柿蒂苦澀而降氣.
　　　　　　⑶人參所以輔眞氣，使得展布.
　　　　　　⑷生薑去痰開鬱而散寒.
　　　　　　⑸火呃亦可用者，蓋從治之法也.
　　·變化方：⑴本方除人參，生薑，亦名丁香柿蒂湯，治同.
　　　　　　⑵本方除人參，生薑，加竹茹，橘紅，名丁香柿蒂竹茹湯，又名橘紅竹茹湯.
　　　　　　⑶寶鑑去人參，加青皮，陳皮；三因去人參，加良薑，甘草，名丁香散. 治同.
　　·來源：嚴氏

11. Ju Pi Zhu Ru Tang. Tangerine Peel and Bamboo Shaving Decoction. 橘皮竹茹湯

·**ACTIONS**：retching and hiccup

·**COMPOSITION**：Ban Xia, Ju Pi, Pi Pa Ye, Mai Men Dong, Zhu Ru, Chi Fu Ling, Ren Shen, Gan Cao

·**INDICATIONS**：(1) treats enduring disease, emaciation, and incessant retching.

(2) also treats hiccup due to stomach vacuity after vomiting and

diarrhea.

·**MODIFICATIONS**：(1) for stomach cold, eliminate Zhu Ru and Mai M
en Dong and add Ding Xiang.

(2) for replete fire, eliminate Ren Shen.

·**CHANNELS ENTERED**：The foot yang brightness channel.

·**Analysis of Formula**：When stomach fire surges upward, the fire of the
liver and gall bladder assists the stomach fire, then the metal qi of the lung cann
ot descend, therefore retching occurs.

(1) Er Chen Tang disperses counterfolw qi.

(2) Zhu Ru, Pi Pa Ye, and Mai Men Dong can clear the lung and
harmonize the stomach. When lung metal is clear, liver qi also gets calm.

(3) Chi Fu Ling descends heart fire.

(4) Sheng Jiang is holy medicinal for retching domain.

(5) for enduring disease and emaciation, therefore Ren Shen, Ga
n Cao, and Da Zao are used to supports stomach qi.

·Another Side Formula：in Jin Gui Yao Lue, Ju Pi Zhu Ru Tang, ：Ju Pi,
Zhu Ru, Ren Shen, Gan Cao, Sheng Jiang, and Da Zao, ; treats retching.

11. 橘皮竹茹湯

·總結：嘔逆呃逆

·組成：半夏, 橘皮, 枇杷葉, 麥冬, 竹茹, 赤茯苓, 人參, 甘草

·主治：(1)治久病虛贏, 嘔逆不已.

(2)亦治吐利後胃虛呃逆.

·加減：(1)胃寒者, 去竹茹, 麥冬, 加丁香.

(2)實火去人參.

·歸經：足陽明藥也

·方義：胃火上衝, 肝膽之火助之, 肺金之氣不得下降, 故嘔.

(1)二陳所以散逆氣.

(2)竹茹, 枇杷葉, 麥門冬, 皆能清肺而和胃, 肺金清則肝氣
亦平矣.

(3)赤茯苓所以降心火.

(4)生薑嘔家之聖藥.

(5)久病虛贏, 故以人參, 甘草, 大棗, 扶其胃氣也.

·又附方：金匱橘皮竹茹湯：橘皮, 竹茹, 人參, 甘草, 生薑, 大棗 治
噦逆.

175

12. Ding Chuan Tang. Arrest Wheezing Decoction. 定喘湯

·**ACTIONS**：wheezing and panting

·**COMPOSITION**：Ma Huang, Xing Ren, Sang Bai Pi, Huang Qin, Ban Xia, Su Zi, Kuan Dong Hua, Bai Guo, Gan Cao

·**INDICATIONS**：treats lung vacuity with contracting to cold, qi counter folw with heat in the diaphragm, wheezing and panting.

·**CHANNELS ENTERED**：The hand greater yin channel.

·**Analysis of Formula**：(1) Exterior cold should be treated with dispersing, ：Gan Cao, Ma Huang, Sang Pi, and Xing Ren are pungent and sweet, they dis perse, drain the lung, and resolve the exterior.

(2) Interior vacuity should be treated with constraining.

① Kuan Dong Hua is warm and moisture.

② Bai Guo is astringent medicinal, stabilizes panting and clears metal.

③ Huang Qin clears lung heat.

④ Su Zi descends lung qi.

⑤ Ban Xia dries damp and phlegm.

12. 定喘湯

·總結：哮喘

·組成：麻黃, 杏仁, 桑白皮, 黃芩, 半夏, 蘇子, 款冬花, 白果, 甘草

·主治：治肺虛感寒, 氣逆膈熱而作哮喘.

·歸經：手太陰藥也

·方義：(1)表寒宜散：甘草, 麻黃, 桑皮, 杏仁, 辛甘發散瀉肺而解表.

(2)裡虛宜斂：

①款冬溫潤.

②白果收濇定喘而清金.

③黃芩清肺熱.

④蘇子降肺氣.

⑤半夏燥溼痰.

Chapter 8. Blood-Rectifying Formulas. 理血之劑

1. Si Wu Tang. Four-Substance Decoction. 四物湯

·**ACTIONS**：nourishes blood

·**COMPOSITION**：Dang Gui, sheng Di Huang, Shao Yao, Chuan Xiong.

·**INDICATIONS**：treats all kinds of vacuous blood and menstrual disease.

·**MODIFICATIONS**：(1) Generally blood pattern is usually treated with Si Wu Tang.

(2) To cool blood： for the heart, add Huang Lian, for the liver, add Huang Qin, for the lung, add Huang Qin, for replete large intestine, add Huang Qin, for the gall bladder, add Huang Lian, ; for the kidney and bladder, add Huang Bai, for the spleen, add Sheng Di Huang, ;for the stomach, add Da Huang, for triple burner, add Di Gu Pi, for the pericardium, add Mu Dan Pi, for the small intestine, add Shan Zhi Zi and Mu Tong.

(3) To clear qi： for the heart and pericardium, add Mai Men Dong, for the lung, add Zhi Ke, for the liver, add Chai Hu and Qing Pi, for the spleen, add Bai Shao Yao, for the stomach, add Ge Gen (dry) and Shi Gao, for the large intestine and triple burner, add Lian Qiao, for the small intestine, add Chi Fu Ling, for the bladder, add Hua Shi and Hu Po.

(4) For blood vacuity, add Gui Ban. For dry blood, add breast milk. For static blood, add Tao Ren, Hong Hua, Fei Zhi, and child's urine to move it. For static blood due to violence, add Bo He and Xuan Shen to disperse it. For incessant bleeding, add Pu Huang and Jing Mo. For enduring incessant bleeding, add Sheng Ma to induce blood to return channel.

(5) When the menstrual color is purple with black, and the pulse is rapid, this means heat, add Huang Lian and Huang Qin. When the color is pale and the pulse is slow, this means cold, add Rou Gui and Fu Zi.

(6) For obese person with phlegm, add Ban Xia, Nan Xing, Ju Hong. For thin person with fire, add Zhi Zi, Zhi Mu, and Huang Bai.

(7) For depression, add Mu Xiang, Sha Ren, Cang Zhu, and Shen Qu. For stasis stagnation, add Tao Ren, Hong Hua, Yan Hu Suo, and Rou Gui.

(8) For qi vacuity, add Ren Shen and Huang Qi. For qi repletion, add Hou Po and Zhi Shi.

·**CHANNELS ENTERED**：The hand lesser yin, the foot greater yin and reverting yin channels [The heart, spleen, and liver]

177

·**Analysis of Formula** ：(1) Dang Gui is pungent, bitter, sweet, and warm. It e nters the heart and spleen to engender blood, acting as sovereign.

(2) Sheng Di Huang is sweet and cold. It enters the heart and kid ney to enrich blood, acting as minister.

(3) Shao Yao is sour and cold. It enters the liver and spleen to res train yin, acting as assistant.

(4) Chuan Xiong is pungent and warm. It frees the upper and low er part, moves qi in the middle of blood, acting as courier.

·**RELATED FORMULA** ：(1) When Huang Bai and Zhi Mu are added, t his is called Zhi Bai Si Wu Tang, again if Ren Shen is added, this is called Zi Y in Jiang Huo Tang, treats yin vacuity with fire.

(2) When Zhi Bia Si Wu Tang is made into pills with honey, this is called Kan Li Wan, treats cough with blood in yin vacuity

(3) When Huang Lian and Hu Huang Lian are added, this is call ed Er Lian Si Wu Tang, treats vacuous construction and blood, vexing heat in the chest, palms, and soles, heat entering blood chamber, and heat effusion at night.

(4) When Huang Bai, Huang Qin, and Gan Cao are added, this is called San Huang Si Wu Tang, treats yin vacuity with tidal heat effusion.

(5) When Sheng and Shu Di Huang are used and Huang Qi, Mu Dan Pi, Sheng Ma, and Chai Hu are added, this is called San Huang Bu Xue Ta ng, treats blood collapse and blood vacuity, and six pulses that are all large but are empty and vacuous when pressure is added.

(6) When Tao Ren and Hong Hua are added, this is called Yuan Rong Si Wu Tang, treats visceral bind, constipation, and static blood due to kn ocks and falls.

(7) When Qiang Huo and Fang Feng, this is called Zhi Feng Liu He Tang, treats wind vacuity with dizziness, wind contending with large intesti ne with difficult to defecate, when this is made into pill with Honey, this is call ed Bu Gan Wan.

(8) When Mu Xiang and Bing Lang are added, this is called Zhi Qi Liu He Tang, treats blood vacuity and qi stagnation, or surging upward of bl ood and qi.

(9) When Qiang Huo and Tian Ma are added and made into pills with Honey, this is called Shen Ying Yang Zhgen Dan, treats the foot reverting yin channel which contracts wind, cold, summerheat, and damp, paralysis, slug gish speech, and blood vacuity with leg qi.

(10) When Tao Ren, Hong Hua, Zhu Li, and Jiang Jiang Zhi (juic

e of ginger)are added, treats hemiplegia. Left side weakness belong to static blood.

  ⑾ When Bai Shao Yao is eliminated and Fang Feng are added, this is called Fang Feng Dang Gui San, treats excessive promotion of sweating causing convulsive disease. This should be treated with eliminating wind and nourishing blood.

  ⑿ When Di Huang is eliminated and Gan Jiang are added, this is called Si Shen Tang, treats blood vacuity of women and gripping pain in the heart and abdomen.

  ⒀ When E Jiao, Ai Ye, and Gan Cao are added, this is called Jiao Ai Tang, treats the vacuity and detriment of the thoroughfare and conception vessels, incessant dribble of menstruation, and blood vacuity with diarrhea.

  ⒁ When Ai Ye and Si Zhi Xiang Fu are added and made into pills with vinegar, this is called Ai Fu Wen Gong Wan, treats vacuous cold of uterus, and when E Jiao is added again, this is called Fu Ren Chan Yu Bao Qing Ji Dan, treats vacuous cold and irregularities of menstruation.

  ⒂ When Mu Dan Pi and Di Gu Pi are added, treats steaming bone in woman.

  ⒃ When Shao Yao and Di Huang are eliminated, this is called Xiong Gui Tang, this is called Fo Shou San, also called Qi Qi San, also called Jun Chen San, treats headache due to blood vacuity after childbirth, threatened abortion with bleeding from uterus, taking this brings about spontaneous recover.

  ⒄ When Si Jun Zi Tang is combined, this is called Ba Zhen Tang, treats vacuity and detriment of the heart and lung, both qi and blood vacuity. When Huang Qi and Rou Gui are added again, this is called Shi Quan Da Bu Tang, this assists yang and secures Defense.

  ⒅ When Bai Shao Yao is eliminated and Shan Zhu Yu, Wu Wei Zi, Fang Feng, Rou Cong Rong, Sheng Jiang and Da Zao are added to Shi Quan Da Bu Tang, this is called Da Bu Huang QiTang, treats both qi and blood vacuity, incessant spontaneous sweating, and reversal by yang vacuity.

  ⒆ The combination of Si Wu Tang and Si Jun Tang with Xiao Chai Hu, this is called San He San, treats enduring vacuous taxation after childbirth.

1. 四物湯
 ·總結：養血
 ·組成：當歸, 生地黃, 芍藥, 芎窮

179

·主治：治一切血虛，及婦人經病.

·加減：(1)凡血證通宜四物湯.

(2)如涼血：心加黃連，肝條芩，肺枯芩，大腸實，芩，膽黃連，腎膀胱黃柏，脾生地，胃大黃，三焦地骨皮，心包絡丹皮，小腸山梔，木通.

(3)如清氣：心與包絡加麥冬，肺枳殼，肝柴胡，青皮，脾白芍，胃乾葛，石膏，大腸三焦，連翹，小腸赤茯苓，膀胱滑石，琥珀.

(4)血虛加龜板. 血燥加人乳. 瘀血加桃仁，紅花，菲汁，童便行之. 暴血加薄荷，玄參散之. 血不止加炒蒲黃，京墨. 久不止加升麻，引血歸經.

(5)婦人經血紫黑，脈數爲熱，加芩，連；血淡，脈遲爲寒，加桂，附.

(6)人肥有痰，加半夏，南星，橘紅. 人瘦有火，加黑梔，知母，黃柏.

(7)鬱者加木香，砂仁，蒼朮，神麴. 瘀滯加桃仁，紅花，延胡，肉桂.

(8)氣虛加參，耆. 氣實加枳，朴.

·歸經：手少陰足太陰厥陰藥也

·方義：(1)當歸辛苦甘溫，入心脾生血爲君.

(2)生地甘寒，入心腎滋血篇爲臣.

(3)芍藥酸寒，入肝脾斂陰爲佐.

(4)芎窮辛溫，通上下而行血中之氣爲使也.

·變化方：(1)本次加黃柏，知母，名知栢四物湯；再加亦參，名滋陰降火湯，治陰虛有火.

(2)知蘗四物蜜丸，名坎離丸，治陰虛嗽血.

(3)本方加黃連，胡黃連，名二連四物湯，治虛榮血虛，五心煩熱，熱入血室，夜分發熱.

(4)本方加黃柏，黃芩，甘草，名三黃四物湯，治陰虛潮熱.

(5)本方用生熟二地，加黃耆，丹皮，升麻，柴胡，名三黃補血湯，治七血血虛，六脈俱大，按之空虛.

(6)本方加桃仁，紅花，名元戎四物湯，治臟結便秘，撲損瘀血.

(7)本方加羌活，防風，名治風六合湯，治風虛眩運，風秘便難. 蜜丸，名補肝丸.

(8)本方加木香，檳榔，名治氣六合湯，治血虛氣滯，或血氣上衝.

(9)本方加羌活，天麻，蜜丸，名神應養眞丹，治足厥陰經受風寒暑溼，癱瘓不遂，語言蹇澀，及血虛脚氣.

(10)本方加桃仁，紅花，竹瀝，薑汁，治半身不遂，在左者屬瘀血.

(11)本方去白芍，加防風，名防風當歸散，治發汗過多而成痙證，宜去風養血.

(12)本方去地黃，加乾薑，名四神湯，治婦人血虛，心腹絞痛.

(13)本方加阿膠，艾葉，甘草，名膠艾湯，治衝任虛損，經水淋瀝，及血虛下痢.

(14)本方加艾葉，四製香附，醋丸，名艾附暖宮丸，治子宮虛冷，再加阿膠，名婦寶丹，治虛寒經水不調.

(15)本方加丹皮，地骨，治婦人骨蒸.

(16)本方除芍藥，地黃，名芎歸湯；爲末名佛手散，又名一奇散，又名君臣散. 治產後血虛頭痛，胎動下血，服此自愈.

(17)本方合四君子，名八珍湯，治心肺虛損，氣血兩虛. 再加黃耆，肉桂，名十全大補湯，兼助陽固衞.

(18)十全湯去白芍，加上茱，五味，防風，蓯蓉，入薑，棗煎，名大補黃耆湯，治氣血兩虛，自汗不止，及陽虛發厥.

(19)四物，四君合小柴胡，名三合散，治產後日久虛勞.

2. Dang Gui Bu Xue Tang. Tangkuei Decoction to Tonify the Blood. 當歸補血湯

·**ACTIONS**：supplements blood

·**COMPOSITION**：Huang Qi (one Liang), Dang Gui (two qian)

·**INDICATIONS**：treats damage to taxation, flesh heat, reddish complexion, vexation and thirst with desire to drink water, a pulse that is large and vacuous.

·**CHANNELS ENTERED**：The foot greater yin and reverting yin channels.

·**Analysis of Formula**：(1) both qi and flavor of Dang Gui are thick and this belong to yin in the middle of yin, therefore this can nourish yin and blood. Huang Qi is the medicinal to supplement qi. In this formula, Huang qi is five times more than Dang Gui, how does it call Bu Xue Tang? Generally blood, which is tangible, engenders from qi which is intangible, and also Dang Gui conducts the other herbs to the blood part, then following the character, blood engenders. Nei Jing says that when

181

yang engenders, yin grows,

·**Original Source**：Li Dong Yuan

2. 當歸補血湯

·總結：補血

·組成：黃耆, 當歸

·主治：治傷於勞役, 肌熱面赤, 煩渴引飲, 脈大而虛.

·歸經：此足太陰厥陰藥也.

·方義：(1)當歸氣味俱厚, 爲陰中之陰, 故能滋陰養血. 黃耆乃補氣之藥, 何以五倍於當歸, 而又云補血湯乎?蓋有形之血, 生於無形之氣, 又有當歸爲引, 則從之而生血矣. 經曰：「陽生則陰長.」此其義耳.

·來源：東垣

3. Gui Pi Tang. Restore the Spleen Decoction. 歸脾湯

·**ACTIONS**： conducts blood to return to the spleen.

·**COMPOSITION**：Dang Gui, Mu Xiang, Gan Cao (mix fried), Bai Zhu, Ren Shen, Huang Qi, Fu Shen, Zao Ren, Long Yan Rou, Yuan Zhi

·**INDICATIONS**：(1) treats excessive thinking, taxation damaging the heart and spleen, fearful throbbing and forgetfulness, fright palpitations and night sweating, heat effusion and fatigue, reduced eating, and insomnia.

(2) or vacuous spleen is unable to control blood, this condition causes frenetic movement of blood, and menstrual and vaginal discharge disease. .

·**CHANNELS ENTERED**：The hand lesser yin and the foot greater yin channels.

·**Analysis of Formula**：(1) Dang Gui nourishes yin and tonifies blood.

(2) Mu Xiang moves qi and soothes the spleen. This moves stagnation in the blood, and assists Ren Shen and Huang Qi to supplement qi.

(3) When blood fails to return to the spleen, blood gets to move frenetically, the sweet and warm of Ren Shen and Bai Zhi, Huang Qi, and Gan Cao supplement the spleen.

(4) The sweet, warm, sour, and bitter of Fu Shen, Yuan Zhi, Zao Ren, and Long Yan Rou supplement the heart. The heart is the mother of the spleen.

(5) When qi is invigorate, this can control blood, blood spontaneously returns to the channels, and then every signs are eliminated.

3. 歸脾湯

　·總結：引血歸脾

　·組成：當歸，木香，炙甘草，白朮，人參，炙黃耆，茯神，棗仁，龍眼肉，遠志

　·主治：⑴治思慮過度，勞傷心脾，怔忡健忘，驚悸盜汗，發熱體倦，食少不眠.

　　　　⑵或脾虛不能攝血，致血妄行. 及婦人經帶.

　·歸經：此手少陰足太陰藥也.

　·方義：⑴當歸滋陰而養血.

　　　　⑵木香行氣而舒脾，既以行血中之滯，又以助參，耆而補氣.

　　　　⑶血不歸脾則妄行，參，朮，黃耆，甘草之甘溫，所以補脾.

　　　　⑷茯神，遠志，棗仁，龍眼之甘溫酸苦，所以補心，心者脾之母也.

　　　　⑸氣壯則能攝血，血自歸經，而諸證悉除矣.

　·來源：濟生

4. Yang Xin Tang. Nourish the Heart Decoction. 養心湯

·**ACTIONS**：supplements heart blood

·**COMPOSITION**：Rou Gui, Fu Shen, Yuan Zhi, Bai Zi Ren, Fu Ling, Suan Zao Ren, Chuan Xiong, Dang Gui, Ban Xia, Gan Cao (mix fried), Wu Wei Zi, Ren Shen, Huang Qi

·**INDICATIONS**：treats vacuous heart with scant blood, disquiet spirit qi, fearful throbbing and fright palpitations.

·**CHANNELS ENTERED**：The hand lesser yin channel.

·**Analysis of Formula**：⑴ Rou Gui conducts the other herbs to enter the heart channel.

　　　　⑵ Fu ling, Fu Shen, Yuan Zhi, Bai Zi Ren, and Suan Zao Ren drain heart heat and quiet heart spirit.

　　　　⑶ Chuan Xiong and Dang Gui nourish heart blood.

　　　　⑷ Ban Xia eliminates phlegm harassing the heart. Gan Cao supplements earth to bank up the son of the heart.

　　　　⑸ Wu Wei Zi contracts spirit qi which is dispersing.

183

(6) Ren Shen and Huang Qi supplement heart qi.

(7) nourishing by moistening, supplementing by warming, contracting by sour, and coursing by aroma can make the heart to be nourished.

4. 養心湯
  ·總結：補心血
  ·組成：肉桂，茯神，遠志，柏子仁，茯苓，酸棗仁，川芎，當歸，半夏麴，炙甘草，五味子，人參，黃耆
  ·主治：治心虛血少，神氣不寧，怔忡驚悸.
  ·歸經：此手少陰藥也.
  ·方義：(1)肉桂引藥以入心經.
        (2)二茯，遠志，柏仁，酸棗，以泄心熱而寧心神.
        (3)川芎，當歸以養心血.
        (4)半夏去擾心之痰涎. 甘草補土以培心子.
        (5)五味收神氣之散越.
        (6)人參，黃耆以補心氣.
        (7)潤以滋之，溫以補之，酸以斂之，香以舒之，則心得其養矣.

5. Ren Shen Yang Ying Tang. Ginseng Constrution-Nourishing Decoction. 人參養榮湯

·ACTIONS：nourishes construction

·INDICATIONS：(1) treats the qi vacuity of the spleen and lung, insufficient construction and blood, fright palpitations and forgetfulness, night sweating with heat effusion, reduced eating with inability to taste, generalized fatigue, desiccated complexion, short of breathing, loss of hair, inhibited voiding of reddish urine.

(2) also treats excessive promotion of sweating, quivering and trembling, jerking sinews and twitching flesh.

·COMPOSITION：Ren Shen, Bai Zhu, Fu Ling, Gan Cao, Chen Pi, Huang Qi, Dang Gui, Bai Shao Yao, Shu Di Huang, Wu Wei Zi, Gui Xin , Yuan Zhi

·CHANNELS ENTERED：The qi and blood of the hand lesser yin, and the hand and foot greater yin channels. [The heart, lung, and spleen]

·Analysis of Formula：(1) Shu Di Huang, Dang Gui, and Shao Yao tonif

184

y blood.

(2) Ren Shen, Huang Qi, Fu Ling, Bai Zhu, Gan Cao, and Chen Pi supplement qi. When blood is insufficient, supplement qi. This means that when yang generates, yin grows.

(3) Ren Shen, Huang Qi, and Wu Wei Zi supplement the lung.

(4) Gan Cao, Chen Pi, Fu ling, and Bai Zhu fortify the spleen.

(5) Dang Gui and Shao Yao nourish the liver.

(6) Shu Di Huang enriches the kidney.

(7) Yuan Zhi can free kidney qi to reach upward to the heart.

(8) Gui Xin can conduct the other herbs to enter construction to engender blood.

5. 人參養榮湯
·總結：養榮
·主治：(1)治脾肺氣虛，榮血不足，驚悸健忘，寢汗發熱，食少無味，身倦肌瘦，色枯氣短，毛髮脫落，小便赤澀.

(2)亦治發汗過多，身振振搖，筋惕肉瞤.

·組成：人參，白朮，茯苓，甘草，陳皮，黃耆，當歸，白芍，熟地黃，五味子，桂心 ，遠志
·歸經：此手少陰手足太陰氣血藥也.
·方義：(1)熟地, 歸, 芍, 養血之品.

(2)參, 耆, 苓, 朮, 甘草, 陳皮, 補氣之品, 血不足而補其氣, 此陽生則陰長之義.

(3)且參, 耆, 五味, 所以補肺.

(4)甘, 陳, 苓, 朮, 所以健脾.

(5)歸, 芍所以養肝.

(6)熟地所以滋腎.

(7)遠志能通腎氣上達於心.

(8)桂心能導諸藥入營生血.

6. Long Nao Ji Su Wan. 龍腦雞蘇丸

·ACTIONS：clears heat and rectifies blood.
·COMPOSITION：Ji Su Ye, Huang Qi, Ren Shen, Gan Cao, Yin Chai Hu, sheng Di Huang, Pu Huang, Mu Tong, Mai Men Dong, E Jiao

·**INDICATIONS**：(1) treats depression heat in the lung, cough, hematemesis, epistaxis, and bleeding from lower part.

(2) heat strangury, wasting-thirst, fetid mouth odor, bitter taste in the mouth, clearing the heart and improving vision.

·**CHANNELS ENTERED**：The hand and foot greater yin, and the lesser yang channels. [The lung, spleen, and gall bladder]

·**Analysis of Formula**：The lung originally clears and depurates qi, sometimes this lung takes the flame evil of heart and harmful hyperactivity of the liver, therefore all signs occur.

(1) Bo He is pungent, cool, and light, and has a dispersing action. This drains the lung and clears the liver, disperses heat and rectifies blood, therefore acting as sovereign.

(2) Ren Shen, Huang Qi, and Gan Cao drain fire and harmonize the spleen.

(3) Chai Hu pacifies the liver and resolves liver heat.

(4) Sheng Di Huang cools blood.

(5) Pu Huang (stir-bake) stanches bleeding.

(6) Mu Tong disinhibits water and descends heart fire.

(7) Mai Men Dong and E Jiao moisten dryness and clear the lung. This formula is to treat heat with vacuity, therefore Ren Shen and Huang Qi are used to supplement qi a little.

·Another Side Formula：in another formula, Huang Lian is added.

·**Original Source**：Ju Fang

6. 龍腦雞蘇丸
　·總結：清熱理血
　·組成：雞蘇葉，黃耆，人參，甘草，銀柴胡，生地黃，蒲黃，木通，麥冬，阿膠
　·主治：(1)治肺有鬱熱，咳嗽吐血，衄血下血.
　　　　　(2)熱淋消渴，口臭口苦，清心明目.
　·歸經：此手足太陰少陽藥也.
　·方義：肺本清肅，或受心之邪燄，或受肝之亢害，故見諸證.
　　　　　(1)薄荷辛涼輕揚升發，瀉肺搜肝，散熱理血，故以爲君.
　　　　　(2)參，耆，甘草瀉火和脾.
　　　　　(3)柴胡平肝解肝熱.
　　　　　(4)生地黃涼血.

186

(5)炒蒲黃止血, 以療諸血.

(6)木通利水降心火.

(7)麥冬, 阿膠潤燥清肺. 此亦爲熱而涉虛者設, 故少佐參,
耆也.

·又附方：一方有黃連.

·來源：局方

7. Ke Xue Fang. Coughing of Blood Formula. 欬血方

·**ACTIONS**：hemoptysis

·**COMPOSITION**：Qing Dai, Shan Zhi Zi, Gua Lou Ren, Hai Shi, He Zi Rou

·**INDICATIONS**：treats coughing phlegm and blood.

·**MODIFICATIONS**：for severe cough, add Xing Ren.

·**CHANNELS ENTERED**：The hand greater yin channel.

·**Analysis of Formula**：(1) The liver holds the office of general, liver fire flaming upward can scorch the heart and lung, therefore cough with phlegm and blood occurs.

(2) Qing Dai drains the liver and rectifies blood, and disperses the depressed fire of the five viscera. Zhi Zi cools the heart and clears the lung, and makes evil heat move downward. Qing Dai and Zhi Zi treat fire.

(3) Gua Lou moistens dryness and lubricates phlegm. This is a key medicinal to treat cough. Hai Shi softens hardness and checks cough, and clears the upper origin of water way. Gua Lou and Hai Shi descend fire and move phlegm.

(4) He Zi can restrain the lung and stabilize phlegm with panting. This formula has no herb for treating blood, when fire retreats, bleeding spontaneously stops.

·**Original Source**：Dan Xi

7. 欬血方

·總結：欬血

·組成：青黛, 山梔, 栝蔞仁, 海石, 訶子肉

·主治：治欬嗽痰血.

·加減：嗽甚加杏仁.

·歸經：此手太陰（肺）藥也.

187

·方義：(1)肝者將軍之官，肝火上逆，能爍心肺，故欬嗽痰血也.

　　　　　(2)青黛瀉肝而理血，散五臟鬱火；梔子涼心而清肺，使邪熱
下行；二者所以治火.

　　　　　(3)栝蔞潤燥滑痰，爲治嗽要藥；海石頓堅止嗽，清水之上源
；二者降火而行痰.

　　　　　(4)加訶子者，以能斂肺而定痰喘也. 不用治血之藥者，火退
則血自止也.

·來源：丹溪

8. Du Sheng San. Single Sage Powder. 獨聖散

·**ACTIONS**：lung wilting and hemoptysis

·**COMPOSITION**：Bai Ji

·**INDICATIONS**：treats cough lasting for a few years, lung wilting, hemoptysis with phlegm.

·**CHANNELS ENTERED**：The hand greater yin channel.

·**Analysis of Formula**：(1) In the middle of the five viscera of human, only a lobe of the lung can regenerate when it is broken and rotten.

　　　　　(2) Bai Ji is bitter, pungent, and astringent. This is supplied with metal qi of fall. This can supplement the lung and stanch bleeding, therefore this treats lung detriment with red phlegm. And it can also treat necrosis of the flesh. This is sage medicinal to eliminating of putridity and engendering the new.

8. 獨聖散

　·總結：肺瘻咯血

　·組成：白芨

　·主治：治多年欬嗽，肺瘻，咯血紅痰.

　·歸經：此手太陰（肺）藥也.

　·方義：(1)人之五臟，惟肺葉壞爛者，可以復生.

　　　　　(2)白芨苦辛收濇，得秋金之令，能補肺止血，故治肺損紅痰. 又能蝕敗疽
死肌，爲去腐生新之聖藥.

9. Qing Yan Tai Ping Wan. Throat-Clearing Peace Pills. 清咽太平丸

·**ACTIONS**：hemoptysis

·**COMPOSITION**：Chuan Xiong, Fang Feng, Bo He, Shi Shuang, Jie Geng, Gan Cao, Xi Jiao

·**INDICATIONS**：treats fire above diaphragm, hemoptysis in the morning, always reddish cheeks, and unclear throat.

·**CHANNELS ENTERED**：The hand greater yin channel.

·**Analysis of Formula**：(1) Chuan Xiong is qi medicinal in blood one, raises clear qi and disperses stasis.

(2) Fang Feng conducts blood herbs to act, drains the lung and contracts the liver.

(3) Bo He is pungent, aromatic, and raising and floating. This disperses wind and heat.

(4) Shi Shuang engenders fluid and moistens the lung.

(5) Jie Geng conducts every herbs to float upward.

(6) Gan Cao moderates fire force which flaming upward.

(7) Xi Jiao cools the heart and clears the lung.

(8) The combination of Gan Cao and Jie Geng clears throat and disinhibits diaphragm.

9. 清咽太平丸

·總結：咯血

·組成：川芎, 防風, 薄荷, 柿霜, 桔梗, 甘草, 犀角

·主治：治膈上有火, 早間咯血, 兩頰常赤, 咽喉不清.

·歸經：此手太陰藥也.

·方義：(1)川芎血中氣藥, 升清散瘀.

(2)防風血藥之使, 瀉肺收肝.

(3)薄荷辛香升浮, 消風散熱.

(4)柿霜生津潤肺.

(5)桔梗載諸藥而上浮.

(6)甘草緩炎上之火勢.

(7)犀角涼心清肺.

(8)又甘, 桔相合, 爲清咽利膈之上劑也.

10. Huan Yuan Shui. Origin Restoring Water. 還元水

·**ACTIONS**：fire cough with loss of blood
·**COMPOSITION**：child's urine
·**INDICATIONS**：treats hemoptysis and hematemesis, and blood dizziness after childbirth, yin vacuity with enduring cough, fire steaming.
·**MODIFICATIONS**：for phlegm, add Jiang Zhi (juice of ginger).
·**CHANNELS ENTERED**：The hand greater yin and foot lesser yin channels.
·**Analysis of Formula**：child's urine is salty and cold, this descends fire and nourishes yin, moistens the lung and disperses stasis, therefore treats blood pattern, fire cough, and blood dizziness after childbirth.

10. 還元水
·總結：火嗽失血
·組成：童便
·主治：治欬血吐血，及產後血運，陰虛久嗽，火蒸如燎.
·加減：有痰加薑汁.
·歸經：此手太陰足少陰藥也.
·方義：童便鹹寒，降火滋陰，潤肺散瘀，故治血證火嗽血運如神

11. Ma Huang Ren Shen Shao Yao Tang. Ephedra, Ginseng, and Peony Decoction. 麻黄人參芍藥湯

·**ACTIONS**： hematemesis with internal vacuity and external contraction
·**COMPOSITION**：Ma Huang, Gui Zhi, Gan Cao (mix fried), Mai Men Dong, Bai Shao Yao, Ren Shen, Dang Gui, Huang Qi, Wu Wei Zi.
·**INDICATIONS**：treats hematemesis, cold evil contracting externally, internal vacuity with congested heat.
·**CHANNELS ENTERED**：The foot greater yang, and the hand and foot greater yin channels. [The bladder, lung, and spleen]
·**Analysis of Formula**：Generally this formula is originated form Zhong Jing's Ma Huang Tang and tonifying medicinal (respectively half).
·**Original Source**：Li Dong Yuan

11. 麻黄人參芍藥湯

·總結：內虛外感吐血
·組成：麻黃，桂枝，炙甘草，麥冬，白芍，人參，當歸，黃耆，五味子
·主治：治吐血外感寒邪，內虛蘊熱.
·歸經：此足太陽手足太陰藥也.
·方義：蓋取仲景麻黃湯與補劑各半服之.
·來源：東垣

12. Xi Jiao Di Huang Tang. Rhinoceros Horn and Rehman nia Decoction. 犀角地黃湯

·**ACTIONS**：cools blood

·**COMPOSITION**：Sheng Di Huang, Bai Shao Yao, Mu Dan Pi, Xi Jiao

·**INDICATIONS**：treats exuberant fire and heat of the stomach in cold da mage, hematemesis, epistaxis, hemoptysis, hematochezia, blood amassment as mania, washing the mouth without desire to swallow it, and yang toxin with ma cula.

·**MODIFICATIONS**：(1) for severe heat as mania, add Huang Qin.

(2) for bleeding by sudden anger, add Zhi Zi and Chai Hu.

·**CHANNELS ENTERED**：The foot yang brightness and greater yin cha nnels.

·**Analysis of Formula**：(1) Blood belongs to yin and is originally tranquil. Fire in every channel gives pressure on blood, the blood is not quiet in its position and ge ts to move frenetically.

(2) Xi Jiao is greatly cold. This resolves stomach heat and clears heart fire.

Shao Yao is sour and cold. This harmonizes yin and bl ood and drains liver fire.

Mu Dan Pi is bitter cold. And this drains the latent fire in the blood.

Sheng Di Huang is greatly cold. This cools blood and enriches water. This formula pacifies excessive counterfolw of every channel.

·**RELATED FORMULA**：Jie An adds Dang Gui, Hong Hua, Jie Geng, Chen Pi, Gan Cao, and Ou Zhi, this is called Jia Wei Xi Jiao Di HuangTang, tre ats same things.

·**Original Source**：Yan Shi Ji Sheng Fang

191

12. 犀角地黃湯

　·總結：涼血

　·組成：生地黃，白芍，丹皮，犀角

　·主治：治傷寒胃火熱盛，吐血衄血，嗽血便血，畜血如狂，漱水不欲嚥．及陽毒發斑．

　·加減：(1)熱甚如狂者，加黃芩一兩．

　　　　　(2)因怒致血者，加梔子，柴胡．

　·歸經：此足陽明太陰藥也．

　·方義：(1)血屬陰，本靜，因諸經火逼，遂不安其位而妄行．

　　　　　(2)犀角大寒，解胃熱而清心火．

　　　　　　　芍藥酸寒，和陰血而瀉肝火．

　　　　　　　丹皮苦寒，瀉血中之伏火．

　　　　　　　生地大寒，涼血而滋水．以共平諸經之僭逆也．

　·變化方：節庵加當歸，紅花，桔梗，陳皮，甘草，藕汁，名加味犀角地黃湯，所治同．

　·來源：濟生

13. Tao Ren Cheng Qi Tang. Peach Pit Decoction to Order the Qi. 桃仁承氣湯

·**COMPOSITION**：Tao Ren, Da Huang, Gui Zhi, Mang Xiao, Gan Cao

·**INDICATIONS**：(1) treats that when a greater yang disease is unresolved and heat binds in the bladder, there is distention and fullness in the lesser abdomen, black stool, uninhibited urination, agitation, thirst, and delirious speech, blood amassment, and heat effusion as mania.

(2) blood stasis, epigastric pain, pain in the abdomen and rib side.

(3) malaria, replete heat effusion at night.

(4) dysentery, blood amassment, acute pain.

·**MODIFICATIONS**：When Qing Pi, Zhi Shi, Dang Gui, Shao Yao, Su Mu Zhi, and Chai Hu are added, this is called Tao Ren Cheng Qi Yin Zi.

·**CHANNELS ENTERED**：The foot greater yang channel.

·**Analysis of Formula**：(1) Da Huang and Mang Xiao flush heat and eliminate the repletion. Gan Cao harmonizes the stomach and moderates the middle. This is Tiao Wei Cheng Qi Tang.

(2) When severe heat binds in the blood part, blood gets to accumulated and the liver gets dry, therefore Tao Ren which is bitter and sweet, is a

192

dded to moisten dryness and moderate the liver. Gui Zhi which is pungent and heat, is added to regulate Construction and resolve the exterior, and to move sta sis through reaching directly where stasis is.

·**Original Source**：Zhong Jing

13. 桃仁承氣湯

　·組成：桃仁, 大黃, 桂枝, 芒硝, 甘草

　·主治：⑴治傷寒外證不解, 熱結膀胱, 小腹脹滿, 大便黑, 小便利, 躁渴譫語, 畜血, 發熱如狂.

　　　　⑵及血瘀胃痛, 腹痛脇痛.

　　　　⑶瘧疾, 實熱夜發

　　　　⑷痢疾, 畜血急痛.

　·加減：本方加青皮, 枳實, 當歸, 芍藥, 蘇木汁, 柴胡, 名桃仁承氣飲子.

　·歸經：此足太陽藥也.

　·方義：⑴大黃, 芒硝, 蕩熱去實, 甘草和胃緩中, 此調胃承氣湯也.

　　　　⑵熱甚搏血, 血聚則肝燥, 故加桃仁之苦甘, 以潤燥而緩肝；加桂枝之辛熱, 以調營而解外, 直達瘀所而行之也.

　·來源：仲景

14. Di Dang Tang. Dead-On Decoction. 抵當湯

·**ACTIONS**：blood amassment in the lower burner

·**COMPOSITION**：Da Huang, Tao Ren, Shui Zhi, Meng Chong

·**INDICATIONS**：⑴ treats that when in greater yang disease that has last ed for six and seven days, the exterior pattern is still present and the pulse is fai nt and sunken, but chest bind is absent.

　　　　⑵ and the person is manic, it is because the heat is in the lower burner, so the lesser abdomen is hard and full.

　⑶ urination is spontaneously uninhibited, there will be blood amassment, this makes one to forget well.

　　　　⑷ Why this is so is because the evil followed the greater yang c hannel, and there is stasis heat in the interior.

·**CHANNELS ENTERED**：The foot greater yang channel.

·**Analysis of Formula**：Cheng Wu Ji says that sweet moderates binds, bit ter drains heat. The sweet and bitter of Tao Ren and Da Huang descend binding

193

heat. The bitter runs to blood and the salty drains blood. The bitter and salty of Meng Chong and Shui Zhi eliminate blood amassment.

·**Original Source**：Zhong Jing

14. 抵當湯

　·總結：血畜下焦

　·組成：大黃，桃仁，水蛭，䗪蟲

　·主治：⑴治太陽病六，七日，表證仍在，脈微而沉，反不結胸.

　　　　　⑵其人發狂者，以熱在下焦，少腹當硬滿.

　　　　　⑶小便自利者，必有畜血，令人善忘.

　　　　　⑷所以然者，以太陽隨經瘀熱在裏故也.

　·歸經：此足太陽藥也.

　·方義：成氏曰：「甘緩結，苦泄熱，桃仁，大黃之甘苦，以下結熱. 苦走血，鹹滲血，䗪蟲，水蛭之苦鹹，以除畜血.

　·來源：仲景

15. Huai Hua San. Sophora Japonica Flower Powder. 槐花 散

·**ACTIONS**：hematochezia

·**COMPOSITION**：. Huai Hua, Ce Bai Ye, Jing Jie Sui, Zhi Ke

·**INDICATIONS**：treats intestinal wind and visceral toxin with bleeding.

·**CHANNELS ENTERED**：The hand and foot yang brightness channels.

·**Analysis of Formula**：(1) Huai Hua courses the liver and drains heat, and this can cool the large intestine.

　　　　　(2) Zhi Ke soothes intestines and disinhibits qi.

　　　　　(3) Ce Bai Ye nourishes dry damp and clears the blood part.

　　　　　(4) Jing Jie disperses stasis and expels wind.

·**RELATED FORMULA**：(1) When Ce Bai Ye and Jing Jie are added and Dang Gui, Huang Qin, Fang Feng, and Di Yu are added, and made into pill with vinegar, this is called Huai Jiao Wan, treats same things.

　　(2) When Dang Gui, Sheng Di Huang, Chuan Xiong, Wu Mei, and Sheng Jiang are added, this is called Jia Jian Si Wu Tang, treats same things.

　　　　(3) When Ce Bai Ye and Zhi Ke are eliminated and Dang Gui, Chuan Xiong, Shu Di Huang, Bai Zhu, Qing Pi, and Sheng Ma are added, this is

also called Huai Hua San, also called Dang Gui He Xue San, treats intestinal af
flux with bleeding and damp toxin with bleeding.

⑷ When Ce Bai Ye and Zhi Ke are eliminated and Qing Pi is ad
ded, this is also called Huai Hua San, treats blood dysentery without abdominal
pain and interior tenesmus.

·**Original Source**：Ben Shi Fang

15. 槐花散

　·總結：便血

　·組成：槐花, 側柏葉, 荊芥穗, 枳殼

　·主治：治腸風臟毒下血.

　·歸經：此手足陽明藥也.

　·方義：⑴槐花疏肝瀉熱, 能涼大腸.

　　　　　⑵枳殼寬腸利氣.

　　　　　⑶側柏養引燥溼, 最清血分.

　　　　　⑷荊芥散瘀搜風.

　·變化方：⑴本方除柏葉, 荊芥, 加當歸, 黃芩, 防風, 地榆, 酒糊丸,
名槐角丸, 治同.

　　　　　⑵本方加當歸, 生地, 川芎, 入烏梅, 生薑煎, 名加減四物湯,
治同.

　　　　　⑶本方除柏葉, 枳殼, 加當歸, 川芎, 熟地, 白朮, 青皮, 升
麻, 亦名槐花散, 又名當歸和血散, 治腸澼下血, 溼毒下血.

　　　　　⑷本方除柏葉, 枳殼, 加青皮等分, 亦名槐花散, 治血痢腹
不痛, 不裏急後重.

　　　　　⑸單用槐花, 荊芥炒研爲末, 酒服, 亦治下血.

　·來源：本事

16. Qin Jiao Bai Zhu Wan. Gentiana Macrophylla and Atr actylodes Macrocephala Pills. 秦艽白朮丸

·**ACTIONS**：blood hemmorhoid

·**COMPOSITION**：Qin Jiao, Tao Ren, Dang Gui Wei, Zao Jiao Zi, Ze X
ie, Zhi Shi , Di Yu, Bai Zhu

·**INDICATIONS**：treats hemorrhoid sore, hemorrhoid, and fistulas with pus and b
lood, dry and hard stool, severe pain where an anal fistula is.

195

·**CHANNELS ENTERED**：The hand and foot yang brightness channels.

·**Analysis of Formula**：Li Dong Yuan says that：(1) Qin Jiao, Tao Ren, and Dang Gui Wei moisten dryness and harmonize blood.

(2) Zao Jiao Ren eliminates dry wind. Di Yu breaks blood and stanches bleeding.

(3) Ze Xie is bland. This makes qi return to anterior yin, and eliminates damp in the large intestine, the damp is taken from the stomach.

(4) Zhi Shi is bitter and cold. This supplements the kidney and drains replete stomach.

(5) The bitter of Bai Zhu supplements insufficient dry qi, the sweet drains fire and boosts source qi, therefore it is said that the combination of sweet and cold drains fire, the cold of Zhi Shi corresponds that example. Constipation is pushed by Da Huang. When the humor and fluid are insufficient, Dang Gui is used to harmonize blood and oily and moisture herbs are added, then the hard stool will be spontaneously disinhibited. .

·**RELATED FORMULA**：(1) When Bai Zhu, Zhi Shi, and Di Yu are eliminated, and Cang Zhu, Huang Bai, Da Huang, Bing Lang, and Fang Feng are added, this is called Qin Jiao Cang Zhu Tang, treats same things.

(2) When Zao Jiao, Zhi Shi, and Di Yu are eliminated and Fang Feng, Sheng Ma, Chai Hu, Chen Pi, Da Huang, Huang Bai, Hong Hua, and Gan Cao are added, this is called Qin Jiao Fang Feng Tang, treats hemorrhoid and fistulas with pain during defecation.

(3) When Di Yu is eliminated and Da Huang and Hong Hua are added, this is called Qin Jiao Dang Gui Tang, treats hemorrhoid and fistulas with hard stool and pain during defecation.

·**Original Source**：Li Dong Yuan

16. 秦艽白朮丸

　·總結：血痔
　·組成：秦艽, 桃仁, 歸尾, 皂角子, 澤瀉, 枳實, 地榆, 白朮
　·主治：治痔瘡痔漏有膿血, 大便燥結, 痛不可忍.
　·歸經：此手足陽明藥也.
　·方義：李東垣曰：(1)秦艽, 桃仁, 歸尾, 潤燥和血.
　　　　　(2)皂角仁以除風燥. 地榆以破血止血.
　　　　　(3)澤瀉淡滲, 使氣歸於前陰, 以補清燥受胃之濕邪也.
　　　　　(4)枳實苦寒, 以補腎而泄胃實.
　　　　　(5)白朮之苦以補燥氣之不足, 其味甘以瀉火而益元氣, 故曰

196

『甘寒瀉火』，乃假枳實之寒也．大便祕澀，以大黃推之，其津液益不足，用當歸和血，加油潤之劑，自然亹利矣．

　·變化方：(1)本方除白术，枳實，地榆，加蒼术，黃柏，大黃，檳榔，防風，名秦艽蒼术湯，治同．

　　　　(2)本方除皂角，枳實，地榆，加防風，升麻，柴胡，陳皮，大黃，黃柏，紅花，炙草，名秦艽防風湯，治痔漏大便時疼痛．

　　　　(3)本方除地榆，加大黃，紅花，名秦艽當歸湯，治痔漏大便燥結疼痛．

　·煎服法：麵糊丸

　·來源：東垣

17. Shao Yao Tang. Peony Decoction. 芍藥湯

·**ACTIONS**：blood dysentery

·**COMPOSITION**：Bai Shao Yao, Huang Qin, Gan Cao, Huang Lian, Da Huang, Mu Xiang, Bing Lang, Dang Gui Wei, Rou Gui

·**INDICATIONS**：treats dysentery with sticky and thick pus and blood, abdominal pain.

·**CHANNELS ENTERED**：The foot greater yin, and the hand and foot yang brightness channels.

·**Analysis of Formula**：(1) ①Shao Yao is sour and cold. This drains liver fire, restrains yin qi, and harmonizes Construction and Defense, therefore acting as sovereign.

　　　　② Da Huang and Dang Gui Wei break accumulation and move blood.

　　　　③ Gan Cao harmonizes every herbs.

　　　　④ Huang Qin and Huang Lian dry damp and clear heat.

　　　　⑤ Mu Xiang and Bing Lang free stagnation and move qi.

　　　　(2) Generally dysentery is originated from the depression and accumulation of damp heat in the stomach and intestines, qi cannot be free, therefore there is abdominal urgency and rectal heaviness during defecation and inhibited voidings of reddish urine. Pungent disperses stagnation, bitter dries damp, cold clears heat, and sweet regulates it.

　　　　(3) Rou Gui which is pungent and heat, is used as counteracting

197

assistant.

    ·RELATED FORMULA：When Rou Gui and Gan Cao is eliminated and Zhi Ke is added, this is called Dao Zhi Tang, treats the above pattern with thirst.

    ·Original Source：Jie Gu

17. 芍藥湯

    ·總結：血痢

    ·組成：白芍, 黃芩, 甘草, 黃連, 大黃, 木香, 檳榔, 當歸尾, 桂皮

    ·主治：治下痢膿血稠粘, 腹重後痛.

    ·歸經：此足太陰手足陽明藥也.

    ·方義：⑴①芍藥酸寒, 瀉肝火, 斂陰氣, 和營衛, 故以爲君.

              ②大黃, 歸尾, 破積而行血.

              ③甘草和之.

              ④黃芩, 黃連, 燥濕而清熱.

              ⑤木香, 檳榔, 通滯而行氣.

        ⑵蓋下痢由濕熱鬱積於腸胃, 不得宣通, 故大便重急, 小便赤濇也. 辛以散之, 苦以燥之, 寒以清之, 甘以調之.

        ⑶加肉桂者, 假其辛熱以爲反佐也.

    ·變化方：本方除桂, 甘草, 加枳殼, 名導滯湯, 治前證兼渴者.

    ·來源：潔古

18. Cang Zhu Di Yu Tang. Atractylodes and Sanguisorba Decoction. 蒼朮地楡湯

    ·ACTIONS：blood dysentery

    ·COMPOSITION：Cang Zhu, Di Yu

    ·INDICATIONS：treats the spleen channel contracting damp, dysentery with bleeding.

    ·CHANNELS ENTERED：The foot greater yin and yang brightness channels.

    ·Analysis of Formula：(1) Cang Zhu dries damp and strengthens the spleen, raises yang and opens depression.

        (2) Di Yu clears heat and cools blood, the sour and astringent can stop dysentery.

        (3) This formula treats blood dysentery and intestinal wind, but d

o not use in initial time.

·**RELATED FORMULA**：When Shao Yao, E Jiao, and Juan Bai are add
ed, this is called Shao Yao Di Yu Tang, treats dysentery with pus and blood an
d prolapse of the rectum.

·**Original Source**：Jie Gu

18. 蒼朮地榆湯

　·總結：血痢

　·組成：蒼朮，地榆

　·主治：治脾經受濕，痢疾下血.

　·歸經：此足太陰陽明藥也.

　·方義：⑴蒼朮燥溼强脾，升陽而開鬱.

　　　　　⑵地榆清熱涼血，酸收能斷下.

　　　　　⑶爲治血痢腸風之平劑，初起者勿用.

　·變化方：本方加芍藥，阿膠，卷柏，名芍藥地榆湯，治泄痢膿血，乃
至脫肛.

　·來源：潔古

19. Xiao Ji Yin Zi. Cephalanoplos Decoction. 小薊飲子

·**ACTIONS**：blood strangury

·**COMPOSITION**：Xiao Ji Gen, sheng Di Huang, Pu Huang, Ou Jie, Mu
Tong, Dan Zhu Ye, Shan Zhi Ren, Hua Shi, Gan Cao, Dang Gui

·**INDICATIONS**：treats binding heat in the lower burner and this causes
blood strangury.

·**CHANNELS ENTERED**：The hand and foot greater yang channels.

·**Analysis of Formula**：(1) Xiao Ji and Ou Jie abate heat and disperse stas
is.

　　　　　(2) Pu Huang stanches bleeding.

　　　　　(3) Mu Tong descends the fire of the heart and lung and sends th
e fire to the small intestine.

　　　　　(4) Hua Shi drains heat and lubricates orifice.

　　　　　(5) Gan Cao boosts yang and can regulate the middle and harmo
nize qi.

　　　　　(6) Sheng Di Huang cools blood.

　　　　　(7) Dang Gui nourishes yin, and can conduct the blood to return

199

channel.

(8) Zhi Zi disperses the depressed fire in triple burner by letting f
ire out through urine.

(9) Zhu Ye cools the heart and clears the lung.

19. 小薊飲子
　　·總結：血淋
　　·組成：小薊根，生地黃，蒲黃，藕節，木通，淡竹葉，山梔仁，滑石，
甘草，當歸
　　·主治：治下焦結熱而成血淋.
　　·歸經：此手足太陽藥也.
　　·方義：(1)小薊，藕節，退熱散瘀.
　　　　　　(2)蒲黃止血.
　　　　　　(3)木通降心肺之火，下達小腸.
　　　　　　(4)滑石瀉熱而滑竅.
　　　　　　(5)甘草益陽，能調中和氣.
　　　　　　(6)生地涼血.
　　　　　　(7)當歸養陰，能引血歸經.
　　　　　　(8)梔子散三焦鬱火，由小便出.
　　　　　　(9)竹葉涼心而清肺.

20. Fu Yuan Qiang Huo Tang. Notopterygium Decoction to Restore the Origin. 復元羌活湯

·**ACTIONS**：detriment damage and accumulated blood

·**COMPOSITION**：Chai Hu, Gan Cao, Dang Gui, Da Huang, Hong Hua,
Gua Lou Gen, Tao Ren, Chuan Shan Jia

·**INDICATIONS**：treats falling from high, malignant blood which retained below
the heart, pain.

·**CHANNELS ENTERED**：The foot reverting yin channel.

·**Analysis of Formula**：in text; the liver and gall bladder channels move b
elow the heart and belong to reverting yin and lesser yang.

(1) therefore Chai Hu is used as channel conductor, acting as sov
ereign.

(2) Dang Gui activates blood vessels and Gan Cao moderates the

200

urgency, acting as minister, they also can engender new blood, when yang engende
rs, yin grows.

       (3) Da Huang flushes vanquished blood, acting as courier.

       (4) Chuan Shan Jia, Tian Hua Fen, Tao Ren, and Hong Hua brea
k blood and moisten blood, acting as assistant.

       (5) The combinations of the qi and flavors of every herbs have a
place where they return to respectively, pain will be eliminated spontaneously.

20. 復元羌活湯
  ·總結：損傷積血
  ·組成：柴胡, 甘草, 當歸, 大黃, 紅花, 栝蔞根, 桃仁, 穿山甲
  ·主治：治從高墜下, 惡血留於脇下, 疼痛不可忍者.
  ·歸經：此足厥陰藥也.
  ·方義：原文曰：「肝膽之經, 行於脇下, 屬厥陰少陽.
     (1)故以柴胡引用爲君.
     (2)以當歸活血脈, 以甘草緩其急爲臣, 亦能生新血, 陽生則
陰長也.
     (3)以大黃蕩滌敗血爲使.
     (4)以穿山甲, 花粉, 桃仁, 紅花, 破血潤血爲佐.
     (5)氣味相合, 各有攸歸, 痛自去矣.

Chapter 9. Wind-Dispelling Formulas. 祛風之劑

1. Xiao Xu Ming Tang. Minor Prolong-Life Decoction. 小續命湯

·**ACTIONS**：common formula for six channels stricken by wind.

·**COMPOSITION**：Ma Huang, Gui Zhi, Fang Feng, Fang Ji, Xing Ren, Huang Qin, Ren Shen, Gan Cao, Da Zao, Chuan Xiong, Bai Shao Yao, Fu Zi, Sheng Jiang

·**INDICATIONS**：(1) treats stroke with loss of consciousness, derangement of spirit qi, hemiplegia, hypertonicity and tense of sinew, deviated eye and mouth, sluggish speech.

(2) lumbar pain due to wind-damp, exuberance of phlegm and fire.

(3) six channels stricken by wind, and hard tetany and soft tetany.

·**MODIFICATIONS**：(1) for hypertonicity of sinew, sluggish speech, and a pulse that is string-like, double the dose of Ren Shen and add Yi Yi Ren and Dang Gui.

(2) eliminate Shao Yao, when there is interior cold.

(3) for vexation with difficulty to defecate, eliminate Gui Zhi and Fu Zi, and double the dose of Shao Yao and add Zhu Li.

(4) for enduring absence of defecation and unpleasant in the chest, add Da Huang and Zhi Ke.

(5) for vacuous cold of the large intestine with diarrhea, eliminate Fang Ji and Huang Qin, double **Fu Zi**, and add Bai Zhu.

(6) for retching, add Ban Xia.

(7) for sluggish speech and wriggle of the limbs, add Shi Chang Pu and Zhu Li.

(8) for generalized pain and convulsions, add Qiang Huo.

(9) for thirst, add Mai Men Dong and Tian Hua Fen.

(10) for vexation, thirst, and often fright, add Xi Jiao and Ling Yang Jiao.

(11) for profuse sweating, eliminate Ma Huang and Xing Ren and add Bai Zhu.

(12) for dry tongue, eliminate Gui Zhi and Fu Zi and add Shi Gao.

202

·**Analysis of Formula** : common formula for six channels stricken by win
d..

        Wu He Gao says that Ma Huang and Xing Ren are the main her
bs in Ma Huang Tang that treats greater yang cold damage ;

        Gui Zhi and Shao Yao are the main herbs in Gui Zhi Tang that tr
eats greater yang wind strike.

        Therefore this formula is used to the pattern that is damaged by
wind and cold, and there will be exterior pattern.

        Ren Shen and Gan Cao supplement qi.

        Chuan Xiong and Shao Yao supplement blood.

        Therefore this formula treats exterior pattern of wind and cold w
ith qi and blood vacuity.

        Excessive wind is controlled with Fang Feng.

        For excessive damp, Fang Ji acts as assistant

        For excessive cold, Fu Zi acts as assistant

        For excessive heat, Huang Qin acts as assistant. The cause of a d
isease is too complicated, therefore herbs are also.

·**RELATED FORMULA** : Zhang Yuan Su's Six Channel

MODIFICATION :

        (1) When Ma Huang, Xing Ren, and Fang Feng are doubled, this
is called Ma Huang Xu Ming Tang, treats greater yang wind strike with absenc
e of sweating and aversion to cold.

        (2) When Gui Zhi, Shao Yao, and Xing Ren are doubled, this is
called Gui Zhi Xu Ming Tang, treats greater yang wind strike with sweating an
d aversion to wind.

        (3) When Fu Zi is eliminated and add Shi Gao and Zhi Mu are a
dded, this is called Bai Hu Su Ming Tang, treats yang brightness wind strike wi
th absence of sweating, generalized heat effusion, and absence of aversion to co
ld.

        (4) When Ge Gen is added and Gui Zhi and Huang Qin are doubl
ed, this is called Ge Gen Su Ming Tang, treats yang brightness wind strike with
generalized heat effusion, sweating, and absence of aversion to wind.

        (5) When Fu Zi is doubled and Gan Jiang and Gan Cao are adde
d, this is called Fu Zi Su Ming Tang, treats greater yin wind strike with absence
of sweating and cool body.

        (6) When Gui Zhi, Fu Zi, and Gan Cao are added, this is called
Gui Fu Xu Ming Tang, treats lesser yin wind strike with sweating and absence
of heat effusion.

1. 小續命湯
    ·總結：六經中風通劑
    ·組成：麻黃, 桂枝, 防風, 防己, 杏仁, 黃芩, 人參, 甘草, 大棗, 川芎, 白芍, 大附子, 生薑
    ·主治：⑴治中風不省人事, 神氣潰亂, 半身不遂, 筋急拘攣, 口眼喎邪, 語言蹇澀.
            ⑵風溼腰痛, 痰火併多.
            ⑶六經中風, 及剛柔二痙.
    ·加減：⑴筋急語遲脈弦者, 倍人參, 加薏仁, 當歸.
            ⑵去芍藥, 以避中寒.
            ⑶煩燥不大便, 去桂, 附, 倍芍藥, 加竹瀝.
            ⑷日久不大便, 胸中不快, 加大黃, 枳殼.
            ⑸臟寒下利, 去黃己, 黃芩, 倍附子, 加白朮.
            ⑹嘔逆加半夏.
            ⑺語言蹇澀, 手足戰掉, 加石菖蒲, 竹瀝.
            ⑻身痛發搐, 加羌活.
            ⑼口渴加麥冬, 花粉.
            ⑽煩渴多驚, 加犀角, 羚羊角.
            ⑾汗多去麻黃, 杏仁, 加白朮.
            ⑿舌燥去桂, 附, 加石膏.
    ·方義：此六經中風之通劑也.
                        吳鶴皋曰：「麻黃, 杏仁, 麻黃湯也, 治太陽傷寒
    ；

            桂枝, 芍藥, 桂枝湯也, 治太陽中風；
            此中風寒, 有表證者所必用也.
            人參, 甘草補氣.
            川芎, 芍藥補血.
            此中風寒, 氣血虛者所必用也.
            風淫故主以防風.
            溼淫佐以防己.
            寒淫佐以附子.
            熱淫佐以黃芩. 病來雜擾, 故藥亦兼該也.
    ·變化方：易老六經加減法：

(1)本方倍麻黃，杏仁，防風，名麻黃續命湯，治太陽中風，無汗惡寒．

(2)本方倍桂枝，芍藥，杏仁，名桂枝續命湯，治太陽中風，有汗惡風．

(3)本方去附子，加石膏，知母，名白虎續命湯，治陽明中風，無汗身熱，不惡寒．

(4)本方加葛根，倍桂枝，黃芩，名葛根續命湯，治陽明中風，身熱有汗，不惡風．

(5)本方倍附子，加乾薑，甘草，名附子續命湯，治太陰中風，無汗身涼．

(6)本方倍桂，附，甘草，名桂附續命湯，治少陰中風，有汗無熱．

·來源：千金

2. Hou Shi Hei San. Hou's Black Powder. 侯氏黑散

·**ACTIONS**：wind strike

·**COMPOSITION**：Ju Hua, Xi Xin, Fang Feng, Bai Zhu, Ren Shen, Dang Gui, Chuan Xiong, Fu Ling, Jie Geng, Gan Jiang, Fan Shi, Mu Li, Gui Zhi

·**INDICATIONS**：(1) treats wind strike, vexation and heaviness of the limbs, fear of cold in the heart, and insufficiency.

(2) Wai Tai Mi Yao uses this formula to treat wind madness.

·**CHANNELS ENTERED**：The hand greater and lesser yin and the foot reverting yin channels.

·**Analysis of Formula**：(1)① Ju Hua grows in fall, this is supplied with the essence of metal and water, this can restrict fire and pacify wood, when wood pacifies, wind gets extinguished, when fire descends, heat is eliminated, therefore this acts as sovereign.

② Fang Feng and Xi Xin eliminate wind.

③ Ren Shen and Bai Zhu supplement qi. Huang Qin clears lung heat.

④ Dang Gui and Chuan Xiong tonify blood.

⑤ Fu Ling frees heart qi and moves spleen damp.

⑥ Jie Geng harmonizes diaphragm qi.

⑦ Gan Jiang and Gui Zhi assist yang part and reach the limbs.

205

⑧ Mu Li and Bai Fan promote contraction with sour and astringe, and also can transform stubborn phlegm.

⑵ Taking this with wine makes the force of medicinal move.

·**Original Source**：Jin Gui Yao Lue

2. 侯氏黑散

·總結：中風

·組成：菊花, 細辛, 防風, 白朮, 人參, 當歸, 川芎, 茯苓, 桔梗, 乾薑, 礬石, 牡蠣, 桂枝

·主治：⑴治中風四肢煩重, 心中惡寒不足者.

⑵外臺用治風癲.

·歸經：此手太陰少陰足厥陰藥也.

·方義：⑴①菊花秋生, 得金水之精, 能制火而平木, 木平則風息, 火降則熱除, 故以爲君.

②防風, 細辛以祛風.

③人參, 白朮以補氣. 黃芩以清肺熱.

④當歸, 川芎以養血.

⑤茯苓通心氣而行脾溼.

⑥桔梗以和膈氣.

⑦薑, 桂助陽分而達四肢.

⑧牡蠣, 白礬, 酸斂濇收, 又能化頑痰.

⑵加酒服者, 以行藥勢也.

·來源：金匱

3. Da Qin Jiao Tang. Major Gentiana Macrophylla Decoction. 大秦芃湯

·**ACTIONS**：tracks down wind, activates blood, and descends fire

·**COMPOSITION**：Qin Jiao, Qiang Huo, Bai Shao Yao, Chuan Xiong, Xi Xin, Du Huo, Fang Feng, Dang Gui, Shu Di Huang, Sheng Di Huang, Bai Zhu, Gan Cao, Shi Gao, Huang Qin, Bai Zhi

·**INDICATIONS**：treats wind stroke, inability of moving the limbs, stiff tongue, impending speech, wind evil that is seen in every six channel not in only one channel.

·**MODIFICATIONS**：⑴ in humid weather, add Sheng Jiang.

(2) in spring and summer, add Zhi Mu.

(3) for glomus below the heart, add Zhi Ke.

·**Analysis of Formula**： This is common formula to treat slight wind stri ke in the six channel.

(1) Qin Jiao acts as sovereign, eliminate wind in whole body.

Shi Gao acts as minister, disperses fire in the chest.

Qiang Huo disperses wind in greater yang.

Bai Zhi disperses wind in yang brightness.

Chuan Xiong disperses wind in reverting yin.

Xi Xin and Du Huo disperse wind in lesser yin.

Fang Feng is like a soldier, this can reach everywhere following channel conductor.

(2) Wind herbs tend to be dry, exterior herbs tend to disperse, the refore to course wind, one should first tonify blood, and to resolve the exterior, also one should secure the interior.

Dang Gui tonifies blood, Sheng Di Huang enriches blood, Chua n Xiong activates blood, Shao Yao restrains yin and harmonizes blood.

When blood is active, wind disperses and the root of t ongue gets soft.

(3) and qi can engender blood, therefore Bai Zhu, Fu Ling, and Gan Cao are used to supplement qi through invigorating the middle. When the spleen moves and damp is eliminated, the hand and foot get strong.

(4) and wind can generate heat, therefore Huang Qin is used to cl ear the upper part, Shi Gao drains the middle, Sheng Di Huang cools the lower part. They pacifies fire which counterfolws upward.

·**Original Source**：Huo Fa Ji Yao

3. 大秦艽湯

·總結：搜風活血降火

·組成：秦艽，羌活，白芍，川芎，細辛，獨活，防風，當歸，熟地，生地，白朮，甘草，石膏，黃芩，白芷

·主治：治中風手足不能運掉，舌強不能言語，風邪散見，不拘一經者.

·加減：(1)雨溼加生薑.

(2)春夏加知母.

(3)心下痞加枳殼.

·方義：此六經中風輕者之通劑也.

(1)以秦艽爲君者，袪一身之風也.

207

以石膏爲臣者, 散胸中之火也.

羌活散太陽之風.

白芷散陽明之風.

川芎散厥陰之風.

細辛, 獨活散少陰之風.

防風爲風藥卒徒, 隨所引而無所不至者也.

(2)風藥多燥, 表藥多散, 故疏風必先養血, 而解表亦必固裏.

當歸養血, 生地滋血, 芎藭活血, 芍藥斂陰和血.

血活則風散, 而舌本柔矣.

(3)又氣能生血, 故用白朮, 茯苓, 甘草, 補氣以壯中樞, 脾運溼除, 則手足健矣.

(4)又風能生熱, 故用黃芩清上, 石膏瀉中, 生地涼下, 以共平逆上之火也.

·來源：機要

4. San Sheng Yin. Three Raw Agents Beverage. 三生飲

·**ACTIONS**：sudden stroke

·**COMPOSITION**：Sheng Chuan Wu, Sheng Fu Zi, Sheng Nan Xing, Mu Xiang

·**INDICATIONS**：treats wind stroke, sudden clouding, loss of consciousness, phlegm-drool congestion, sluggish speech, and so on.

·**CHANNELS ENTERED**：The foot greater yin, yang brightness, reverting yin, and hand lesser yang channels. [The spleen, stomach, liver, and triple burner]

·**Analysis of Formula**：(1)① Wu Tou clears and course, warms the spleen and expels wind.

② Fu Zi is drastic, warms the spleen and expels cold. The reason of using of raw herbs is to make the force of medicinal move fast.

(2) Ren Shen (large dose) is used to support the right qi. Mu Xiang (small dose) acting as assistant, is used to move the counterfolw qi.

4. 三生飲

·總結：卒中

·組成：生川烏, 生附子, 生南星, 木香

·主治：治中風卒然昏憒, 不省人事, 痰涎壅盛, 語言蹇澀等證.

208

·歸經：此足太陰陽明厥陰手少陽藥也.

·方義：(1)①烏頭清疏，溫脾逐風.

②附子猛峻，溫脾逐寒. 皆用生者，取其力峻而行速也.

(2)重用人參，所以扶其正氣. 少佐木香，所以行其逆氣也.

5. Di Huang Yin Zi. Rehmannia Decoction. 地黃飲子

·ACTIONS：wind disablement

·COMPOSITION：Shu Di Huan, Rou Cong Rong, Rou Gui, Fu Zi, Ba Ji Tian, Shan Zhu Yu, Shi Hu, Fu Ling, Yuan Zhi, Shi Chang Pu, Mai Men Dong, Wu Wei Zi

·INDICATIONS：treats wind stroke, impeding speech, lameness with in ability of move, this is that the qi of lesser yin is reversed so that cannot reach, t his is called wind disablement, sudden onset should be treated with warming.

·MODIFICATIONS：(1)① Shu Di Huang enriches yin.

② Ba Ji Tian, Rou Cong Rong, Rou Gui, and Fu Zi ret urn the origin fire.

③ Shan Zhu Yu warms the liver and secures essence.

④ Shi Hu quiets the spleen and keeps qi.

⑤ Shi Chang Pu, Yuan Zhi, and Fu Ling supplement t he heart and free the kidney.

⑥ Mai Men Dong and Wu Wei Zi preserve the lung t o enrich the source of water.

(2) When water and fire interact, essence qi gradually gets effulg ent and wind fire spontaneously gets distinguished.

·CHANNELS ENTERED：The hand and foot lesser and greater yin, and the foot reverting yin channels. [The heart, kidney, lung, spleen, and liver]

·Original Source：Liu He Jian's formula

5. 地黃飲子

·總結：風痱

·組成：熟地黃，肉蓯蓉，官桂，附子，巴戟，山茱萸，石斛，茯苓，遠志，石菖蒲，麥冬，五味子

·主治：治中風舌瘖不能言，足廢不能行，此少陰氣厥不至，名曰風痱，急發溫之.

209

·加減：(1)①熟地以滋根本之陰.
②巴戟，蓯蓉，官桂，附子，以返真元之火.
③山茱溫肝而固精.
④石斛安脾而祕氣.
⑤菖蒲，遠志，茯苓，補心而通腎臟.
⑥麥冬，五味，保肺以滋水源.
(2)使水火相交，精氣漸旺，而風火自息矣.
·歸經：此手足少陰太陰足厥陰藥也.
·來源：河間

6. Shun Feng Yun Qi San. Wind Normalizing Qi Equating Powder. 順風勻氣散

·**ACTIONS**：deviation and hemiplegia.

·**COMPOSITION**：Tian Ma, Bai Zhi, Su Ye, Wu Yao, Chen Xiang, Qing Pi, Ren Shen, Gan Cao (mix fried), Bai Zhu, Mu Gua

·**INDICATIONS**：treats wind stroke, hemiplegia, deviated eye and mouth.

·**CHANNELS ENTERED**：The foot reverting yin and yang brightness channels. [The liver and stomach]

·**Analysis of Formula**：(1) qi in the place where evil gathers will be vacuous, hemilateral withering and deviation in left or right are generally due to irregularity of blood and vessels and inequality of qi.

(2) Tian Ma, Su Ye, and Bai Zhi course wind qi. Wu Yao, Qing Pi, and Chen Xiang move stagnated qi. Ren Shen, Bai Zhu, and Gan Cao supplement the right qi. This formula courses, moves, and supplements qi to equate qi. When qi is equated, wind gets normalized.

(3) Mu Gua can drain wood in earth, regulates the construction and defense and stretches sinew.

6. 順風勻氣散
·總結：喎邪不遂
·組成：天麻，白芷，蘇葉，烏藥，沉香，青皮，人參，炙甘草，白朮，木瓜
·主治：治中風半身不遂，口眼喎邪.
·歸經：此足厥陰陽明藥也.

·方義：(1)邪之所湊，其氣必虛，偏枯喎僻，或左或右，蓋血脈不周，而氣不勻也.

      (2)天麻，蘇，芷，以疏風氣. 烏藥，青，沉，以行滯氣. 參，朮，炙草，以補正氣. 疏之行之補之，而氣勻矣，氣勻則風順矣.

      (3)用木瓜者，能於土中瀉木，調榮衛而伸筋也.

7. Xi Xian Wan. Siegesbeckia Pill. 豨薟丸

·**ACTIONS**：wind impediment

·**COMPOSITION**：**Xi Xian Cao.**

·**INDICATIONS**：(1) treats wind stroke, deviation, difficult sluggish speech, weak limbs, and bone pain.

(2) and wind impediment, wandering pain, or numbness of ten fingers.

(3) wind qi in the liver and kidney, wind-damp with every sores.

·**CHANNELS ENTERED**：The foot lesser yin and reverting yin. [The kidney and liver]

·**Analysis of Formula**：(1) Xi Xian Cao can eliminate wind, disperse damp, and move the qi of the large intestine.

·**Original Source**：Zhang Yong

7. 豨薟丸

  ·總結：風痺

  ·組成：豨薟草.

  ·主治：(1)治中風喎僻，語言蹇澁，肢緩骨痛

      (2)及風痺走痛，或十指麻木.

      (3)肝腎風氣，風溼諸瘡.

  ·歸經：此足少陰厥陰藥也.

  ·方義：(1)豨薟能祛風散溼，行大腸之氣.

  ·來源：張詠

8. Qian Zheng San. Pull Aright Powder. 牽正散

·**ACTIONS**：qian wind

·**COMPOSITION**：Jiang Can, Quan Xie, Bai Fu Zi

211

·**INDICATIONS**：treats wind stroke, deviated eye and mouth.

·**CHANNELS ENTERED**：The foot yang brightness and reverting yin channels. [The stomach and liver]

·**Analysis of Formula**：(1) Wu He Gao says that Qin Jiao and Fang Feng expel exterior wind but do not treat wind which is engendered in the interior. Dan Xing and Ban Xia treat damp phlegm but do not treat phlegm which belongs to vacuous wind. Jiang Can, Quan Xie, and Bai Fu Zi treat wind that is engendered in the interior and phlegm that belongs to vacuous heat. This formula with wine can enter channel and brings the mouth and eye to rights.

(2) also says that the pungent of Bai Fu can eliminate wind, the salty of Jiang Can and Quan Xie can soften phlegm.

·**Original Source**：Zhi Zhi Fang

8. 牽正散

·總結：牽風

·組成：殭蠶，全蠍，白附子

·主治：治中風口眼喎邪，無他證者.

·歸經：此足陽明厥陰藥也.

·方義：(1)吳鶴皋：「芃，防之屬，可以驅外風，而內生之風非其治也. 星，夏之屬，可以治溼痰，而風虛之痰非其治也. 三藥療內生之風，治虛熱之痰. 得酒引之，能入經而正口眼. 」

(2)又曰：「白附辛可祛風，蠶，蠍鹹能輭痰.

·來源：直指方

9. Ru Sheng San. Sagely Powder. 如聖飲

·**ACTIONS**：hard and soft tetany.

·**COMPOSITION**：Fang Feng, Chuan Xiong, Bai Zhi, Gan Cao, Chai Hu, Qiang Huo, Wu Yao, Ban Xia, Dang Gui, Shao Yao, Huang Qin

·**INDICATIONS**：treats hard and soft tetany, reddish complexion, stiff nape, shaking of the head, clenched jaw, arched back rigidity, convulsions.

·**MODIFICATIONS**：(1) for febrile convulsion without chills, add Bai Zhu and Gui Zhi.

(2) for febrile convulsion with chills, add Cang Zhu and Ma Huang.

(3) for clenched jaw, grinding of the teeth, and constipation, add

212

Da Huang.

·**CHANNELS ENTERED**：The foot greater yang and reverting yin channels. [The bladder and liver].

·**Analysis of Formula**：(1) The pungent and sweet of Qiang Huo, Fang Feng, Chuan Xiong, Bai Zhi, Chai Hu, and Gan Cao disperse wind evil.

(2) Wu Yao is used because when treating wind, normalizing of qi is needed.

(3) Ban Xia, Zhu Li, and Jiang Zhi (juice of ginger) are used because wind tends to be with phlegm.

(4) Dang Gui and Shao Yao are used because when treating wind, activating blood should be first used.

(5) Huang Qin is used because wind tends to engender heat.

(6) for febrile convulsion without chills, add Bai Zhu and Gui Zhi.

(7) for febrile convulsion with chills, add Cang Zhu and Ma Huang.

(8) the mouth and teeth belong to yang brightness, when yang brightness is replete, clenched jaw, grinding of the teeth, and constipation occur, therefore add Da Huang to drain stomach heat.

·**Original Source**：Jie An

9. 如聖飲
·總結：剛柔二痙
·組成：防風, 川芎, 白芷, 甘草, 柴胡, 羌活, 烏藥, 半夏, 當歸, 芍藥, 黃芩
·主治：治剛柔二痙, 面赤項強, 頭搖口噤, 角弓反張, 與瘈瘲同法.
·加減：(1)柔痙加白朮, 桂枝.
　　　　(2)剛痙加蒼朮, 麻黃.
　　　　(3)口噤咬牙, 大便實, 加大黃.
·歸經：足太陽, 厥陰藥.
·方義：(1)羌, 防, 芎, 芷, 柴胡, 甘草, 辛甘以發散風邪.
　　　　(2)用烏藥者, 治風須順氣也.
　　　　(3)用半夏, 竹瀝, 薑汁者, 風必挾痰也.
　　　　(4)用歸, 芍者, 治風先活血也.
　　　　(5)用黃芩者, 風必生熱也.
　　　　(6)柔痙加白朮, 桂枝.

213

(7)剛痓加蒼朮，麻黃.

(8)口齒屬陽明，陽明實則口噤咬牙而便祕，故加大黃以泄胃
熱也.

·來源：節庵

10. Du Huo Tang. Angelica Pubescens Decociton. 獨活湯

·**ACTIONS**：convulsions and clouding.

·**COMPOSITION**：Du Huo, Qiang Huo, Fang Feng, Ren Shen, Bai Wei, Dang Gui, Chuan Xiong, Fu Shen, Yuan Zhi, Xi Xin, Gui Xin, Shi Chang Pu, Ban Xia, Gan Cao (mix fried)

·**INDICATIONS**：treats convulsions with wind vacuity, clouding, or aversion to cold and heat effusion.

·**CHANNELS ENTERED**：The hand lesser yin and foot reverting yin channels. [The heart and liver]

·**Analysis of Formula**：(1) The liver governs wind wood and sinew, therefore convulsions is related with liver evil. The liver [qi] longs for dispersion. [In case of a disease in the liver], quickly consume pungent [flavor] to disperse its [qi]. Du Huo, Qiang Huo, and Fang Feng eliminate wind. Xi Xin and Gui Xin warm channel. Ban Xia eliminates phlegm. The pungent of Chuan Xiong and Dang Gui disperses wind and warms and harmonizes blood. When blood is activated, wind disperses. Wind is dispersed by pungent, this means that pungent supplements qi.

(2) The heart is the son of the liver, when the liver passes the heat to the heart, clouding occurs, therefore Ren Shen supplements heart qi, Shi Chang Pu opens orifices of the heart, Fu Shen and Yuan Zhi quiet heart spirit, the salty and cold of Bai Wei abates heat and treats reverting. When wind is calm and fire is distinguished, blood gets activated, spirit quiets, and convulsions spontaneously disappears.

·**Original Source**：Dan Xi

10. 獨活湯

·總結：瘈瘲昏憒

·組成：獨活，羌活，防風，人參，白薇，當歸，芎藭，伏神，遠志，細辛，桂心，菖蒲，半夏，炙甘草

·主治：治風虛瘈瘲，昏憒不覺，或爲寒熱.

·歸經：手少陰，足厥陰藥.

214

·方義：(1)肝主風木而主筋，故瘛瘲爲肝邪. 肝欲散，急食辛以散之.
二活，防風祛風；細辛，桂心溫經；半夏除痰；芎，歸辛散風而溫和血，
血活則風散. 辛以散之，卽辛以補之也.

(2)心爲肝子，肝移熱於心則昏憒，故以人參補心氣；菖蒲開
心竅；茯神，遠志安心神；白薇鹹寒，退熱而治厥. 使風靜火息，血活神
寧，而瘛瘲自已矣.

·來源：丹溪

11. Huo Luo Dan. Network-Quickening Elixir. 活絡丹

·ACTIONS：damp, phlegm, and dead blood

·COMPOSITION：Chuan Wu, Cao Wu, Mo Yao, Ru Xiang, Dan Nan Xing, Di Long

·INDICATIONS：treats wind stroke, numbness of the hand and foot, no recover for long time, damp, phlegm, dead blood in the channels and networks, sudden pain in the one or two spot in the legs and arms.

·CHANNELS ENTERED：The foot greater yin and reverting yin channels. [The spleen and liver]

·Analysis of Formula：Wu He Gao says that (1)Dan Nan Xing is pungent and harsh, therefore this dries damp phlegm. Chuan Wu and Cao Wu are pungent and heat, therefore they disperse cold d amp.

(2) when wind evil wanders in the limbs and joints for long time, blood and vessels congeal, gather, and do not move, therefore Ru Xiang and Mo Yao are used to disperse static blood.

(3) Di Long is engendered from damp earth, this is used to conduct Chuan Wu, Cao Wu, and Dan Nan Xing directly to the place where damp- phlegm gathers.

11. 活絡丹
·總結：溼痰死血
·組成：川烏，草烏，沒藥，乳香，膽星，地龍
·主治：治中風手足不仁，日久不愈，經絡中有溼痰死血，腿臂間忽有
一，二點痛.
·歸經：足太陰，厥陰藥.
·方義：吳鶴皋曰：「(1)膽星辛烈，所以燥溼痰. 二烏辛熱，所以散寒
溼.

(2)風邪注於肢節，久則血脈凝聚不行，故用乳香，沒藥以消瘀血.

(3)蚯蚓溼土所生，欲其引烏星直達溼痰所結之處，大易所謂『同氣相求』也.」

12. Xiao Feng San. Eliminate Wind Powder. 消風散

·**ACTIONS**：wind heat

·**COMPOSITION**：Jing Jie, Fang Feng, Chan Tui, Ren Shen, Gan Cao, Chuan Xiong, Qiang Huo, Jiang Can, Hou Po, Huo Xiang, Fu Ling, Chen Pi.

·**INDICATIONS**：(1) treats wind heat attacking upward, headache, blurred vision, pain in the nape, back, and eyes, contracture, Sneezing, and deep voice.

(2) and severe numbness of the skin, eruption with itch, blood wind in woman.

·**CHANNELS ENTERED**：The foot greater yang and the hand greater yin channels. [The bladder and lung]

·**Analysis of Formula**：(1) The pungent and floating of Qiang Huo, Fang Feng, Jing Jie, and Chuan Xiong treats wind in the head, eyes, and nape.

(2) Jiang Can and Chan Tui are clear and tend to ascend. They eliminate wind in the skin.

(3) Huo Xiang and Hou Po eliminate malign and disperse fullness.

(4) Ren Shen, Fu Ling, Gan Cao, and Chen Pi supplement the right qi and regulate the middle. Then wind evil is unable to stay.

12. 消風散

·總結：風熱

·組成：荊芥，防風，蟬蛻，人參，甘草，川芎，羌活，殭蠶，厚朴，藿香，茯苓，陳皮.

·主治：(1)治風熱上攻，頭目昏痛，項背拘急，鼻嚏聲重.

(2)及皮膚頑麻，癮疹瘙癢，婦人血風.

·歸經：此足太陽手太陰藥

·方義：(1)羌，防，荊，芎之辛浮，以治頭目項背之風.

(2)殭蠶，蟬蛻之清揚，以去皮膚之風.

(3)藿香，厚朴；以去惡散滿.

(4)參，苓，甘，橘；以輔正調中，使風邪無留壅也.

216

13. Qing Kong Gao. Clear Sky Paste. 清空膏

·**ACTIONS**：head wind and headache

·**COMPOSITION**：Qiang Huo, Chuan Xiong, Chai Hu, Fang Feng, Huang Qin, Huang Lian, Gan Cao

·**INDICATIONS**：(1) treats unbiased and hemilateral headache for long time.

(2) and wind damp and heat that are congested in the head and eyes.

(3) and incessant brain pain.

·**MODIFICATIONS**：(1) for lesser yin headache, add Xi Xin.

(2) for greater yin headache, a pulse that is moderate, and phlegm, eliminate Qiang Huo, Fang Feng, Chuan Xiong, and Gan Cao, and add Ban Xia.

(3) for no recover of hemilateral headache after taking of decoction, reduce Qiang Huo, Fang Feng, Chuan Xiong to the half, and add Chai Hu (double).

(4) if there is spontaneous sweating, heat effusion, aversion to heat, and thirst, this is yang brightness headache, just give Bai Hu Tang with Bai Zhi.

·**CHANNELS ENTERED**：The foot greater yang and lesser yang channels. [The bladder and gall bladder]

·**Original Source**：Dan Xi

13. 清空膏

·總結：頭風頭痛

·組成：羌活, 川芎, 柴胡, 防風, 黃芩, 黃連, 甘草

·主治：(1)治正偏頭痛, 年深不愈.

(2)及風濕熱上壅頭目.

(3)及腦苦痛不止.

·加減：(1)少陰頭痛：加細辛.

(2)太陰頭痛, 脈緩有痰：去羌活, 防風, 川芎, 甘草 加半夏.

(3)如偏頭痛服之不愈：減羌活, 防風, 川芎一半, 加柴胡一倍.

(4)如自汗發熱惡熱而渴, 此陽明頭痛：只與白虎湯加白芷.

·歸經：此足太陽少陽藥.

217

·煎服法：茶調如膏，白湯送下．

·來源：丹溪

14. Wei Feng Tang. Stomach Wind Decociton. 胃風湯

·**ACTIONS**：stomach wind

·**COMPOSITION**：Ren Shen, Bai Zhu, Fu Ling, Dang Gui, Chuan Xiong, Shao Yao, Rou Gui.

·**INDICATIONS**：(1) treats wind-cold exploiting vacuity, wind cold visiting the stomach and intestines, swill diarrhea, non-transformation of food, and intestinal wind with blood.

(2) also treats that wind vacuity in that case one can eat, clenched jaw, convulsions, muscular cramp, face swelling, this is called stomach wind.

·**CHANNELS ENTERED**：The foot yang brightness and reverting yin channels. [The stomach and liver]

·**Analysis of Formula**：(1) Stomach wind means that when the stomach is vacuous, wind evil exploits the vacuity.

(2) Wind is related with liver wood. Wind can restrain spleen earth, therefore Ren Shen, Bai Zhu, and Fu Ling are used to supplement spleen qi and boost the stomach.

(3) Dang Gui and Chuan Xiong nourish liver blood and regulate construction.

(4) Shao Yao drains the liver and can harmonize the spleen.

(5) Rou Gui disperses wind and can pacify wood, therefore this can check diarrhea and treat wind damp.

(6) Bai Zhu and Fu Ling can invigorate the spleen and eliminate damp.

(7) Chuan Xiong and Rou Gui can enter blood and expel wind.

14. 胃風湯

·總結：胃風

·組成：人參, 白朮, 茯苓, 當歸, 川芎, 芍藥, 肉桂．

·主治：(1)治風冷乘虛, 客於腸胃, 飧泄注下, 完穀不化及腸風下血．

(2)又治風虛能食, 牙關緊閉, 手足瘈瘲, 肉瞤面腫, 名曰胃風．

·歸經：此爲足陽明厥陰藥．

218

·方義：(1)胃風者：胃虛而風邪乘之也.

(2)風屬肝木，能剋脾土，故用參，朮，茯苓以補脾氣而益胃.

(3)當歸，川芎：以養肝血而調榮.

(4)芍藥：瀉肝而能和脾.

(5)肉桂：散風而能平木，故能住瀉泄而療風濕也.

(6)又曰：白朮. 茯苓：能壯脾而除濕.

(7)川芎，肉桂：能入血而驅風.

15. Shang Zhong Xia Tong Yong Tong Feng Wan. Upper, Middle and Lower General Use Pills for Wind-Pain. 上中下通用痛風丸

·ACTIONS：pain wind

·COMPOSITION：Huang Bai, Cang Zhu, Long Dan Cao, Fang Ji, Tao Ren, Hong Hua, Chuan Xiong, Qiang Huo, Bai Zhi, Wei Ling Xian, Nan Xing, Gui Zhi, Shen Qu.

·INDICATIONS：pain wind, this could with cold, damp, heat, phlegm, blood. This formula can treat all of them.

·CHANNELS ENTERED：This formula generally treats pain wind.

·Analysis of Formula：(1) Huang Bai clears heat. Cang Zhu dries damp. Long Dan Cao drains fire. Fang Ji moves water. The four herbs treat damp with heat.

(2) Nan Xing dries phlegm and disperses wind. Tao Ren and Hong Hua activate blood and transform stasis. Chuan Xiong is qi medicinal in blood. Therefore this treats phlegm with blood.

(3) Qiang Huo eliminates wind in one hundred joints. Bai Zhi eliminates wind in the head and face. Gui Zhi and Wei Ling Xian eliminate wind in the arms and legs. The four herbs treat wind.

(4) Shen Qu disperse old and accumulated qi in the middle.

(5) this formula disperses wind to diffuse the upper part, drains heat and disinhibits damp to treat diarrhea in the lower part, activates blood and disperses stagnation to regulates the middle. Therefore this formula is generally used to treat pain wind with various patterns.

·Original Source：Dan Xi

15. 上中下通用痛風丸

·總結：痛風

·組成：黃柏，蒼朮，龍膽草，防己，桃仁，紅花，川芎，羌活，白芷，威靈仙，南星，桂枝，神麴，麵糊丸．

·主治：痛風有寒，有濕，有熱，有痰，有血之不同，此爲通治．

·歸經：此治痛風之通劑也．

·方義：(1)黃柏：清熱；蒼朮：燥濕；龍膽：瀉火；防己：行水．　四者所以治濕與熱也．

　　　　(2)南星：燥痰散風；桃仁，紅花：活血化瘀；川芎：爲血中氣藥，所以治痰與血也．

　　　　(3)羌活：祛百節之風；白芷：祛頭面之風；桂枝，威靈仙：祛臂脛之風；四者所以治風也．

　　　　(4)加神麴者：所以消中州陳積之氣也．

　　　　(5)疏風以宣於上，瀉熱利濕以泄瀉於下，活血.消滯以調其於中，所以能兼治而通用也，證不兼者，以意消息可矣．

·來源：丹溪

16. Shi Guo Gong Yao Jiu Fang. Statesmam Shi's Medicinal-Wine Formula. 史國公藥酒方

·**ACTIONS**：wind impediment

·**COMPOSITION**：Qin Jiao, Song Jie, Cang Er Zi, Jia Gen, Qiang Huo, Wan Can sha, Chuan Bi Xie, Fang Feng, Du Zhong, chuan Niu Xi, Gou Qi, Dang Gui, Bie Jia, Hu Jing Gu, Bai Zhu.

·**INDICATIONS**：treats wind stroke, difficult sluggish speech, spasm of the limbs, hemiplegia, wilting, impediment, and numbness.

·**CHANNELS ENTERED**：The foot reverting yin channel. [The liver]

·**Analysis of Formula**：(1) Fang Feng, Qiang Huo, Cang Er Zi, Qin Jiao, Song Jie, Jia Gen, Can Sha, and Bi Xie eliminate wind with drying damp.

　　　　(2) Dang Gui, Gou Qi, Du Zhong, and Niu Xi supplement yin, moisten dryness, tonify blood, and nourish sinew.

　　　　(3) Bai Zhu supplements qi and fortifies the spleen.

　　　　(4) Hu Jing expels wind and invigorates bone.

　　　　(5) Bie Jia also is the herb of blood part of reverting yin. This can boost yin blood and eliminate liver wind. When wind-damp are eliminated, qi and blood get effulgent, then, disease removes.

220

16. 史國公藥酒方
　·總結：風痺
　·組成：秦艽，松節，蒼耳子，茄根，羌活，晚蠶砂，川萆薢，防風，杜仲，川牛膝，枸杞，當歸，鱉甲，虎脛骨，白朮.
　·主治：治中風言語蹇澀，手足拘攣，半身不遂，癱瘓不仁.
　·歸經：此足厥陰藥.
　·方義：(1)防風，羌活，蒼耳，秦艽，松節，茄根，蠶砂，萆薢：既以祛風，兼以燥濕.
　　　　(2)當歸，枸杞，杜仲，牛膝：補陰潤燥，養血營筋.
　　　　(3)白朮：補氣而健脾.
　　　　(4)虎脛：驅風而壯骨.
　　　　(5)鱉甲：亦厥陰血分之藥，能益陰血而去肝風，風濕去，氣血旺，則病除.
　·煎服法：爲粗末，絹袋盛，浸無灰酒，煮熟退火服，每日數次，常令醺醺不斷.

17. Juan Bi Tang. Remove Painful Obstruction Decoction.
蠲痺湯

·**ACTIONS**：wind impediment

·**COMPOSITION**：Gan Cao, Jiang Huang, Huang Qi, Dang Gui, Chi Shao, Fang Feng, Qiang Huo.

·**INDICATIONS**：treats wind stroke, generalized vexed pain, tensed nape and back, cold impediment of the limbs, heaviness of the lumbus and knees, difficulty to move.

·**CHANNELS ENTERED**：The foot greater yang and reverting yin channels. [The bladder and liver].

·**Analysis of Formula**：(1) Pungent can disperse cold, wind can overcome damp. Fang Feng and Qiang Huo eliminate damp and course wind.

　　　　(2) When qi frees, blood is activated, and when blood is activated, wind disperses. Huang Qi and Gan Cao supplement qi and replete Defense.

　　　　(3) Dang Gui and Chi Shao activate blood and harmonize construction.

　　　　(4) Jiang Huang rectify qi in the blood. This can enter the hand and foot and eliminate cold damp.

·**Original Source**：Yan Shi

221

17. 蠲痺湯

　·總結：風痺

　·組成：甘草，片子薑黃，黃耆，當歸，赤芍，防風，羌活.

　·主治：治中風身體煩痛，項背拘急，手足冷痺，腰膝沉重，舉動艱難.

　·歸經：此足太陽陰厥陰藥.

　·方義：(1)辛能散寒，風能勝濕，防風，羌活，除濕而疏風.

　　　　　(2)氣通則血活，血佸則風散，黃耆，炙草補氣而實衛.

　　　　　(3)當歸，赤芍：活血而和營.

　　　　　(4)薑黃理血中之氣，能入手足而袪寒濕.

　·煎服法：加薑棗煎.

　·來源：嚴氏

18. San Bi Tang. Three-Painful Obstruction Decoction. 三痺湯

　·**ACTIONS**：wind, cold, and damp impediment

　·**COMPOSITION**：Huang Qi, Xu Duan, Ren Shen, Fu Ling, Gan Cao, Dang Gui, Chuan Xiong, Bai Shao Yao, Sheng Di Huang, Du Zhong, chuan Niu Xi, Gui Xin, Xi Xin, Qin Jiao, Du Huo, Fang Feng, Sheng Jiang, Da Zao

　·**INDICATIONS**：treats congealed and stagnated qi and blood, spasm of the hand foot, wind, cold, and damp impediment.

　·**CHANNELS ENTERED**：The foot three yin channels.

　·**Analysis of Formula**：(1) 喻嘉言 says that this formula uses Ren Shen and Huang Qi and Si Wu Tang.

　　　　　(2) Fang Feng and Qin Jiao overcome wind damp.

　　　　　(3) Gui Xin overcomes cold.

　　　　　(4) Xi Xin and Du Huo free kidney qi.

　　　　　(5) This formula treats impediment which is caused by the attacking of wind, cold, and damp into vacuous person.

18. 三痺湯

　·總結：風寒溼痺

　·組成：黃耆，續斷，人參，茯苓，甘草，當歸，川芎，白芍，生地，杜仲，川牛膝，桂心，細辛，秦艽，川獨活，防風，生薑，大棗

　·主治：治氣血凝滯，手足拘攣，風寒濕三痺.

222

·歸經：此足三陰藥.

·方義：(1)喻嘉言曰：此方用參者四物一派補藥.

(2)內加防風，秦芁以勝風濕.

(3)桂心以勝寒.

(4)細辛，獨活以通腎氣.

(5)凡治三氣襲虛而成庫患者，宜準諸此.

19. Du Huo Ji Sheng Tang. Angelica Pubescens and Taxillus Decoction. 獨活寄生湯

·**ACTIONS**：wind, cold, and damp impediment

·**COMPOSITION**：Du Huo, Sang Ji Sheng, Ren Shen, Fu Ling, Gan Cao, Dang Gui, Shao Yao, Chuan Xiong, Shu Di Huang, Gui Xin, Du Zhong, Niu Xi, Xi Xin, Fang Feng, Qin Jiao.

·**INDICATIONS**：treats vacuity heat of the liver and kidney, wind-damp attacking the interior, pain in lumbus and knees, cold impediment with forceless, difficulty in bending and stretching.

·**CHANNELS ENTERED**：The foot lesser yin and reverting yin channels. [The kidney and liver]

·**Analysis of Formula**：(1) Du Huo and Xi Xin enters lesser yin to free blood and vessels.

(2) Qin Jiao and Fang Feng course channel and raise yang to eliminate wind.

(3) Sang Ji Sheng boosts qi and blood and eliminates wind-damp.

(4) Du Zhong and Niu Xi fortify bones, strengthens sinew, and secures the lower part.

(5) Chuan Xiong, Dang Gui Shao Yao, and Shu Di Huang activate blood and supplement yin.

(6) Ren Shen, Gui Xin, Fu ling, and Gan Cao boost qi and supplement yang. Pungent and warm supplement qi. When qi and blood are sufficient and wind–damp removes, the liver and kidney get strong and numbness and pain recover.

·**RELATED FORMULA**：Qiang Huo Xu Duan Tang：Du Huo and Sang Ji Sheng are eliminated and Qiang Huo and Xu Duan are added. This treats same things.

·Original **Source**：Tian Jin Yao Fang

223

19. 獨活寄生湯

·總結：風寒溼痺

·組成：獨活，桑寄生，人參，茯苓，甘草，當歸，芍藥，川芎，熟地，桂心，杜仲，牛膝，細辛，防風，秦艽．

·主治：治肝腎虛熱，風濕內攻，腰膝作痛，冷痺無力，屈伸不便．

·歸經：此足少陰厥陰藥．

·方義：(1)獨活，細辛：入少陰通血脈．

(2)偕秦艽，防風：疏經升陽以祛風．

(3)桑寄生：益氣血，祛風濕．

(4)偕杜仲，牛膝：健骨強筋而固下．

(5)芎，歸，芍，地：所以活血而補陰．

(6)參，桂，苓，草：所以益氣而補陽，辛溫以補之，使氣血足而風濕除，則肝腎強而庫痛癒矣．

·變化方：羌活續斷湯：除獨活，寄生，加羌活，續斷，治同．

·來源：千金

20. Chen Xiang Tian Ma Tang. Aquilariae and Gastrodia Decociton. 沈香天麻丸

·**ACTIONS**：fright wind

·**COMPOSITION**：Qiang Huo, Du Huo, Chen Xiang, Tian Ma, Gan Cao, Dang Gui, Chuan Wu Tou, Jiang Can, **Fu Zi**, Yi Zhi Ren, Ban Xia, Fang Feng.

·**INDICATIONS**：treats convulsions due to fright in child, copious phlegm, white eye, epilepsy, muscular spasm.

·**CHANNELS ENTERED**：The foot reverting yin channel. [The liver]

·**Analysis of Formula**：(1) Bao Jian Says that when one is in fear, then the qi moves down, then the essence withdraws, when it withdraws, then the upper burner becomes closed. Qiang Huo and Du Huo are bitter and warm, they conduct qi to move upward, and enter greater yang as channel conductor, therefore acts as sovereign.

(2) Tian Ma and Fang Feng disperse with pungent and warm. Dang Gui and Gan Cao supplement qi and blood with pungent and warm, and also nourish stomach qi, therefore acts as minister.

(3) Fu Zi and Yi Zhi Ren are great pungent and warm, move yang and retreat yin, and also treat visit-cold invading the stomach. The kidney governs the five humors, enter the spleen to be drool. Sheng Jiang and Ban Xia dry

224

damp and move phlegm, therefore act as assistant. Chen Xiang is pungent, warm, and heavy, but the qi is light. This eliminates timidity and quiets spirit, acting as courier.

·**Original Source**：Bao Jian

20. 沈香天麻丸

·總結：驚風

·組成：羌活，獨活，沉香，天麻，甘草，當歸，川烏頭，僵蠶，附子，益智仁，半夏，防風.

·主治：治小兒因驚發搐，痰多眼白，癇瘲筋攣.

·歸經：此足厥陰藥.

·方義：(1)寶鑑曰：『恐則氣下精怯而上焦閉』；以羌活，　獨活：苦溫引氣上行，又入太陽爲引，故以爲君.

　　　　(2)天麻，防風：辛溫以散之，當歸，甘草辛溫以補氣血不足，又養胃氣，故以爲臣.

　　　　(3)烏附，益智：大辛溫，行陽退陰，又治客寒犯胃，腎主五液，入脾爲涎；以生薑，半夏燥濕行痰，故以爲佐，沉香辛溫體重氣輕，去怯安神爲使.

·來源：寶鑑

21. Tong Ding San. Unblock the Vertex Powder.　通頂散

·**ACTIONS**：wind stroke.

·**COMPOSITION**：Li Lu, Ren Shen, Chuan Xiong, Xi Xin, Shi Gao, Gan Cao.

·**INDICATIONS**：treats initial wind stroke, loss of consciousness, clenched jaw.

·**CHANNELS ENTERED**：The hand greater and lesser yin channels. [The lung and heart]

·**Analysis of Formula**：(1) Wu He Gao says that wind stroke and loss of consciousness mean that the disease is already severe, this cannot be treated with common medicinal to open the congestion.

　　　　(2) therefore Li Lu with Ren Shen and Xi Xin is used. The character between Li Lu and Ren Shen with Xi Xin is different but used together.

　　　　(3) The lung suffers when qi counterfolws upward, therefore Shi Gao is used.

225

(4) The neutral of Gan Cao moderates qi.

(5) Chuan Xiong is used to clear qi and disinhibit orifices.

21. 通頂散

　·總結：中風取嚔

　·組成：藜蘆, 人參, 川芎, 細辛, 石膏, 甘草.

　·主治：治初中風, 不知人事, 口噤不開.

　·歸經：此手太陰少陰藥也.

　·方義：(1)吳鶴皋曰：『中風不省人事, 病已極矣, 非平藥可以開其壅塞.』

　　　　　(2)故用藜蘆與人參, 細辛, 取其相反而相用也.

　　　　　(3)肺苦氣上逆, 故石膏之重以墜之.

　　　　　(4)甘草之平以緩之.

　　　　　(5)芎藭之用取其清氣利竅而已.

22. Wu Mei Ca Ya Fang. Mume Formula to Bore Teeth. 烏梅擦牙方

·**ACTIONS**：clenched jaw

·**COMPOSITION**：Wu Mei

·**INDICATIONS**：treats wind strike and clenched jaw.

·**CHANNELS ENTERED**：The foot yang brightness and reverting yin channels. [The stomach and liver]

·**Analysis of Formula**：The sour first enters sinew, wood can restrain earth.

22. 烏梅擦牙方

　·總結：口噤

　·組成：烏梅

　·主治：治中風口噤不開.

　·歸經：此足陽明厥陰藥也.

　·方義：酸先入筋, 木能尅土.

226

Chapter 10. Cold-Dispelling Formulas. 祛寒之劑

1. Li Zhong Tang. Regulate the Middle Decoction. 理中湯

·**ACTIONS** : warms the middle

·**COMPOSITION** : Ren Shen, Bai Zhu, Gan Cao (mix fried), Gan Jiang

·**INDICATIONS** : (1) treat scold damage greater yin disease, spontaneous ly diarrhea without thirst, aversion to cold [more that heat effusion], retching, a bdominal pain, sloppy stool, a pulse that is sunken and forceless.

(2) or reversal cold and contracture, or chest bind and vomiting of worms, and contracting of cold, sudden turmoil.

·**MODIFICATIONS** : (1) for spontaneous diarrhea and abdominal pain, a dd Mu Xiang.

(2) for curled-up lying, generalized heaviness, incessant diarrhea, add Fu Zi.

(3) for vomiting, eliminate Bai Zhu and add Ban Xia and Jiang Z hi (juice of ginger).

(4) for stirring qi below the umbilicus, eliminate Bai Zhu and ad d Gui Zhi.

(5) for palpitations, add Fu Ling.

(6) for yin jaundice, add Yin Chen.

(7) for cold chest bind, add Zhi Shi.

(8) for often diarrhea without pain, double the dose of Bai Zhu.

(9) for thirst, double the dose of Bai Zhu.

(10) for abdominal fullness, eliminate Gan Cao.

·**CHANNELS ENTERED** : The foot greater yin channel. [The spleen]

·**Analysis of Formula** : (1) Ren Shen supplements qi and boosts the splee n, therefore acts as sovereign.

(2) Bai Zhu fortifies the spleen and dries damp, therefore acts as minister.

(3) Gan Cao harmonizes the middle and supplements earth, there fore acts as courier.

(4) Gan Jiang warms the stomach and disperses cold, therefore a cts as courier.

·**RELATED FORMULA** : (1) When three liang of this formula with Fu

Zi, this is called Fu Zi Li Zhong Tang, treats cold damage with abdominal pain, generalized pain, contracture of the limbs.

⑵ When Zhi Shi and Fu Ling are added and made into Pills with Honey, this is called Zhi Shi Li Zhong Wan, treats cold repletion chest bind, verging on expiry due to pain, distention chest diaphragm, the hand that is not allowed to get near, no recover after using of Da Xian Xiong Tang.

⑶ When Gan Cao is eliminated and Fu Ling, Chuan Jiao, and Wu Mei are added, this is called Li Zhong An Hui Wan, treats stomach cold and vomiting of worms.

⑷ When Gui Zhi is added and Gan Cao is doubled, this is called Gui Zhi Ren Shen Tang, treats that when in greater yang disease, the exterior pattern has not yet been eliminated, and precipitation has been used repeatedly, and consequently, there is incessant complex diarrhea, a hard glomus below the heart, and both the exterior and the interior are not resolved,

⑸ When Huang Lian and Fu Ling are added, this is called Lian Li Tang, treats summerheat damage, diarrhea, and thirst.

⑹ When Chen Pi and Fu Ling are added, this is called Bu Zhong Tang, treats diarrhea. For incessant diarrhea, add Fu Zi. For aversion to eat and no transformation of food, add Sha Ren.

⑺ When Dang Gui, Bai Shao Yao, Chen Pi, Hou Po, and Chuan Xiong are added, this is called Wen Wei Tang, treats anxiety, depression, the congealed qi of the spleen and lung, distention and fullness with qi surging upward, inability to get food down.

⑻ When Huang Qi, Bai Shao Yao, Chen Pi, and Huo Xiang are added, this is called Huang Qi Tang.

⑼ When Qing Pi and Chen Pi are added, this is called Zhi Zhong Tang, treats the above pattern with abdominal fullness, glomus, oppression, and food accumulation.

·**Original Source**：Zhong Jing

1. 理中湯
   ·總結：溫中
   ·組成：人參, 白朮, 炙甘草, 乾薑
   ·主治：⑴治傷寒太陰病, 自利不渴, 寒多而嘔, 腹痛糞溏, 脈沈無力.
   　　　　⑵或厥冷拘急, 或結胸吐蚘, 及感寒霍亂.
   ·加減：⑴自利腹痛者, 加木香.
   　　　　⑵蜷臥沈重, 利不止, 加附子.

228

(3)嘔吐：去白朮, 加半夏, 薑汁.

(4)臍下動氣：去朮, 加桂.

(5)悸：加茯苓.

(6)陰黃：加茵陳.

(7)寒結胸：加枳實.

(8)不痛利多者：倍白朮.

(9)渴者：倍白朮.

(10)腹滿：去甘草.

·歸經：此足太陰之藥也(脾)

·方義：(1)人參：補氣益脾, 故以爲君.

(2)白朮：健脾燥溼, 故以爲臣.

(3)甘草：和中補土, 故以爲使.

(4)乾薑：溫胃散寒, 故以爲使.

·變化方：(1)本方三兩, 加附子一枚, 名附子理中湯, 治中寒腹痛, 身痛, 四肢拘急.

(2)本方加枳實, 茯苓, 蜜丸, 名枳實理中丸, 治寒實結胸欲絶, 胸膈高起, 手不可近, 用大陷胸不瘥者.

(3)本方去甘草, 加茯苓, 川椒, 烏梅, 名理中安蚘丸, 治胃寒吐蚘.

(4)本方加桂枝, 倍甘草, 名桂枝人參湯, 治太陽表證不除, 而數下之, 協熱而利, 利下不止, 心下痞硬, 表裏不解者.

(5)本方加黃連, 茯苓, 名連理湯, 治傷暑瀉而口渴.

(6)本方加陳皮, 茯苓, 名補中湯, 治泄瀉. 瀉不已者, 加附子. 惡食, 食不化, 加砂仁.

(7)本方加當歸, 白芍, 陳皮, 厚朴, 川芎, 入薑煎, 名溫胃湯, 治憂思鬱結, 脾肺氣凝, 脹滿上衝, 飲食不下.

(8)本方加黃耆, 白芍, 陳皮, 藿香, 名黃耆湯.

(9)本方加青皮, 陳皮, 名治中湯, 治前証腹滿痞悶, 兼食積者.

·來源：仲景

2. Si Ni Tang. Counterflow Cold Decoction. 四逆湯

·ACTIONS：yin pattern and reverse flow. Si Ni means reverse flow of the limbs. Again when Gan Jiang (two liang) is added, this is Tong Mai Si Ni Ta

229

ng.

·**COMPOSITION** ： Gan Cao (mix fried), Gan Jiang, Fu Zi

·**INDICATIONS** ： (1) treats three yin cold damage, generalized pain, abd ominal pain, clear-food diarrhea, aversion to cold without thirst, reversal cold o f the limbs.

(2) or instead, there is absence of aversion to cold, reddish compl exion, and vexation and agitation, this means interior cold exterior heat.

(3) or dry retching, or sore throat, a pulse that is sunken, faint, fine, and ver ging on expiry.

·**MODIFICATIONS** ： (1) Sore throat means that yin qi binds in the upper, add Jie Geng (one liang) to disinhibit throat.

(2) Abdominal pain indicates that true yin is insufficient, add Sh ao Yao (two liang) to restrain yin.

(3) When diarrhea stops and a pulse is sunken without coming o ut, add Ren Shen (two liang) to assist yang and supplement qi and blood.

(4) Reddish complexion indicates that repelled yang is in the upp er, add Cong Bai to free yang.

(5) For vomiting, add Sheng Jiang (two liang) to disperses revers al qi.

·**CHANNELS ENTERED** ： The foot lesser yin channel [the kidney]

·**Analysis of Formula** ： (1) Excessive cold in the interior should be treated with sweet and heat, therefore the great heat of Gan Jiang and Fu Zi effuses yan g qi and disperses cold evil in the exterior.

(2) Gan Cao also disperses cold during supplementing the middl e. And also this moderates the action of Gan Jiang and Fu Zi.

·**RELATED FORMULA** ： (1) When Bai Zhu and Da Zao are added, this is called Zhu Fu Tang, treats contention of wind and damp, generalized vexed p ain, and cold strike with reversal heart pain.

(2) When Gan Cao is eliminated, this is called Gan Jiang Fu Zi T ang, treats relapsing sweating after precipitation, agitation in day quiet in night, absence of retching, thirst, and exterior pattern, a pulse that is sunken and faint, absence of great heat effusion. Also treats cold strike, reversal flow, dizziness, absence of sweating, spontaneous sweating as water flows, exterior heat, vexati on and agitation, yin exuberance repelling yang.

(3) Jian Fu Tang with Dang Gui and Rou Gui is called Jiang Fu Gui Tang, again when Ren Shen and Gan Cao added, this is called Jiang Fu Gu i Gui Shen Gan Tang.

230

(4) When Gan Cao is eliminated and Cong Bai are added, this is called Bai Tong Tang. Again when Ren Niao (human urine) and pig's bile are added, this is called Bai Tong Jia Ren Niao Zhu Dan Zhi Tang.

(5) When Ren Shen (one liang) is added, this is called Si Ni Jia Ren Shen Tang, treats when there is aversion to cold and a pulse that is faint, then diarrhea, and the diarrhea stops and there is blood collapse. Again when Fu Ling (Six Liang) is added, this is called Fu Ling Si Ni Tang, treats that after the promotion of sweating, if precipitation is used and the disease still does not resolve, and there is vexation and agitation.

(6) When Gan Jiang is eliminated and Shao Yao (three liang) is added, this is called Shao Yao Gan Cao Fu Zi Tang, treats that when sweating is promoted, if the disease dose not resolve, and instead there is aversion to cold, this is because of vacuity.

(7) When Fu Zi is eliminated, Gan Cao (four Liang) and Gan Jiang (two liang) are used, this is called Gan Cao Gan Jiang Tang, treats that when in cold damage, the pulse is floating and there is spontaneous sweating, frequent urination, heart vexation, mild aversion to cold, and hypertonicity of the feet, but gui zhi [tang] is given in order to attack the exterior, this is an error. If the person is given this formula, there will be reversal, dryness in the throat, vexation and agitation, and counterflow vomiting, so one should use gan cao gan jiang tang to restore yang. If a counterflow patient recovers, and the feet become warm, one can use Shao Yao Gan Cao Tang and the feet will then be able to stretch.

(8) When Wu Zhu Yu is added, this is called Zhu Yu Si Ni Tang, treats abdominal pain in reverting and lesser yin.

(9) When Dang Gui and Mu Tong are added, this is called Dang Gui Si Ni Tang, treats cold contraction, reversal cold of the limbs, a pulse that is fine and verging on expiry, and cold abdominal colic in woman and man, cold below the umbilicus, pain stretching into the lumbus and crotch.

(10) When Yin Chen is added, this is called Yin Chen Si Ni Tang, treats yin jaundice.

(11) When Sheng Mai San and Chen Pi are added, this is called Fui Yang Fan Ben Tang, treats yin exuberance repelling yang.

(12) When Rou Gui, Liang Jiang, and Ban Xia are added, this is called Jiang Shui San, treats vacuous cold, water diarrhea, cold sweating, a pulse that is faint, vomiting in severe case, this is urgent disease.

·**Original Source** ：Zhong Jing

2. 四逆湯

231

·總結：陰證厥逆. 四逆者四肢厥逆也. 再加乾薑二兩則通脈四逆湯.

·組成：炙甘草, 乾薑, 附子

·主治：(1)治三陰傷寒, 身痛腹痛, 下利清穀, 惡寒不渴, 四肢厥冷.

　　　　(2)或反不惡寒, 面赤煩躁, 裏寒外熱.

　　　　(3)或乾嘔, 或咽痛, 脈沈微細欲絕.

·加減：(1)咽痛：陰氣上結也, 加桔梗一兩以利咽.

　　　　(2)腹痛者：真陰不足也, 加芍藥二兩以斂陰.

　　　　(3)利止脈不出：加人參二兩, 以助陽補氣血.

　　　　(4)面赤者：格陽于上也, 加葱九莖以通陽.

　　　　(5)嘔吐：加生薑二兩以散逆氣.

·歸經：此足少陰之藥也(腎)

·方義：(1)寒淫于內, 治以甘熱, 故以薑, 附大熱之劑, 伸發陽氣, 表散寒邪.

　　　　(2)甘草亦補中散寒之品, 又以緩薑, 附上僭也.

·變化方：(1)本方加白朮, 大棗, 名朮附湯, 治風溼相搏, 身體煩疼, 及中寒發厥心痛.

　　　　(2)本方除甘草, 名乾薑附子湯, 治下後復汗, 晝躁夜靜, 不嘔不渴, 無表證, 脈沈微, 無大熱者. 又治中寒厥逆, 眩仆無汗, 或自汗淋漓, 及外熱煩躁, 陰盛格陽.

　　　　(3)薑附湯加當歸, 肉桂, 入蜜和服, 名薑附歸桂湯. 再加人參, 甘草, 名薑附歸桂參甘湯.

　　　　(4)本方除甘草, 加葱四莖, 名白通湯. 再加人尿, 豬膽汁, 名白通加人尿豬膽汁湯.

　　　　(5)本方加人參一兩, 名四逆加人參湯, 治惡寒, 脈微復利, 利止亡血. 再加茯苓六兩, 名茯苓四逆湯, 治汗下後病不解而煩躁.

　　　　(6)本方除乾薑, 加芍藥三兩, 名芍藥甘草附子湯, 治傷寒發汗不解, 反惡寒者, 虛故也.

　　　　(7)本方除附子, 用甘草四兩, 乾薑二兩, 名甘草乾薑湯, 治傷寒脈浮, 自汗, 小便數, 心煩, 微惡寒, 腳攣急, 用桂枝湯誤攻其表, 得之便厥, 咽中乾, 煩躁吐逆, 與此湯以復其陽. 若厥愈足溫者, 更作芍藥湯以和其陰其腳即伸. 芍藥, 甘草各四兩.

　　　　(8)本方加吳茱萸, 名茱萸四逆湯, 治厥陰少陰腹痛.

　　　　(9)本方加當歸, 木通, 名當歸四逆湯. 治感寒手足厥冷, 脈細欲節, 及男婦寒疝, 臍下冷, 引腰胯而痛.

　　　　(10)本方加茵陳, 名茵陳四逆湯, 治陰黃.

232

(11)本方加生脈散，陳皮，名回陽返本湯，治陰盛格陽.

(12)本方加官桂，良薑，半夏，名漿水散，治虛寒水瀉，冷汗，脈微，甚者嘔吐，此為急病.

·來源：仲景

3. Dang Gui Si Ni Tang. Tangkuei Counter Flow Cold Decoction. 當歸四逆湯

·**ACTIONS**： cold reversal in reverting yin

·**COMPOSITION**：Dang Gui, Da Zao, Tong Cao, Gan Cao (mix fried), Gui Zhi, Xi Xin, Shao Yao

·**INDICATIONS**：reverting yin cold damage, reversal cold of the limbs, a pulse that is fine and verging of expiry.

·**CHANNELS ENTERED**：The foot reverting yin channel. [The liver]

·**Analysis of Formula**：(1) Cheng Wu Ji says that vessel is the storehouse of blood. Every blood belongs to the heart. To free vessels, one should first supplement the heart and boost blood.

(2) Bitter first enters the heart. The bitter of Dang Gui assists heart blood.

(3) When the heart suffers from slackening, quickly consume sour [flavor] to contract it again. The sour of Shao Yao contract heart qi.

(4) When the liver suffers from tensions, quickly consume sweet [flavor] to relax [these tensions]. Da Zao, Gan Cao, and Tong Cao relax yin blood.

·**Original Source**：Zhong Jing

3. 當歸四逆湯

·總結：厥陰寒厥

·組成：當歸，大棗，通草，炙甘草，桂枝，細辛，芍藥

·主治：厥陰傷寒，手足厥寒，脈細欲絕

·歸經：此足厥陰藥也(肝)

·方義：(1)成無己曰：「脈者，血之府也. 諸血皆屬于心，通脈者必先補心益血.

(2)苦先入心，當歸之苦，以助心血.

(3)心苦緩，急食酸以收之，芍藥之酸，以收心氣.

(4)肝苦急，急食甘以緩之，大棗，甘草，通草，以緩陰血.

233

4. Si Ni San. Counterflow Cold Powder. 四逆散

·**ACTIONS**：yang pattern and reversal heat. This is cold formula to harm onize and release.

·**COMPOSITION**：Gan Cao (mix fried), Zhi Shi, Chai Hu, Shao Yao

·**INDICATIONS**：(1) in cold damage lesser yin pattern, yang evil enters t he interior, there is counterflow cold of the limbs.

(2) or cough, or palpitations, or inhibited urination, or pain in the abdomen, or diarrhea with rectal heaviness.

·**MODIFICATIONS**：(1) for abdominal pain, add Fu Zi.

(2) for diarrhea with rectal heaviness, add Xie Bai.

(3) for inhibited urination, add Fu Ling.

(4) for palpitations, add Gui Zhi.

(5) for cough, add Wu Wei Zi and Gan Jiang.

·**CHANNELS ENTERED**：The foot lesser yin channel. [The kidney]

·**Analysis of Formula**：(1) In cold damage, yang heat is major pathomechanism, if yang evil passes into the interior and reversal cold of the limbs occurs, this is the i mage of yin progress. This condition cannot be precipitated with herbs with bitter a nd cold, this can damage yang.

(2) Nei Jing says that every counterfolw of the limbs cannot be tr eated with precipitation. Therefore Gan Cao is used to regulate counterfolw qi. Zhi Shi drains bind heat. Chai Hu disperses yang evil. Shao Yao contract origin yin. Herbs with pungent, bitter, sour, and cold are used to harmonize and releas e, then yang qi gets to spread over the limbs.

(3) This formula is same meaning with Xiao Chai Hu Tang whic h treats lesser yang.

·**Original Source**：Zhong Jing

4. 四逆散
·總結：陽證厥熱. 此和解之寒劑.
·組成：炙甘草, 枳實, 柴胡, 芍藥
·主治：(1)傷寒少陰證, 陽邪入裏, 四逆不溫.
　　　　(2)或欬或悸, 或小便不利, 或腹中痛, 或泄利下重.
·加減：(1)腹痛：加附子.

(2)泄利下重：加薤白.

(3)小便不利：加茯苓.

(4)悸：加桂枝.

(5)欬：加五味子, 乾薑, 併主下利.

·歸經：此足少陰藥也(腎)

·方義：(1)傷寒以陽為主, 若陽邪傳裏而成四逆, 有陰進之象, 又不敢以苦寒下之, 恐傷其陽.

(2)經曰：「諸四逆不可下也.」故用甘草調逆氣；枳實泄結熱；柴胡散陽邪；芍藥收元陰. 用辛苦酸寒之藥以和解之, 則陽氣敷布于四末矣.

(3)此與少陽之用小柴胡意同, 有兼證者, 視加法為治.

·煎服法：等分為末, 水調飲.

·來源：仲景

5. Zhen Wu Tang. True Warrior Decoction. 眞武湯

·ACTIONS：disperses cold and disinhibits water.

·COMPOSITION：Fu Ling, Bai Zhu, Sheng Jiang, Fu Zi, Shao Yao

·INDICATIONS：(1) When in lesser yin cold damage, there is abdominal pain, inhibited urination, heaviness and pain in the limbs, and spontaneous diarrhea, it means there is water qi, and the person may cough, or have uninhibited urination, or diarrhea, or retching.

(2) and when in greater yang disease, sweating has been promoted and sweat issues but the disease dose not resolve, the person still has heat effusion, and there is palpitations below the heart, dizzy head, generalized twitching, and the person is quivering and about to fall, qi vacuity with aversion to cold.

·MODIFICATIONS：(1) for contention of water and cold, cough, add Wu Wei Zi, Xi Xin, and Gan Jiang.

(2) for inhibited urination, eliminate Fu Ling.

(3) for diarrhea, eliminate Shao Yao, add Gan Jiang.

(4) for retching, eliminate Fu Zi, add Sheng Jiang (double).

·CHANNELS ENTERED：The foot lesser yin channel. [The kidney].

·Analysis of Formula：(1) Fu Ling and Bai Zhu supplement earth and disinhibit water. They can quell kidney evil and treat heart palpitations.

(2) Sheng Jiang and Fu Zi restore yang and boost defense. They

235

can invigorate true fire and expel vacuous cold.

       (3) The sour of Shao Yao contracts, this can restrain yin, harmonize construction, and allay abdominal pain.

  ·**Original Source**：Zhong Jing

5. 眞武湯

  ·總結：散寒利水.

  ·組成：茯苓, 白朮, 生薑, 附子, 芍藥

  ·主治：(1)少陰傷寒腹痛, 小便不利, 四肢沈重疼痛, 自下利者, 此爲有水氣, 或欬或嘔, 或小便利.

       (2)又太陽病發汗, 汗出不解, 仍發熱, 心悸頭眩, 筋惕肉瞤, 振振欲擗地, 氣虛惡寒.

  ·加減：(1)水寒相博, 咳者：加五味子細辛乾薑.

       (2)小便利：去茯苓.

       (3)下利：去芍藥, 加乾薑.

       (4)嘔：去附子, 加生薑一倍.

  ·歸經：此足少陰藥(腎).

  ·方義：(1)茯苓, 白朮：補土利水, 能伐腎邪而療心悸.

       (2)生薑, 附子：回陽益衛, 能壯眞火而遂虛寒.

       (3)芍藥：酸收, 能斂陰和營, 而止腹痛.

  ·來源：仲景

6. Bai Tong Jia Ren Niao Zhu Dan Zhi Tang. Scallion Yang -Freeing Decoction Plus Pig's Bile. 白通加人尿豬膽汁湯

  ·**ACTIONS**：yin pattern with reverse flow.

  ·**COMPOSITION**：Cong Bai, Gan Jiang, Fu Zi, Rn Niao (human urine), Zhu Dan Zhi (pig's bile)

  ·**INDICATIONS**：(1) treats that when in lesser yin disease there is diarrhea and the pulse is faint, give Bai Tong Tang. When there is incessant diarrhea, reverse-flow, an absent pulse, dry retching, and vexation, Bai Tong Jia Zhu Dan Tang governs.   (2) If after taking the decoction, the pulse suddenly moves outward, this means death, but if the pulse continues to be faint, this means life.

236

·**MODIFICATIONS**：(1) abdominal pain indicates that true yin is insuffi
cient. Eliminate Cong Bai and add Shao Yao to contract yin.

(2) for retching, add Sheng Jiang to disperse counterfolw qi.

(3) for sore throat, add Jie Geng to disinhibit throat.

(4) when diarrhea stops and a pulse does not come out, add Ren
Shen to assist yang.

·**CHANNELS ENTERED**：The lesser yin channel. [The kidney]

·**Analysis of Formula**：(1) Cong Bai is pungent and assists yang qi.

(2) The heat of Gan Jiang and Fu Zi disperses yin cold.

(3) After taking of Bai Tong Tang, if there is no response, this in
dicates that yin exuberance repels yang, heat medicinal cannot reach lesser yin,
therefore Ren Niao and Zhu Dan Zhi are added as channel conductor.

(4) Ren Niao and Zhu Dan Zhi are same family with yin. Bitter e
nters the heart and frees vessels, cold supplements the liver and harmonizes yin.
After taking this formula, cold qi of medicinal are already dispersed and heat qi
of medicinal act.

·**Original Source**：Zhong Jing

6. 白通加人尿豬膽汁湯

·總結：陰證厥逆.

·組成：葱白, 乾薑, 附子, 人尿, 豬膽汁

·主治：(1)治少陰病下利脈微者, 與白通湯；利不止, 厥逆無脈, 乾嘔
而煩, 白通加人尿豬膽汁湯主之.

(2)服此湯後, 脈暴出者死, 微續者生.

·加減：(1)腹痛者 真陰不足也：去葱 加芍藥以斂陰.

(2)嘔者：加生薑以散逆.

(3)咽痛者：加桔梗以利咽.

(4)利止脈不出：加人參以助陽.

·歸經：此足少陰藥. (腎)

·方義：(1)葱白：之辛以助陽氣.

(2)薑附之熱以散陰寒.

(3)白通湯服而不應者, 乃陰盛格拒乎陽藥, 不能達於少陰,
故加人尿, 豬膽汁爲引.

(4)取其陰同類, 苦入心而通脈, 寒補肝而和陰, 下咽之後冷
體旣消, 熱性便發, 性且不違, 而致大益.

·來源：仲景

237

7. Wu Zhu Yu Tang. Evodia Decoction. 吳茱萸湯

·**ACTIONS** ： vomiting, diarrhea, and cold reverse.

·**COMPOSITION** ： Wu Zhu Yu, Sheng Jiang, Da Zao, Ren Shen

·**INDICATIONS** ： (1) treats that when in yang brightness pattern, there is a desire to retch after eating, Evodia Decoction (wu zhu yu tang) governs. But when taking the decoction makes the retching more severe, this pattern belongs to the upper burner.

(2) When in lesser yin disease there is vomiting and diarrhea, counterflow cold of the extremities, and vexation and agitation, as if the person is about to die

(3) When in reverting yin pattern, there is dry retching, ejection of drool and foam, and headache.

·**CHANNELS ENTERED** ： The foot reverting and lesser yin and yang brightness channels. [The liver, Kidney, and stomach]

·**Analysis of Formula** ： (1) A desire to retch after eating in yang brightness pattern is treated with the pungent of Wu Zhu Yu and Sheng Jiang by warming the stomach, dispersing cold, and descend qi downward.

(2) The sweet of Ren Shen and Da Zao moderate the spleen, boost qi, and harmonize the middle.

(3) 喻嘉言 says that I already explained that retching and vomiting are in both greater yang and yang brightness. If a desire to retch after eating belongs to stomach cold, this is different with the heat pattern of greater yang with aversion to cold and retching. I am anxious that one treats cold retching and vomiting with cold herbs. And after taking of Wu Zhu Yu Tang, if the pattern gets severe, this belongs to greater yang heat evil.

(4) If in lesser yin pattern there is vomiting and reverse qi, and vexation and agitation on the verge of expiry, this means that the qi in the kidney counterfolws upward, this is urgent sign.

(5) Therefore Wu Zhu Yu is used to disperse cold and descend counterfolw.

(6) Ren Shen, Sheng Jiang, and Da Zao assist yang and supplement earth. This prevents yin cold from invading the upper and warms the channel and the middle.

(7) Wu Zhu Yu is the original herb of reverting yin, therefore this treats the counterfolw of liver qi, vomiting of drool, and headache.

·**RELATED FORMULA** ： Wu Zhu Yu Jia Fu Zi Tang, treats cold abdominal colic, lumbar pain, pain stretching and pulling into the balls, and a pulse i

238

n cubit that is sunken and slow.
　　·**Original Source**：Zhong Jing

7. 吳茱萸湯
　　·總結：吐利寒厥.
　　·組成：吳茱萸, 生薑, 大棗, 人參
　　·主治：(1)治陽明證食穀欲嘔, 吳茱萸湯主之, 若得湯反劇者, 則屬上
焦.
　　　　　(2)少陰證吐利, 手足厥冷, 煩躁欲死.
　　　　　(3)厥陰證, 乾嘔吐涎, 頭痛.
　　·歸經：此足厥陰少陰陽明藥.(肝腎胃)
　　·方義：(1) 治陽明食穀欲嘔者 吳茱, 生薑之辛以溫胃散寒下氣.
　　　　　(2)人參, 大棗之甘以緩脾益氣和中.
　　　　　(3)喻嘉言曰：『此明嘔有太陽, 亦有陽明, 若食穀而嘔者屬
胃寒, 與太陽之惡寒嘔逆原爲熱證之不同. 恐誤以寒藥治寒嘔也, 若服吳
茱萸反劇者, 則仍屬太陽熱邪, 而非胃寒明矣.』
　　　　　(4)若少陰證吐逆厥逆, 至於煩燥欲死, 腎中之氣上逆, 將成
危候.
　　　　　(5)故用吳茱萸散寒降逆.
　　　　　(6)人參, 薑, 棗助陽補土, 使陰寒不得上干溫經而兼溫中也.
　　　　　(7)吳茱萸爲厥陰本藥, 故又治肝氣上逆, 嘔涎頭痛.
　　·變化方：吳茱萸加附子湯：加附子；治寒疝腰痛, 牽引睪丸, 尺脈沉
遲.
　　·來源：仲景

8. Da Jian Zhong Tang. Major Center fortifying Decoction.
　　大建中湯

　　·**ACTIONS**：cold strike and abdominal pain
　　·**COMPOSITION**：Gan Jiang, Shu Jiao, Ren Shen, Yi Tang.
　　·**INDICATIONS**：treats great cold pain in the heart and chest, retching w
ith inability to eat food, surging upward of cold qi in the abdomen, which reach
es to abdominal skin, upper and lower abdominal pain with not allowing anyon
e even to get near.
·**CHANNELS ENTERED**：The foot greater yin and yang brightness channels. [T

he spleen and stomach]

  ·**Analysis of Formula**：(1) Gan Jiang is pungent and heat. This frees the heart, assists yang, expels cold, and disperses counterfolw qi.

  (2) Shu Jiao is pungent and heat, enters the lung to disperse cold, enters the spleen to warm the stomach, and enters life gate to supplement fire.

  (3) The sweet of Yi Tang can supplement earth, the relaxing character can harmonize the middle.

  (4) Ren Shen is sweet and warm, this greatly supplements the qi of the spleen and lung.

  (5) Generally in human, the middle qi is considered as main, herbs with pungent, sweet, and heat are used to warm and fortify the middle organ, greatly eliminate the yin of the lower burner, and restore the yang of the upper burner.

  ·**Original Source**：Jin Gui Yao Lue

8. 大建中湯

  ·總結：中寒腹痛

  ·組成：乾薑, 蜀椒, 人參, 飴糖.

  ·主治：治心胸中大寒痛, 嘔不能飲食, 腹中寒氣上衝, 皮起出見, 有頭足上下痛不可觸近者.

  ·歸經：此足太陰陽明藥.(脾胃)

  ·方義：(1)乾薑辛熱通心, 助陽逐冷散逆.

  (2)蜀椒辛熱, 入肺散寒, 入脾暖胃, 入腎命補火.

  (3)飴糖甘能補土, 緩可和中.

  (4)人參甘溫, 大補脾肺之氣.

  (5)蓋人之一身以中氣爲主, 用辛辣甘熱之藥, 溫建其中臟, 以大祛下焦之陰, 而復其上焦之陽也.

  ·煎服法：煎去渣, 內飴糖一升, 微煎溫服.

  ·來源：金匱

9. Shi Si Wei Jian Zhong Tang. Fourteen-Ingredient Center fortifying Decoction. 十四味建中湯

·**ACTIONS**：vacuity detriment and yin macula.

·**COMPOSITION**：Ban Xia, Fu Zi, Rou Cong Rong, Mai Men Dong, Ren Shen, Bai Zhu, Fu Ling, Gan Cao (mix fried), Dang Gui, Shu Di Huang, Bai

240

Shao Yao, Chuan Xiong, Huang Qi, Rou Gui

·**INDICATIONS**：(1) treats insufficient qi and blood, vacuity detriment, consumption, shortness of breath, a tendency to lie down, and consumption.

(2) and yin pattern with macula, severe cold, and a pulse that is faint.

·**CHANNELS ENTERED**：The foot three yin and yang brightness channels. [The spleen, kidney, liver, and stomach]

·**Analysis of Formula**：(1) Ban Xia harmonizes the stomach and fortifies the spleen.

(2) Huang Qi boosts the stomach, fortifies the spleen, and supplements the middle.

(3) Si Jun Zi Tang supplements yang, therefore this boosts qi.

Si Wu Tang supplements yin therefore this tonifies blood. When yin and yang are regulated and harmonious, blood and qi quiet in their position.

(4) Mai Men Dong clears the heart and moistens the lung.

(5) Rou Cong Rong supplements life gate and insufficient ministerial fire.

(6) Gui Zhi and Fu Zi conduct vacuous fire to return the origin.

(7) This formula is modified from Shi Quan Da Bu Tang. This formula strengthens the middle and treats macula in the exterior.

·**RELATED FORMULA**：(1) Ba Wei Da Jian Zhong Tang, ：Fu Ling, Bai Zhu, Mai Men Dong, Chuan Xiong, Shu Di Huang, Rou Cong Rong are eliminated, treats same things.

9. 十四味建中湯

·總結：虛損陰斑

·組成：半夏, 附子, 肉蓯蓉, 麥冬, 人參, 白术, 茯苓, 炙甘草, 當歸, 熟地, 白芍, 川芎, 黃耆, 肉桂

·主治：(1)治氣血不足, 虛損勞瘠, 短氣嗜臥, 欲成勞瘵.

(2)及陰證發斑, 寒甚脈微.

·歸經：此足三陰陽明氣血藥也.

·方義：(1)半夏：和胃健脾.

(2)黃耆：益胃健脾, 補中首藥.

(3)四君：補陽所以益氣,

四物：補陰所以養血, 陰陽調和則血氣各安其位矣.

241

(4)麥冬：清心潤肺.

(5)菠蓉：補命門相火之不足.

(6)桂附：引失守之火歸元.

(7)於十全大補中而有加味，要以強中而戰外也.

·變化方：(1)八味大建中湯：除茯苓，白朮，麥冬，川芎，熟地，菠蓉
治同.

10. Xiao Jian Zhong Tang. Minor Center fortifying Decocti on. 小建中湯

·**ACTIONS**：warms the middle and disperses cold

·**COMPOSITION**：Gui Zhi, Shao Yao, Gan Cao (mix fried), Sheng Jian g, Da Zao.

·**INDICATIONS**：(1) When in cold damage, the yang pulse is rough and the yin pulse is string like, as a rule, there should be acute pain in the abdomina l

(2) When in cold damage that has lasted for two of three days, th ere is palpitation and vexation in the heart.

(3) generally treats vacuity taxation, palpitations, epistaxis, interi or acute abdominal pain, dream emission, consumption of essence, aching pain of the limbs, vexed heat in the hand and foot, dry throat and mouth, vacuity tax ation, and jaundice.

·**CHANNELS ENTERED**：The foot greater yin and yang brightness channels. [The spleen and stomach]

·**Analysis of Formula**：(1) Zhun Sheng says that the spleen resides in the center of four organs, engenders and brings up the construction and defense, frees and moves the humor and liquid. When this gets irregulartied, this fails to bring up and move t he construction and defense. This formula warms and fortifies the middle organ, th erefore this is called Jian Zhong.

(2) When the spleen has a desire to relax, quickly consume sweet [flavor] to relax [these tensions]. Therefore Yi Tang acts as sovereign and Gan Cao acts as minister.

(3) Gui Zhi is pungent and heat. The pungent disperses and mois tens the insufficient construction and defense. Shao Yao is sour and cold, the so ur can both contract and drain. In this disease, the humor does not free, therefor e Shao Yao is used to free the fluid and make the fluid move, therefore Gui Zhi and Shao Yao act as assistant.

(4) Sheng Jiang is pungent and warm, Da Zao is sweet and warm, the stomach is the origin of the defense, the spleen is the root of the construction. Zhen Jing says that construction comes out from the middle burner, defense engenders in the upper burner, therefore defense is related with yang and is boosted by pungent, construction is related with yin and is supplemented with sweet, when pungent and sweet combine, the spleen and stomach get strong and the construction and defense free, therefore Sheng Jiang and Da Zao act as courier.

·**RELATED FORMULA**：Huang Qi Jian Zhong Tang is Xiao Jian Zhong Tang with Huang Qi. This treats vacuity taxation and insufficiency, also treats that when in scold damage after promotion of sweating, there is generalized pain, exterior vacuity, aversion to cold, and a pulse that is slow and weak.

·**Original Source**：Zhong Jing

10. 小建中湯

　·總結：溫中散寒

　·組成：桂枝, 芍藥, 炙甘草, 生薑, 大棗.

　·主治：(1)傷寒陽脈濇, 陰脈弦, 腹中急痛.

　　　　　(2)傷寒二, 三日, 心悸而煩.

　　　　　(3)通治虛勞悸衄, 裏急腹痛, 夢遺失精, 四肢酸痛, 手足煩熱, 咽燥口乾, 虛勞黃疸.

　·歸經：此足太陰陽明藥.(脾胃)

　·方義：(1)準繩曰：脾居四臟之中, 生育榮衛通行津液, 一有不調, 則失所育所行也. 必以此湯溫建中臟, 故名建中.

　　　　　(2)脾欲緩急食甘以緩之, 故以飴糖爲君, 甘草爲臣.

　　　　　(3)桂枝辛熱, 辛散也, 潤也榮衛不足, 潤而散之, 芍藥酸寒, 酸收也, 泄也津液不通, 收而行之, 故以桂芍爲佐.

　　　　　(4)生薑辛溫, 大棗甘溫, 胃者.胃之源, 脾者榮之本. 鍼經曰：榮出中焦, 衛生上焦, 是以衛爲陽, 益之必以辛, 榮爲陰, 補之必以甘, 辛甘相合, 脾胃建而榮衛通, 故以薑棗爲使.

　·變化方：黃耆建中湯...加黃耆. 治虛勞不足, 亦治傷寒汗後身痛, 表虛惡寒, 脈遲弱者.

　·來源：仲景

11. Bai Zhu Fu Zi Tang. Ovate Atratylodes and Aconite Decoction. 白朮附子湯

·**ACTIONS**：wind vacuity and dizziness.

·**COMPOSITION**：Bai Zhu, **Fu Zi**, Gan Cao

·**INDICATIONS**：treats wind vacuity, dizziness, extreme pain, inability to taste food. This formula is used to warm the flesh, supplement the middle, and boost essence qi.

·**CHANNELS ENTERED**：The foot greater yin and lesser yin channels. [The spleen and kidney]

·**Analysis of Formula**：⑴ 喻嘉言 says that when kidney qi is vacuous, external wind invades, wind with yin turbid-qi in the kidney counterflows upward and attacks the upper part, therefore heavy head, dizziness, and pain that is unendurable occur, and if this pattern combines with spleen vacuity, inability to taste food occurs. This indicates that the spleen and kidney are vacuous and external wind enters the organs.

⑵ Fu Zi warms the water organ, Bai Zhu warms the earth organ, once water and earth get warm, the qi of turbid yin goes downward and the vacuity of the spleen and kidney spontaneously disappear.

·**RELATED FORMULA**：⑴ Gan Cao Fu Zi Tang. This formula is Bai Zhu Fu Zi Tang with Gui Zhi, but Sheng Jiang and Da Zao are not used. This treats the contention of wind and damp, generalized vexed pain, sweating, aversion to wind, inhibited urination, or generalized mild swelling.

⑵ Chuang Xiong Chu Shi Tang.：This is Bai Zhu Fu Zi Tang with Rou Gui and Chuan Xiong. This treats cold-damp, headache, and dizziness.

·**Original Source**：Jin Xiao Fang

11. 白朮附子湯

·總結：風虛頭眩

·組成：白朮, 附子, 甘草

·主治：治風虛頭眩, 苦極, 食不知味, 用此暖肌補中, 益精氣.

·歸經：此足太陰少陰藥. (脾腎)

·方義：⑴喻嘉言曰：腎氣空虛, 外風入之, 風夾腎中陰濁之氣, 厥逆上攻, 頭間重眩, 極苦難耐, 兼以脾虛不知食味, 以脾腎兩虛, 風以入臟.

⑵但用附子暖其水臟, 白朮暖其土臟, 水土一暖則濁陰之氣盡趨於下, 而二虛自止.

·變化方：⑴甘草附子湯：加桂枝, 不用薑棗. 治風濕相博, 一身煩痛, 汗出惡風, 小便不利或身微腫.

　　　　　⑵芎朮除濕湯：加官桂, 川芎. 治寒濕頭痛眩運.

·煎服法：薑棗煎.

·來源：近效方

12. Yi Yuan Tang. Benefit the Basal Decoction. 益元湯

·**ACTIONS**：yin agitation

·**COMPOSITION**：Gan Cao, Gan Jiang, Fu Zi, Ren Shen, Mai Men Dong, Wu Wei Zi, Ai Ye, Cong Bai, Huang Lian, Zhi Mu

·**INDICATIONS**：treats reddish complexion, generalized heat effusion, agitation without vexation, desire to drink water with inability to swallow, this is called Dai Yang (upcast yang) pattern.

·**CHANNELS ENTERED**：The foot lesser yin channel. [The kidney]

·**Analysis of Formula**：(1) Fu Zi, Gan Jiang, and Ai Ye return yang.

　　　　(2) Ren Shen and Gan Cao supplement yang vacuity and retreat yin fire, because Gan Cao eliminates great heat.

　　　　(3) Huang Lian breaks fire that floods upward.

　　　　(4) Zhi Mu enriches yin in the lower.

　　　　(5) Mai Men Dong and Wu Wei Zi supplement the lung and clears the heart.

　　　　(6) with Ren Shen engenders the vessel.

·**Original Source**：Huo Ren

12. 益元湯

·總結：陰躁

·組成：甘草, 薑, 附子, 人參, 麥冬, 五味子, 艾葉, 葱白, 黃連, 知母

·主治：治面赤身熱, 不煩而躁, 飲水不入口, 名戴陽證.

·歸經：此足少陰藥. (腎)

·方義：⑴附子, 乾薑, 艾葉：回陽之藥.

　　　　⑵協以人參, 甘草：補其陽虛, 退其陰火, 所謂甘草除大熱.

　　　　⑶黃蓮：以折泛上之火.

245

(4)知母：以滋在下之陰.

(5)麥冬, 五味：補肺清心.

(6)合人參：以生其脈.

·來源：活人

13. Hui Yang Jiu Ji Tang. Restore and Revive the Yang Decoction. 回陽救急湯

·**ACTIONS**：cold reversal in three yin.

·**COMPOSITION**：Fu Zi, Gan Jiang, Rou Gui, Ren Shen, Bai Zhu, Fu Ling, Ban Xia, Chen Pi, Gan Cao, Wu Wei Zi

·**INDICATIONS**：(1) treats cold strike in three yin at early stage, absence of generalized heat effusion, absence of headache, aversion to cold, chilling, reversal cold of the limbs, pulling clothes and covering oneself with it spontaneously, curled-up lying posture, abdominal pain, vomiting, and diarrhea, absence of thirst.

(2) or blue colored nails and lip, drool foaming at the mouth, a pulse that is not felt or is sunken, slow, and forceless.

·**MODIFICATIONS**：(1) for no feeling of pulse, add Zhu Dan Zhi.

(2) for diarrhea, add Sheng Ma and Huang Qi.

(3) for vomiting, add Jiang Zhi (juice of ginger).

(4) for vomiting of drool foaming, add Wu Zhu Yu (stir-bake with salt).

·**CHANNELS ENTERED**：The foot three yin channels. [The liver, kidney, and spleen]

·**Analysis of Formula**：(1) When cold strikes in three yin, yin gets exuberant and yang gets weak, therefore the heat of Fu Zi, Gan Jiang, and Rou Gui eliminates yin cold.

(2) Liu Jun Zi Tang is the formula for warming and supplementing, this assists yang qi.

(3) Wu Wei with Ren Shen can generate the vessels.

(4) She Xiang frees orifices.

13. 回陽救急湯

·總結：三陰寒厥

·組成：附子, 乾薑, 肉桂, 人參, 白朮, 茯苓, 半夏, 陳皮, 甘草, 五

味子

　　·主治：⑴治三陰中寒，初病身不熱，頭不痛，惡寒戰慄，四肢厥冷，引衣自蓋，踡臥沈重，腹痛吐瀉，口中不渴.

　　　　　　⑵或指甲唇青，口吐涎沫，無脈，或脈沈遲無力.

　　·加減：⑴無脈：加豬膽汁.

　　　　　　⑵泄瀉：加升麻，黃耆.

　　　　　　⑶嘔吐：加薑汁.

　　　　　　⑷吐涎沫：加鹽炒吳茱萸.

　　·歸經：此足三陰藥.(肝腎脾)

　　·方義：⑴寒中三陰，陰盛則陽微，故以附子，薑，桂辛熱之劑祛其陰寒.

　　　　　　⑵而以六君溫補之藥助其陽氣.

　　　　　　⑶五味和人參可以生脈.

　　　　　　⑷加麝香者通其竅也.

14. Si Shen Wan. Four-Miracle Pill. 四神丸

·**ACTIONS**：kidney diarrhea and spleen diarrhea.

·**COMPOSITION**：Po Gu Zhi, Rou Dou Kou, Wu Wei Zi, Wu Zhu Yu

·**INDICATIONS**：treats kidney diarrhea and spleen diarrhea.

·**CHANNELS ENTERED**：The foot lesser yin channel. [The kidney]

·**Analysis of Formula**：⑴ Po Gu Zhi is pungent, bitter, and great warm, this can supplement ministerial fire to free sovereign fire, then exuberant fire can engender earth, therefore acts as sovereign.

　　⑵ Rou Dou Kou is pungent and warm. This can move qi, disperse food, warm the stomach, and secure the intestines. The salty of Wu Wei Zi can supplement the kidney and the sour can astringe essence.

　　⑶ Wu Zhu Yu is pungent and heat. This eliminates damp and dries the spleen, this can enter the qi part of lesser and reverting yin and supplements fire.

　　⑷ Sheng Jiang warms the stomach. Da Zao supplements earth, therefore they block water.

　　⑸ Generally enduring diarrhea is due to debilitated fire in kidney life, this is not only due to the spleen and stomach, therefore if the original yang of the lower burner is greatly supplemented, fire will be exuberant and earth strong, then water is controlled and is unable to move frenetically again.

·**RELATED FORMULA**：(1) Wu Wei Zi Sa, this is composed of Wu W
ei Zi and Wu Zhu Yu. This treats same things.

(2) Er Shen Wan, this is composed of Po Gu Zhi and Rou Dou K
ou. This treats same things.

14. 四神丸
　·總結：腎瀉脾瀉
　·組成：破故紙，肉荳蔻，五味子，吳茱萸
　·主治：治腎瀉脾瀉.
　·歸經：此足少陰藥也.(腎)
　·方義：(1)破故紙：辛苦大溫，能補相火以通君火，火旺乃能生土，故
以爲君.

(2)肉蔻：辛溫能行氣消食，暖胃固腸，五味鹹能補腎，酸能
澀精.

(3)吳茱：辛熱除濕燥脾，能入少陰厥陰氣分而補火.

(4)生薑：暖胃；大棗：補土，所以防水.

(5)蓋久瀉皆由於腎命火衰，不能專責脾胃，故大補下焦元陽，
使火旺土强，則能制水而不復妄行矣.
　·變化方：(1)五味子散：單用五味子，吳茱萸. 治同.

(2)二神丸：單用破故紙，肉豆蔻. 治同.

15. Gan Ying Wan. Response Pills. 感應丸

·**ACTIONS**：cold accumulation, and diarrhea and dysentery
·**COMPOSITION**：Ding Xiang, Mu Xiang, Xing Ren, Rou Dou Kou, G
an Jiang, Ba Dou, Bai Chao Shuang
·**INDICATIONS**：treats old or new cold accumulation, diarrhea, and dys
entery.
·**CHANNELS ENTERED**：The hand and foot yang brightness channels.
[The large intestine and stomach]
·**Analysis of Formula**：(1) Rou Dou Kou repels cold, disperses food, desc
ends qi, and harmonizes the middle.

(2) Ding Xiang warms the stomach, assists yang, diffuses conges
tion, and eliminates aggregation.

(3) Mu Xiang ascends and descends every qi, harmonizes the spl
een, and courses the liver.

248

(4) Xing Ren descends qi, disperses cold, moistens dryness, and dissipates accumulation.

(5) Bao Jiang can expels intractable cold and disperse glomus.

(6) Ba Dou is good at breaking deep cold, attacking hardness, and diffusing stagnation

(7) Bai Chao Shuang harmonizes the middle and disperses with warm. This also can disperse accumulation and treat dysentery. This acts as assistant.

15. 感應丸
　·總結：寒積瀉痢
　·組成：丁香, 木香, 杏仁, 肉豆蔻, 乾薑, 巴豆, 百草霜
　·主治：治新舊冷積瀉痢等證.
　·歸經：此手足陽明藥. (大腸胃)
　·方義：(1)肉蔻：逐冷消食, 下氣和中.
　　　　　(2)丁香：暖胃助陽, 宣壅除癖.
　　　　　(3)木香：升降諸氣, 和脾疏肝.
　　　　　(4)杏仁：降氣散寒, 潤燥消積.
　　　　　(5)炮薑：能逐錮冷而散痞通關.
　　　　　(6)巴豆：善破沉寒而奪門宣滯.
　　　　　(7)百草霜：和中溫散亦能消積治痢爲佐也.

16. Dao Qi Tang. Conduct the Qi Decoction. 導氣湯

·ACTIONS：cold abdominal colic

·COMPOSITION：Wu Zhu Yu, Xiao Hui Xiang, Mu Xiang, Chuan Lian Zi

·INDICATIONS：treats cold abdominal colic with pain.

·CHANNELS ENTERED：The foot reverting yin and lesser yin channels. [The liver and kidney]

·Analysis of Formula：(1) Chuan Lian Zi is bitter and cold. This can enter the liver and soothe sinew, so this treats hypertonicity. And this also can abduct the heat of the small intestine and bladder to move downward through urination, this is main herb to treat mounting (Shan).

(2) Mu Xiang ascends and descends every qi, frees and disinhibits triple burner, courses the liver, and harmonizes the spleen.

249

(3) Xiao Hui Xiang can enter the kidney and the bladder to warm cinnabar field and eliminate cold qi.

(4) Wu Zhu Yu enters the qi part of the liver and kidney qi to dry damp and eliminate cold.

(5) The three of them are pungent and warm. They are used to diffuse and free qi and disinhibit urination, then cold removes and damp eliminates.

16. 導氣湯
　·總結：寒疝
　·組成：吳茱萸, 茴香, 木香, 川楝子
　·主治：治寒疝疼痛.
　·歸經：此足厥陰少陰藥. (肝腎)
　·方義：(1)川楝：苦寒, 能入肝舒筋, 使無攣急之苦, 又能導小腸膀胱之熱, 從小水下行, 爲治疝之主藥.
　　　　(2)木香：升降諸氣, 通利三焦, 疏肝而和脾.
　　　　(3)茴香：能入腎與膀胱, 暖丹田而祛冷氣.
　　　　(4)吳茱萸：入肝腎氣分, 燥濕而除寒.
　　　　(5)三者皆辛溫之品, 用以宣通其氣, 使小便小利, 則寒去而濕除也.

17. Tian Tai Wu Yao San. Top-Quality Lindera Powder. 天臺烏藥散

·**ACTIONS**： small intestinal mounting (shan) qi

·**COMPOSITION**：Wu Yao, Bing Lang, Mu Xiang, Qing Pi, Xiao Hui Xiang, Liang Jiang, Ba Dou, Chuan Lian Zi.

·**INDICATIONS**：treats small intestinal mounting (shan) qi, its pain stretching to the umbilicus and abdomen.

·**CHANNELS ENTERED**：The foot reverting yin and the hand greater yin channels. [The liver and lung]

·**Analysis of Formula**：(1) Wu Yao disperses cold qi of the bladder and can disperse swelling and relieve pain.

(2) Chuan Lian Zi can abduct the evil heat of the small intestine to move downward through urination.

(3) Mu Xiang and Qing Pi move qi and pacify the liver.

250

(4) Liang Jiang and Xiao Hui Xiang disperse cold and warm the kidney.

(5) Bing Lang can descend water and promote rupture.

(6) Ba Dou is pungent, heat, and harsh. This breaks blood accumulation and cold accumulation.

(7) This formula move qi, eliminate damp, and disperse cold.

17. 天臺烏藥散
　·總結：小腸疝氣
　·組成：烏藥，檳榔，木香，青皮，茴香，良薑，巴豆，川楝子.
　·主治：治小腸疝氣，牽引臍腹疼痛.
　·歸經：此足厥陰手太陰藥.(肝肺)
　·方義：(1)烏藥：散膀胱冷氣，能消腫止痛.
　　　　　(2)川楝：能導小腸邪熱，由小便下行.
　　　　　(3)木香，青皮：行氣而平肝.
　　　　　(4)良薑，茴香：散寒而暖腎.
　　　　　(5)檳榔：性如鐵石，能下水，潰堅.
　　　　　(6)巴豆：辛熱. 破血瘕，寒積.
　　　　　(7)皆行氣祛濕散寒之品也.

18. Shan Qi Fang. Mounting Qi Formula. 疝氣方

·**ACTIONS**：mounting(shan)qi with pain.
·**COMPOSITION**：Wu Zhu Yu, Zhi Zi, Shan Zha, Zhi Ke, Li Zhi He.
·**INDICATIONS**：mounting(shan) qi with pain.
·**CHANNELS ENTERED**：The foot reverting yin channel. [The liver]
·**Analysis of Formula**：(1) Wu Zhu Yu enters the qi part of reverting yin qi to warm the liver and expel.

(2) Shan Zhi Zi drains the fire heat of triple burner through the bladder.

(3) Zhi Ke moves qi and breaks concretion.

(4) Shan Zha disperses stasis and rubs accumulation.

(5) Li Zhi He looks like the balls. This can enter the liver and kidney to repel cold and disperse stagnation, therefore this is used as channel conductor.

251

18. 疝氣方
　　·總結：疝氣疼痛
　　·組成：吳茱萸, 梔子, 山楂, 枳殼, 荔枝核.
　　·主治：疝氣疼痛.
　　·歸經：此足厥陰藥.(肝)
　　·方義：(1)吳茱：入厥陰氣分, 溫肝逐寒.
　　　　　　(2)山梔：瀉三焦之火熱, 由膀胱出.
　　　　　　(3)枳殼：行氣而破癥.
　　　　　　(4)山楂：散瘀而磨積.
　　　　　　(5)荔枝：雙結, 行類睪丸, 能入肝腎辟寒散滯, 故假之以爲
引也.
　　·來源：丹溪

Chapter 11. Summerheat-Clearing Formulas. 清暑 之劑

1. Si Wei Xiang Ru Yin. Four Ingredient Elsholtzia Beverage. 四味香薷飲

·**ACTIONS**：disperses summerheat and harmonizes the spleen

·**COMPOSITION**：Huang Lian, Bian Dou, Xiang Ru, Hou Po

·**INDICATIONS**：treats all kinds of common cold and summerheat qi, steaming heat effusion in the skin, headache, heavy-head, spontaneous sweating, fatigued and cumbersome limbs, or vexation and thirst, or vomiting and diarrhea.

·**CHANNELS ENTERED**：The hand lesser yin, the hand and foot greater yin, and the foot yang brightness channels. [The kidney, lung, spleen, and stomach]

·**Analysis of Formula**：(1) Huang Lian is bitter and cold, can enter the heart and spleen to clear heat and eliminate vexation.

(2) Bian Dou is sweet and bland, can disperse the summerheat and damp of the spleen and stomach, descend turbid, and raise clear [qi].

(3) Xiang Ru is pungent, warm, and aromatic, can enter the qi part of the spleen and lung to effuse yang qi through dispersing steaming heat of the skin.

(4) Hou Po is bitter and warm, eliminates damp and disperses fullness through resolving congealing binds in the heart and abdomen.

·**RELATED FORMULA**：(1) When Bian Dou is eliminated, this is called Huang Lian Xiang Ru Yin, treats damage to summerheat with exuberant heat, thirst, heart vexation, or defecation with flesh blood.

(2) When Huang Lian is eliminated, this is called San Wu Xiang Ru Yin, treats damage to summerheat with retching and diarrhea.

Again Fu Ling and Gan Cao are added to this, this is called Wu Wu Xiang Ru Yin, expels summerheat and harmonizes the middle.

Again Mu Gua is added, this is called Lie Wei Xiang Ru Yin, treats damage to summerheat with damp exuberance.

Again Ren Shen, Huang Qi, Bai Zhu, and Chen Pi are added, this is called Shi Wei Xiang Ru Yin, treats summerheat and damp with internal damage, heavy-headedness, vomiting and diarrhea, generalized fatigue,

253

loss of consciousness.

        (3) San Wu Xiang Ru Yin with Qiang Huo and Fang Feng treats summerheat with wind strike, falling dawn with rigidity, and convulsion.

        (4) San Wu Xiang Ru Yin with Ge Gen, this is called Xiang Ru Ge Gen Tang, treats damage to wind with cough in summerheat.

        (5) when Fu Shen is added, this treats malaria.

        (6) When Xiang Ru, Bian Dou, Hou Po, Mu Gua, and Gan Cao [in this this formula] are added with Xiang Fu, Chen Pi, Cang Zhu, and Zi Su Ye, this is called Er Xiang San, treats external contraction internal damage, generalized heat effusion, and abdominal distention.

1. 四味香薷飲
   ·總結：散暑和脾
   ·組成：黃連, 扁豆, 香薷, 厚朴
   ·主治：治一切感冒暑氣, 皮膚蒸熱, 頭痛頭重, 自汗肢倦, 或煩渴, 或吐瀉.
   ·歸經：手少陰手足太陰足陽明藥也
   ·方義：(1)黃連苦寒, 能入心脾清熱而除煩也.
        (2)扁豆甘淡, 能消脾胃之暑溼, 降濁而升清.
        (3)香薷辛溫香散, 能入脾肺氣分, 發越陽氣, 以散皮膚之蒸熱.
        (4)厚朴苦溫, 除溼散滿, 以解心腹之凝結.
   ·變化方：(1)本方除扁豆, 名黃連香薷飲, 治中暑熱盛, 口渴心煩, 或下鮮血.
        (2)本方除黃連, 名三物香薷飲, 治傷暑嘔逆泄瀉.
            再加茯苓, 甘草, 名五物香薷飲, 驅暑和中.
            再加木瓜, 名六味香薷飲, 治中暑溼盛.
            再加人參, 黃耆, 白朮, 陳皮, 名十味香薷飲, 治暑溼內傷, 頭重吐利, 身倦神昏.
        (3)三物香薷飲加羌活, 防風, 治中暑兼中風, 僵仆搐搦.
        (4)三物香薷飲加乾葛, 名香薷葛根湯, 治暑月傷風欬嗽.
        (5)本方加茯神, 治瘴瘧.
        (6)本方用香薷, 扁豆, 厚朴, 木瓜, 甘草, 加香附, 陳皮, 蒼朮, 紫蘇, 名二香散, 治外感內傷, 身熱腹脹.

2. Qing Shu Yi Qi Tang. Clear Summerheat and Augment t he Qi Decoction. 清暑益氣湯

·**ACTIONS**：clears summerheat and boosts qi

·**COMPOSITION**：Qing Pi, Chen Pi, Ge Gen, Sheng Ma, Gan Cao (mix fried), Mai Men Dong, Wu Wei Zi, Huang Bai, Ren Shen, Huang Qi, Dang Gui, Shen Qu, Ze Xie, Cang Zhu, Bai Zhu

·**INDICATIONS**：(1) treats the flaming and steaming of damp and heat in long su mmer, cumbersome and fatigue of the limbs, devitalized essence and spirit.

(2) thoracic fullness and hasty breathing, generalized heat effusio n and heart vexation, thirst and aversion to food, spontaneous sweating and gen eralized heaviness, pain in the limbs and body.

(3) rough voidings of reddish urine, sloppy and yellow stool, and pulse that is vacuity.

·**CHANNELS ENTERED**：The hand and foot greater yin, and the foot y ang brightness channels. [The lung, spleen, and stomach]

·**Analysis of Formula**：(1)① Qing Pi pacifies the liver and breaks stagnat ion.

② Chen Pi rectifies qi.

③ Ge Gen raises and resolves fleshy heat and raises cl ear [qi].

④ Gan Cao harmonizes the middle.

⑤ when fire is exuberant, metal gets sick and water de bilitated, therefore Mai Men Dong and Wu Wei Zi are used to preserve the lung an d generate the fluids. Huang Bai drains heat and enriches water.

⑥ Heat damages qi, Ren Shen and Huang Qi boost qi and secure exterior.

⑦ Dang Gui tonifies blood and harmonizes yin.

⑧ Shen Qu digests food and disperses accumulation.

⑨ Ze Xie drains damp-heat and descends turbid.

⑩ Damp damages the spleen, Cang Zhu and Bai Zhu dry damp and strengthen the spleen.

(2) The combination of them boosts qi, strengthens the spleen, el iminates damp, and clears heat.

·**RELATED FORMULA**：(1) When Qing Pi, Ze Xie, and Ge Gen (dry) a re eliminated, this is called Huang Qi Ren Shen Tang, treats summerheat dama ging source qi, fatigue in long summer, thoracic fullness, spontaneous sweating,

255

periodic headache.

      (2) When Bai Zhu, Qing Pi, Mai Men Dong, and Wu Wei Zi are eliminated, Fu Ling, Zhu Ling, Chai Hu, Fang Feng, Qiang Huo, Lian Qiao, and Zhi Mu are added, this is called Bu Gan Tang, treats yin sweating as water, the coldness of anterior part as ice, leg wilting with forceless.

   ·Original Source：Li Dong Yuan

2. 清暑益氣湯
   ·總結：清暑益氣
   ·組成：青皮，陳皮，葛根，升麻，炙甘草，麥冬，五味，黃柏，人參，黃者，當歸，神麴，澤瀉，蒼朮，白朮
   ·主治：⑴治長夏溼熱炎蒸，四肢困倦，精神減少.
          ⑵胸滿氣促，身熱心煩，口渴惡食，自汗身重，肢體疼痛.
          ⑶小便赤濇，大便溏黃而脈虛者.
   ·歸經：手足太陰足陽明藥也
   ·方義：⑴①青皮平肝而破滯.
            ②陳皮理氣.
            ③葛，升解肌熱而升清.
            ④甘草和中.
            ⑤火盛則金病而水衰，故用麥冬，五味以保肺而生津，用黃柏以瀉熱而滋水.
            ⑥熱傷氣，參，者益氣而固表.
            ⑦當歸養血而和陰.
            ⑧神麴化食而消積.
            ⑨澤瀉瀉溼熱而降濁.
            ⑩溼傷脾，二朮燥溼而強脾.
          ⑵合之以益氣強脾，除溼清熱也.
   ·變化方：⑴本方除青皮，澤瀉，乾葛，名黃者人參湯，治暑傷元氣，長夏倦怠，胸滿自汗，時作頭痛.
          ⑵本方除白朮，青皮，麥冬，五味，加茯苓，豬苓，柴胡，防風，羌活，連翹，知母，名補肝湯，治陰汗如水，陰冷如冰，腳痿無力.
   ·來源：東垣

256

3. Sheng Mai San. Generate the Pulse Powder. 生脈散

·**ACTIONS**：preserves the lung and generates vessels.

·**COMPOSITION**：Ren Shen, Mai Men Dong, Wu Wei Zi

·**INDICATIONS**：heat damaging source qi, shortness of breath, fatigue, t hirst, profuse sweating, and lung vacuity with cough.

·**CHANNELS ENTERED**：The hand greater yin and lesser yin channels

·**Analysis of Formula**：(1) The lung controls qi, when lung qi is effulgent, the qi of the four organs are effulgent. Because it is vacuous. Therefore the pulse is verging on expiry and there is shortness of breath.

(2) Ren Shen is sweet and warm, greatly supplements the lung qi, acting as sovereign. Mai Men Dong checks sweating, moistens the lung, enriches water, clears the heart, and drains heat, acting as minister. Wu Wei Zi is sour and warm, restrains the lung, generates the fluids, and gathers dispersed qi, acting as assistant.

(3) Generally the heart controls vessels, the lung faces the hundred vessels, when the lung is supplemented and the heart is cleared, qi gets to be full and the vessels becomes restored, therefore it is said that this generates the vessels.

(4) Flaming and hot weather in summer, effulgent fire overwhelms metal, this is treated with mainly preserving the lung. Taking this in the morning when the temperature is rather clear, can boost qi and eliminate summerheat.

·**RELATED FORMULA**：(1) When Chen Pi and Gan Cao (mix fried) are added, this is called Wu Wei Zi Tang. When this is made into pills, this is Bu Qi Wan, treats lung vacuity, shortage of qi, cough, and spontaneous sweating.

(2) When Huang Q is added as sovereign, and Gan Cao and Jie Geng are added as assistant, this is called Bu Qi Tang, treats qi vacuity, spontaneous sweating, and fearful throbbing. And again when Fu Shen, Yuan Zhi, and Mu Tong are added, this is called Fu Shen Tang, treats vessel vacuity, cough with causing heat pain, inhibited throat with swelling.

·**Original Source**：Tian Jin Yao Fang

3. 生脈散
　·總結：保肺生脈
　·組成：人參, 麥冬, 五味子
　·主治：熱傷元氣, 氣短倦怠, 口渴多汗, 肺虛而欬.
　·歸經：手太陰少陰藥也

·方義：(1)肺主氣，肺氣旺則四臟之氣皆旺，虛故脈絕短氣也.

(2)人參甘溫，大補肺氣爲君. 麥冬止汗，潤肺滋水，清心瀉熱爲臣. 五味酸溫，斂肺生津，收耗散之氣爲佐.

(3)蓋心主脈，肺朝百脈，補肺清心，則氣充而脈腹，故曰生脈也.

(4)夏月炎暑，火旺剋金，當以保肺爲主. 清晨服此，能益氣而袪暑也.

·變化方：(1)本方加陳皮，炙甘草，名五味子湯. 蒸餅爲丸，名補氣丸. 治肺虛少氣，咳嗽自汗.

(2)本方加黃耆者爲君，甘草，桔梗爲佐，名補氣湯，治氣虛自汗怔忡. 再加茯神，遠志，木通，名茯神湯，治脈虛咳則心痛，喉中介介或腫.

·來源：千金

4. Liu Yi San. Six-to-One Powder. 六一散

·**ACTIONS**：disinhibits water and drain fire

·**COMPOSITION**：Hua Shi (six liang), Gan Cao (one liang)

·**INDICATIONS**：(1) treats cold damage and summerheat strike, heat of both exterior and interior, vexation and agitation, thirst, and urinary stoppage.

(2) diarrhea and heat malaria, sudden turmoil with vomiting and diarrhea. This also can promote lactation, treat habitual abortion, and resolve the to xin of wine and food, stone strangury.

·**MODIFICATIONS**：If there is cold in the middle burner, add Liu Huan g (a little bit).

·**CHANNELS ENTERED**：The foot greater yang and the hand greater yi n channels. [The bladder and lung]

·**Analysis of Formula**：(1) The qi of Hua Shi is light, this can resolve the flesh, the material of this is heavy, this can clear and descend, the cold can drain heat, the sli ppery can free orifice, the bland can move water, and makes lung qi to descend and free to the bladder, therefore this can eliminate summerheat, check diarrhea, allay v exation and thirst, and move urine.

(2) Gan Cao is added to harmonizes the middle qi, and also mod erate the cold and slippery character of Hua Shi.

(3) if Chen Sha is added, this settles heart spirit and drains evil h eat of Bing Ding.

(4) Six liang of Hua Shi and One liang of Gan Cao are used, and the numbers of six and one are used to the name of this formula, the meaning is taken from 'one heaven engendering water of six earth'.

·**RELATED FORMULA**：(1) When Chen Sha is added, this is called Yi Yuan San. When Bo He is added, this is called Ji Su San. Qing Dai is added, this is called Bi Yu San, treats same things.

(2) When Hong Qu (five qian) is added, this is called Qing Liu Wan, treats red dysentery. When Gan Jiang (five qian) is added, this is called Wen Liu Wan, treats white dysentery.

(3) When Ce Bai Ye, Che Qian Zi, and Ou Jie (respectively raw) are added, this is called San Sheng Yi Yuan San, treats blood stranguary.

(4) When Niu Huang is added, this treats vacuity vexation and inability to sleep.

(5) When Gan Cao is eliminated and Wu Zhu Yu (one liang) is added, this is called Zhu Yu Liu Yi San, treats damp heat and acid regurgitation.

(6) When Hua Shi is eliminated and Huang Qi (six liang) and Da Zao are added, this is called Huang Qi Liu Yi San, treats every vacuity and insufficiency, night sweating, and wasting-thirst.

·**Original Source**：Liu He Jian's formula

4. 六一散
　·總結：利水瀉火
　·組成：滑石, 甘草
　·主治：(1)治傷寒中暑, 表裏俱熱, 煩躁口渴, 小便不通.
　　　　　(2)瀉痢熱瘧, 霍亂吐瀉, 下乳滑胎, 解酒食毒, 偏主石淋.
　·加減：中寒者, 加硫黃少許.
　·歸經：足太陽手太陰藥也
　·方義：(1)滑石氣輕能解肌, 質重能清降, 寒能瀉熱, 滑能通竅, 淡能行水, 使肺氣降而下通膀胱, 故能袪暑住瀉, 止煩渴而行小便也 .
　　　　　(2)加甘草者, 和其中氣, 又以緩滑石之寒滑也.
　　　　　(3)加辰砂者, 以鎮心神, 而瀉丙丁之邪熱.
　　　　　(4)其數六一者, 取天一生水地六成之之義也.
　·變化方：(1)本方加辰砂少許, 名益元散；　加薄荷少許, 名雞蘇散；加青黛少許, 名碧玉散, 治同.
　　　　　(2)本方加紅麴五錢, 名清六丸, 治赤痢；　加乾薑五錢, 名溫六丸, 治白痢.

259

(3)本方加生柏葉，生車前，生藕節，名三生益元散，治血淋.

(4)本方加牛黃，治虛煩不得眠.

(5)本方除甘草，加吳茱萸一兩，名茱萸六一散，治溼熱吞酸.

(6)本方除滑石，加黃耆六兩，大棗煎，熱服，名黃耆六一散，治諸虛不足，盜汗消渴.

·來源：河間

5. Suo Pi Yin. Amomum Splenic Beberage. 縮脾飲

·**ACTIONS**：rectifies the spleen and clears summerheat

·**COMPOSITION**：Ge Gen (dry), Wu Mei, Sha Ren, Cao Guo, Gan Cao (mix fried), Bian Dou

·**INDICATIONS**：clears summerheat qi, eliminates vexation and thirst, stops vomiting, diarrhea, and sudden turmoil, and damage to wine and food in summerheat.

·**CHANNELS ENTERED**：The foot greater yin and yang brightness channels

·**Analysis of Formula**：In summerheat with damp, damp belongs to spleen earth, summerheat combining with damp evil causes the disease of the spleen and stomach, therefore when treating summerheat, first of all, eliminate the damp.

(1) Ge Gen can raise the clear yang of the stomach and engender the fluid.

(2) Wu Mei clears heat and allays thirst.

(3) Sha Ren and Cao Guo are pungent, aromatic, and warm, and tend to disperse. They disinhibit qi and gratify the spleen, digest wind and food, and disperse damp.

5. 縮脾飲

·總結：理脾清暑

·組成：乾葛，烏梅，砂仁，草果，炙甘草，扁豆

·主治：清暑氣，除煩渴，止吐瀉霍亂，及暑月酒食所傷.

·歸經：足太陰陽明藥也

·方義：暑必兼溼，而溼屬脾土，暑溼合邪，脾胃病矣，故治暑必先去溼.

(1)葛根能升胃中清陽而生津.

260

(2)烏梅清熱解渴.

(3)砂仁, 草果, 辛香溫散, 利氣快脾, 消酒食而散溼.

6. Xiao Shu Wan. Summerheat-Dispersing Wan. 消暑丸

·**ACTIONS**：disinhibits damp and clears summerheat

·**COMPOSITION**：Fu Ling, Ban Xia, Gan Cao

·**INDICATIONS**：treats latent summerheat, vexation and thirst, heat effu
sion, headache, and inhibited spleen and stomach.

·**CHANNELS ENTERED**：The foot greater yin and greater yang channe
ls. [The spleen and bladder]

·**Analysis of Formula**：(1) When the weather is flaming and steaming in long sum
mer, damp-earth governs the weather, therefore summerheat is always with damp.
When there is constipation, vexation and thirst, or vomiting, or diarrhea, this is bec
ause excessive damp makes qi not to diffuse and transform.

(2) This formula does not treat the summerheat but treats the da
mp. Ban Xia and Fu Ling are used to move water. Gan Cao is used to harmoniz
e the middle. Ban Xia is boiled with vinegar, vinegar can open the stomach and
disperse water, this restrains heat and resolves toxin. If both summerheat qi and
damp qi descend through urine, the spleen and stomach get harmonious and ve
xation and thirst spontaneously get to be allayed.

(3) Ju Fang takes the name of this formula as Xiao Shu Wan. Thi
s is called Summerheat-Dispersing Pills, the meaning is profound. This is very
good at damage to summerheat with heat effusion and headache.

·**RELATED FORMULA**：When this formula (one liang) is added with
Huang Lian (two qian), this is called Huang Lian Xiao Shu Wan, treats latent s
ummerheat, vexation and thirst, and lots of heat phlegm.

·**Original Source**：Wang Hai Zang

6. 消暑丸

·總結：利溼清暑

·組成：茯苓, 半夏, 甘草

·主治：治伏暑煩渴, 發熱頭痛, 脾胃不利.

·歸經：足太陰太陽藥也

·方義：(1)長夏炎蒸, 溼土司令, 故暑必兼溼. 證見便祕煩渴, 或吐或
利者, 以溼勝則氣不得施化也.

(2)此方不治其暑而治其溼. 用半夏，茯苓行水之藥. 少佐甘草，以和其中. 半夏用醋煮者，醋能開胃散水，是欲熱解毒也. 使暑氣溼氣俱從小便下降，則脾胃和而煩渴自止矣.

(3)局方取此名消暑丸，意甚深遠. 傷暑而發熱頭痛者，服此尤良.

·變化方：本方一兩，加黃連二錢，名黃連消暑丸，治伏暑煩渴而多熱痰.

·來源：海藏

7. Da Shun San. Great Rectifying Powder. 大順散

·**ACTIONS**：warms the middle and disperses summerheat

·**COMPOSITION**：Gan Jiang, Rou Gui, Xing Ren, Gan Cao

·**INDICATIONS**：treats contracting to summerheat, latent heat, excessive drinking, the spleen and stomach that contract dampness, unseparated water and grain, mutual struggle of the clear and turbid, the counterflow of yin, yang, and qi, sudden turmoil, vomiting, and diarrhea, irregularities of the viscera and bowels.

·**CHANNELS ENTERED**：The foot greater yang channel. [The bladder]

·**Analysis of Formula**：(1) In summer, if drinks cold beverage and eats cold fool too much, this prevents qi diffusing, therefore qi gets to counterfolw and this brings about sudden turmoil, vomiting, and diarrhea.

(2) The spleen and stomach like dryness and are averse to damp, and like warm and are averse to cold.

(3) Gan Jiang and Rou Gui disperse cold and dry damp. Xing Ren and Gan Cao disinhibit qi and regulate the spleen. Generally herbs with pungent, sweet, and a character of dispersing, raises latent yang in yin.

(4) In case of damage summerheat without cold pattern, there is no need to adhere to this formula.

7. 大順散

·總結：溫中散暑

·組成：乾薑, 桂, 杏仁, 甘草

·主治：治冒暑伏熱，引飲過多，脾胃受溼，水穀不分，清濁相干，陰陽氣逆，霍亂吐瀉，臟腑不調.

·歸經：足太陽藥也

262

·方義：(1)夏月過於飲冷食寒，陽氣不得伸越，故氣逆而霍亂吐瀉也.

(2)脾胃者，喜燥而惡溼，喜溫而惡寒.

(3)乾薑，肉桂，散寒燥溼. 杏仁，甘草，利氣調脾. 皆辛甘發散之藥，升伏陽於陰中，亦從治之法也.

(4)如傷暑無寒證者，不可執泥.

·煎服法：等分，先將甘草用白砂炒，次入薑，杏炒過，去砂，合桂爲末，每服二錢.

8. Wu Ling San. Five-Ingredient Powder with Poria. 五苓散

·ACTIONS：contending of summerheat and damp.

·INDICATIONS：treats summerheat entered the heart, heat effusion, great thirst, inhibited urination, contending of summerheat and damp, spontaneous sweating, generalized heaviness.

·MODIFICATIONS：for thirst, eliminate Gui Zhi and add Huang Lian.

·see number 1 in chapter 12. Dampness Rectifying Formulas.

8. 五苓散
·總結：暑溼相搏
·主治：治暑毒入心，發熱大渴，小便不利，及暑溼相搏，自汗身重.
·加減：渴者去桂加黃連.
·見 第12章 利濕之劑 1番

9. Ren Shen Bai Hu Tang. Ginseng White Tiger Decoction. 人參白虎湯

·ACTIONS：summerheat damage in greater yang.

·INDICATIONS：treats summerheat stroke in greater yang, generalized heat effusion, sweating, coldness of the lower limbs, aversion to cold, a pulse that is faint, and thirst.

· see number 4 in chapter 14. Fire Draining Formulas

9. 人參白虎湯
·總結：太陽中暑

263

·主治：治太陽中暍，身熱汗出，足冷惡寒，脈微而渴.
·見 第14章 瀉火之劑 4番 變化方

10. Zhu Ye Shi Gao Tang. Lophatherum and Gypsum Decoction. 竹葉石膏湯

·**ACTIONS**： summerheat damage with thirst

·**INDICATIONS**： summerheat damage with thirst and a pulse that is vacuous.

· see number 5 in chapter 14. Fire Draining Formulas

10. 竹葉石膏湯
   ·總結：傷暑發渴
   ·主治：傷暑發渴脈虛.
   ·見 第14章 瀉火之劑 5番

Chapter 12. Dampness Rectifying Formulas. 利濕之劑

1. Wu Ling San. Five-Ingredient Powder with Poria. 五苓散

·**ACTIONS**：disinhibits damp and drains heat

·**COMPOSITION**：Zhu Ling, Fu Ling, Ze Xie, Bai Zhu, Gui Zhi

·**INDICATIONS**：(1) treats that when in greater yang disease, after sweating is promoted and great sweating issues, if there is dryness in the stomach, vexation and agitation with insomnia, and a desire to drink water, giving a small amount of water will harmonize the stomach qi so that recovery will ensue. If the pulse is floating and there is inhibited urination, mild heat, and dispersion-thirst, Wu Ling San governs.

(2) and when in wind strike the person has heat effusion unresolved after six or seven days and vexation, so that there is an exterior and an interior pattern marked by thirst with a desire to drink water and immediate vomiting of ingested fluids, this is called water counterflow.

(3) and when in cold damage there is a glomus and fullness below the heart, give Heart-Draining Decoction (xie xin tang). If the glomus dose not resolve, and the person is thirsty, has a dry mouth, vexation, and inhibited urination, Wu Ling San governs.

(4) generally treats all kinds of damp and abdominal fullness, water rheum, water swelling, retching, diarrhea, water-cold shooting into the lung, of panting, or cough, summerheat strike, vexation, thirst, generalized heat effusion, headache, accumulated heat in the bladder, constipation, thirst, sudden turmoil, vomiting, diarrhea, phlegm, damp malaria, generalized pain and heaviness.

·**MODIFICATIONS**： for summerheat damage, add Zhu Sha and Deng Xin Cao. ·**CHANNELS ENTERED**：The foot greater yang channel.

·**Analysis of Formula**：(1) The heat of greater yang enters the storehouse of the bladder, therefore thirst and urinary stoppage occur.

(2) Nei Jing says that :

'bland flavor causes seeping and outflow and is yang'. The sweet and bland of Fu Ling and Zhu Ling enter the lung and free the bladder, acting as sovereign.

'the salty flavor causes gushing up and outflow and is yin'. Ze

Xie is sweet and salty, enters the kidney and bladder to disinhibit water, acting as minister.

'Boosting earth is to control water'. Therefore the bitter and warm of Bai Zhu fortifies the spleen and eliminates damp, acting as assistant.

'the bladder stores the fluid and humor'. When the qi transforms, urine can come out.' therefore Gui Zhi that is pungent heat is used and acts as courier. Heat is treated with heat, this enter the bladder to transform the qi, and makes damp and heat evil to come out through urine.

·RELATED FORMULA ： (1) When Gui Zhi is eliminated, this is called Si Ling San. When Chen Sha is added, this is called Chen Sha Wu Ling San. They treat inhibited urination.

(2) When Cang Zhu is added, this is called Chang Gui Wu Ling San, treats cold with damp.

(3) When Yin Chen is added, this is called Yin Chen Wu Ling San, treats damp heat with yellowing, constipation, vexation, and thirst.

(4) When Qiang Huo is added, this is called Yuan Rong Wu Ling San, treats accumulated heat in the middle burner

(5) When Shi Gao, Hua Shi, and Han Shui Shi are added, this clears the heat of the six bowels, this is called Gui Ling Gan Lu Yin.

(7) When only Gui Zhi and Fu Ling (respectively same dose) are used and made into pills with honey, this is called Gui Ling Wan, treats summerheat, vexation, thirst, excessive drinking of water, abdominal distention, and reddish urine.

(8) When only Ze Xie and Bai Zhu are used, this is called Ze Xie Tang, treats propping rheum below the heart and dizziness.

(9) When only Fu Ling and Bai Zhu are used, this is called Fu Ling Bai Zhu Tang, treats inability to control water due to spleen vacuity, diarrhea due to exuberant damp. Again Yu Li Ren is added to this, this is called Bai Fu Ling Tang, treats water swelling.

(10) When Chuan Lian Zi is added, this treats water mounting(shan).

(11) When Ren Shen is added, this is called Chun Ze Tang. Again Gan Cao is added, this is also called Chun Ze Tang, treats absence of disease with thirst, and thirst after recovering from disease.

(12) When Gui Zhi is eliminated and Cang Zhu, Gan Cao, Shao Yao, Zhi Zi, Huang Qin, and Qiang Huo are added, this is called Er Zhu Si Ling Tang, generally treats damp evil in the exterior and interior, and clears summer heat and heat.

⒀ When Gui Zhi is doubled and Huang Qi is added, treats summerheat damage with incessant profuse sweating.

⒁ When Gan Cao, Hua Shi, Zhi Zi, salt, and Deng Xin Cao are added, this is called Jie An Dao Chi San, treats heat amassment in the bladder, constipation, and thirst. For damp strike with yellowing, add Yin Chen. For water chest bind, add Mu Tong.

⒂ When this formula is combined with Yi Yuan San, treats all kinds of damp strangury. Again Hu Po is added, this is called Fu Ling Hu Po Tang, treats strangury.

⒃ When this formula is combined with Ping Wei San, this is called Wei Ling San and also called Dui Jin Yin Zi, treats summerheat strike and damp damage, retention food and drink, abdominal pain, diarrhea, thirst, and constipation.

⒄ When this formula is combined with Huang Lian Xiang Ru Yin, this is called Xiang Ling Tang, treats summerheat damage with diarrhea.

⒅ When this formula is combined with Xiao Chai Hu Tang, this is called Chai Ling Tang, treats heat effusion, diarrhea, thirst, malaria with the heat effusion more pronounced than the aversion to cold, dry mouth, and heart vexation.

·**Original Source**：Zhong Jing

1. 五苓散
　·總結：利溼瀉熱
　·組成：豬苓, 茯苓, 澤瀉, 白朮, 桂枝
　·主治：(1)治太陽病發汗後, 大汗出, 胃中乾, 煩躁不得眠, 欲飲水者, 少少與之, 令胃氣和則愈. 若脈浮, 小便不利, 微熱消渴者, 此湯主之.

　　　(2)及中風發熱, 六, 七日不解而煩, 有表裡證, 渴欲飲水, 水入即吐, 名曰水逆.

　　　(3)及傷寒痞滿, 服瀉心湯不解, 渴而煩躁, 小便不利.

　　　(4)通治諸濕腹滿, 水飲水腫, 嘔逆泄瀉, 水寒射肺, 或喘或欬, 中暑煩渴, 身熱頭痛, 膀胱積熱, 便秘而渴, 霍亂吐瀉, 痰飲溼瘧, 身痛身重.

　·加減：傷暑者加硃砂, 燈心煎.
　·歸經：足太陽藥（膀胱)
　·方義：(1)太陽之熱, 傳入膀胱之腑, 故口渴而便不通.

　　　(2)經曰：

「淡味滲泄爲陽.」二苓甘淡入肺, 而通膀胱爲君.

「鹹味湧泄爲陰.」澤瀉甘鹹入腎膀胱, 同利水道爲臣.

「益土所以制水.」故以白朮苦溫, 健脾去濕爲佐.

「膀胱者津液藏焉, 氣化則能出矣.」故以肉桂辛熱爲使.

熱因熱用, 引入膀胱以化其氣, 使濕熱之邪, 皆從小水而出也.

·變化方: (1)本方去桂, 名四苓散. 本方加辰砂, 名辰砂五苓散. 並治小便不利.

(2)本方加蒼朮, 名蒼桂五苓散, 治寒濕.

(3)本方加茵陳, 名茵陳五苓散, 治濕熱發黃, 便祕煩渴.

(4)本方加羌活, 名元戎五苓散, 治中焦積熱.

(5)本方加石膏, 滑石, 寒水石, 以清六腑之熱, 名桂苓甘露飲.

(7)本方單用肉桂, 茯苓等分, 蜜丸, 名桂苓丸, 治冒暑煩渴, 引飲過多, 腹脹便赤.

(8)本方單用澤瀉, 白朮, 名澤瀉湯, 治心下支飲, 常苦眩冒.

(9)本方單用茯苓, 白朮等分, 名茯苓白朮湯, 治脾虛不能制水, 濕盛泄瀉. 再加郁李仁, 入薑汁服, 名白茯苓湯, 治水腫.

(10)本方加川楝子, 治水疝.

(11)本方加人參, 名春澤湯. 再加甘草, 亦名春澤湯. 治無病而渴, 與病瘥後渴者.

(12)本方去桂, 加蒼朮, 甘草, 芍藥, 梔子, 黃芩, 羌活, 名二朮四苓湯, 通治表裡濕邪, 兼清暑熱.

(13)本方倍桂, 加黃耆如朮之數, 治傷暑大汗不止.

(14)本方加甘草, 滑石, 梔子, 入食鹽, 燈草煎, 名節庵導赤散, 治熱畜膀胱, 便祕而渴. 如中濕發黃, 加茵陳; 水結胸, 加木通.

(15)本方合益元散, 治諸濕淋瀝. 再加琥珀, 名茯苓琥珀湯, 治小便數而欠.

(16)本方合平胃散, 名胃苓湯, 一名對金飲子, 治中暑傷濕, 停飲夾食, 腹痛泄瀉, 及口渴便祕.

(17)本方合黃連香薷飲, 名薷苓湯, 治傷暑泄瀉.

(18)本方合小柴胡湯, 名柴苓湯, 治發熱泄瀉口渴, 瘧疾熱多寒少, 口燥心煩.

·來源: 仲景

2. Zhu Ling Tang. Polyporus Decoction. 豬苓湯

·**ACTIONS**：disinhibits damp and drains heat

·**COMPOSITION**：Zhu Ling, Fu Ling, Ze Xie, Hua Shi, E Jiao

·**INDICATIONS**：(1) treats when in yang brightness disease, if the pulse is floating and there is heat effusion, thirst with a desire to drink water, and inhibited urination.

(2) When in lesser yin disease there is spontaneous diarrhea for six or seven days, cough, retching, thirst, heart vexation, and inability to sleep.

(3) generally treats jaundice due to damp-heat, thirst, and reddish urine.

·**CHANNELS ENTERED**：The foot greater yang and yang brightness channels [the bladder and the stomach]

·**Analysis of Formula**：(1) When heat congests in the upper part, the lower part does not free, when the lower part does not free, heat gets to congest more in the upper part. And damp depression brings about heat and steaming heat causes damp, therefore the heart vexation, retching, thirst, constipation and yellowing occur.

(2) Bland can drain damp, cold can overcome heat. The sweet and bland of Fu Ling drains the damp of the spleen and lung. The sweet and bland of Zhu Ling and the salty and cold of Ze Xie drain the damp of the kidney and bladder. Hua Shi is sweet, bland, and cold, the heaviness descends fire, the light qi resolves the flesh, this makes the damp of the exterior and interior to free and move upward and downward. E Jiao is sweet, neutral, moisture, and slippery, this treats vexation, thirst, and insomnia. The key point of this formula is in freeing and disinhibiting of water way, heat evil descends through urine, then all of triple burner get clear.

(3) Wu He Gao says that because herbs that disinhibiting water are too dry, therefore E Jiao is added to preserve the fluid and humor.

·**Original Source**：Zhong Jing

2. 豬苓湯
　·總結：利溼瀉熱
　·組成：豬苓, 茯苓, 澤瀉, 滑石, 阿膠
　·主治：(1)治陽明病脈浮發熱, 渴欲飲水, 小便不通
　　　　　(2)少陰病下利六, 七日, 欬而嘔渴, 心煩不得眠.
　　　　　(3)通治溼熱黃疸, 口渴溺赤.
　·歸經：足太陽陽明藥也 (膀胱, 胃)

·方義：(1)熱上壅則下不通，下不通熱益上壅．又溼鬱則爲熱，熱蒸更爲溼，故心煩而嘔渴，便祕而發黃也．

(2)淡能滲溼，寒能勝熱．茯苓甘淡，滲脾肺之溼．豬苓甘淡，澤瀉鹹寒，瀉腎與膀胱之溼．滑石甘淡而寒，體重降火，氣輕解肌，通行上下表裡之溼．阿膠甘平潤滑，以療煩渴不眠．要使水道通利，則熱邪皆從小便下降，而三焦俱清矣．

(3)吳鶴臯曰：「以諸藥過燥，故又加阿膠以存津液.」

·來源：仲景

3. Fu Ling Gan Cao Tang. Poria and Licorice Decoction. 茯苓甘草湯

·**ACTIONS**： Water rheum with palpitations and reverse flow.

·**COMPOSITION**： Gui Zhi, Sheng Jiang, Fu Ling, Gan Cao

·**INDICATIONS**： (1) treats when in water qi overwhelming the heart in cold damage, there is reversal and palpitations below the heart, it is appropriate to first treat the water. One should take Fu Ling Gan Cao Tang which will treat reversal. If not treated in that way, the water will soak into the stomach and there will be diarrhea.

(2) also treats cold damage with sweating and absence of thirst.

(3) also treats bladder cough, incontinence during coughing.

·**CHANNELS ENTERED**： The foot greater yang channel.

·**Analysis of Formula**： (1) Pungent can disperse rheum, warm can promote sweating and resolve the flesh, therefore Gui Zhi and Sheng Jiang are used.

(2) Bland can drain water, sweet can quiet the heart and assist yang, therefore Fu Ling is used.

(3) Boosting of earth can control water, the sweet and neutral can supplement qi and harmonize the middle, therefore Gan Cao is used.

·**RELATED FORMULA**： When Sheng Jiang is eliminated and Bai Zhu is added, this is called Fu Ling Gui Zhi Bai Zhu Gan Cao Tang.

1　treats when, in cold damage, after vomiting or precipitation, there is counterflow fullness below the heart, the qi surges upward to the chest, the person experiences dizzy head upon standing, and the pulse is sunken and tight, if sweating is promoted, the channels will be stirred and there will be quivering and trembling.

(2) Jin Gui Yao Lue uses this formula to treat phlegm below the heart, propping fullness in the chest and rip-side, and dizzy vision.

·**Original Source**：Zhong Jing

3. 茯苓甘草湯

　·總結：水飲悸厥

　·組成：桂枝, 生薑, 茯苓, 甘草

　·主治：(1)治傷寒水氣乘心, 厥而心下悸者. 先治其水, 當服茯苓甘草湯, 卻治其厥, 不爾水漬入胃, 必作利也.

　　　　(2)亦治傷寒汗出不渴者.

　　　　(3)亦治膀胱腑欬, 欬而遺溺.

　·歸經：足太陽藥也 (膀胱)

　·方義：(1)辛能散飲, 溫能發汗解肌, 故用桂, 薑.

　　　　(2)淡能滲水, 甘能寧心助陽, 故用茯苓.

　　　　(3)益土可以制水, 甘平能補氣和中, 故用甘草.

　·變化方：本方去生薑, 加白朮, 名茯苓桂枝白朮甘草湯(苓桂朮甘湯)

　　　　　(1)治傷寒吐下後, 心下逆滿, 氣上衝胸, 起則頭眩, 脈沈緊, 發汗則動經, 身為振搖者.

　　　　　(2)金匱用治心下有痰飲, 胸脇支滿, 目眩.

　·來源：仲景

4. Xiao Ban Xia Jia Fu Ling Tang. Minor Pinellia Decoction Plus Poria. 小半夏加茯苓湯

·**ACTIONS**：　water rheum with glomus and dizziness.

·**COMPOSITION**：Ban Xia, Sheng Jiang, Fu Ling

·**INDICATIONS**：treats sudden vomiting, glomus below the heart, water between diaphragm, dizziness, and palpitation.

·**CHANNELS ENTERED**：The foot greater yang and yang brightness channels

　·**Analysis of Formula**：(1) Ban Xia and Sheng Jiang move water and qi and disperse counterfolw qi, can check vomiting.

　　　　　2　Fu Ling quiets heart qi and drains kidney evil, can disinhibit urination.

　　　　　3　If fire moves downward with the help of water, palpitation

271

and dizziness will disappear and glomus disperses.

·**RELATED FORMULA**：⑴ When Fu Ling is eliminated, this is called Xiao Ban Xia Tang, treats propping rheum and vomiting without thirst, and also treats Jaundice.

⑵ When Fu Ling and Sheng Jiang are eliminated and Ren Shen and honey are added, this is called Da Ban Xia Tang, treats stomach reflux and immediate vomiting of ingested food.

·**Original Source**：Jin Gui Yao Lue

4. 小半夏加茯苓湯
　·總結：水飲痞眩
　·組成：半夏, 生薑, 茯苓
　·主治：治卒嘔吐, 心下痞, 膈間有水, 眩悸.
　·歸經：足太陽陽明藥也
　·方義：⑴半夏, 生薑行水氣而散逆氣, 能止嘔吐.
　　　　　⑵茯苓寧心氣而泄腎邪, 能利小便.
　　　　　⑶火因水而下行, 則悸眩止而痞消矣.
　·變化方：⑴本方除茯苓, 名小半夏湯, 治支飲嘔吐不渴, 亦治黃疸.
　　　　　⑵本方除茯苓, 生薑, 加人參, 白蜜, 名大半夏湯, 治反胃,
食入卽吐.
　·來源：金匱

5. Jia Wei Shen Qi Wan. Modified Kidney Qi Pill. 加味腎氣丸

·**ACTIONS**：water drum distention and lower wasting-thirst

·**COMPOSITION**：Shu Di Huang, Fu Ling, Shan Yao, Mu Dan Pi, Shan Yu Rou, Ze Xie, Chuan Niu Xi, Che Qian Zi, Rou Gui, Fu Zi

·**INDICATIONS**：⑴ treats great vacuity of the spleen and kidney, distention and enlargement of the abdomen, edema in the limbs, panting, exuberant phlegm, inhibited urination, sloppy stool with drum distention pattern.

⑵ also treats wasting-thirst, the volume of drinking and urine is same.

·**CHANNELS ENTERED**：The foot greater yin and lesser yin channels

·**Analysis of Formula**：⑴ Earth is the mother of all things, when the sple

272

en vacuous, earth is unable to control water and the water gets to overflow. Water is the origin of all things, when the kidney is vacuous, water is disquiet and moves frenetically, and then water gets to overflows among the flesh, the limbs, and the body. If this is treated with attacking of precipitation, this make vacuous pattern to be more vacuous.

(2) Gui Fu Ba Wei Wan enriches yin, can move water, and strengthens the spleen with supplementing life fire. Che Qian Zi is added to disinhibit urination without draining qi.

(3) Niu Xi is added to boost the liver and kidney and moves downward, therefore this makes water way to free and then swelling gets disappear. This does not damage the true origin of the kidney.

5. 加味腎氣丸
　·總結：水蠱下消
　·組成：熟地黃，茯苓，山藥，丹皮，山萸肉，澤瀉，川牛膝，車前子，肉桂，附子
　·主治：(1)治脾腎大虛，肚腹脹大，四肢浮腫，喘急痰盛，小便不利，大便溏黃已成蠱證.
　　　　　(2)亦治消渴，飲一溲一.
　·歸經：足太陰少陰藥也
　·方義：(1)土爲萬物之母，脾虛則土不能制水而洋溢；水爲萬物之源，腎虛則水不安其位而妄行；以致泛濫，皮膚肢體之間，因而攻之，虛虛之禍，不待言矣.
　　　　　(2)桂附八味丸，滋眞陰而能行水，補命火因以強脾. 加車前利小便，則不走氣.
　　　　　(3)加牛膝益肝腎，藉以下行. 故使水道通而腫脹已. 又無損於眞元也.

6. Yue Bi Tang. Maidservant from Yue Decoction. 越婢湯

·**ACTIONS**：wind water

·**COMPOSITION**：Ma Huang, Shi Gao, Sheng Jiang, Gan Cao, Da Zao

·**INDICATIONS**：treats wind water, aversion to wind, generalized edema, a pulse that is floating without thirst, incessant spontaneous sweating, and absence of great heat effusion.

·**MODIFICATIONS**：for aversion to wind, add Fu Zi.

273

·CHANNELS ENTERED：The foot greater yang channel

·Analysis of Formula：(1) for wind water between the flesh and skin, the pungent and heat of the Ma Huang is used to drain the lung.

(2) Shi Gao is sweet and cold, clears the stomach.

(3) Gan Cao makes water to come out through pores, acting as as sistant. (4) Sheng Jiang and Da Zao, acting as courier, regulate and harmonize the construction and defense, and make effusing action of the other herbs not to exhaust the fluid and humor.

·Original Source：Jin Gui Yao Lue

6. 越婢湯

·總結：風水

·組成：麻黃, 石膏, 生薑, 甘草, 大棗

·主治：治風水惡風, 一身悉腫, 脈浮不渴, 續自汗出, 無大熱者.

·加減：惡風者, 加附子.

·歸經：足太陽藥也

·方義：(1)風水在肌膚之間, 用麻黃之辛熱以瀉肺.

(2)石膏之甘寒以清胃.

(3)甘草佐之, 使風水從毛孔中出.

(4)又以薑, 棗爲使, 調和榮衛, 不使其太發散耗津液也.

·來源：金匱

7. Fang Ji Huang Qi Tang. Stephania and Astragalus Deco ction. 防己黃耆湯

·ACTIONS：wind water with every damp

·COMPOSITION：Fang Ji, Huang Qi, Bai Zhu, Gan Cao, Sheng Jiang, Da Zao

·INDICATIONS：(1) treats wind water, sweating, aversion to wind, a pul se that is floating, and generalized heaviness.

(2) and all kinds of wind and damp, numbness, and generalized p ain.

·MODIFICATIONS：(1) for abdominal pain, add Shao Yao.

(2) for panting, add Ma Huang.

(3) for cold pattern, add Xi Xin.

(4) for qi surging upward, add Gui Zhi.

(5) for heat swelling, add Huang Qin.

(6) for pulling pain with cold, add Gan Jiang and Gui Zhi.

(7) for damp exuberance, add Fu Ling, Cang Zhu.

(8) for qi fullness and hard pain, add Chen Pi, Zhi Ke, Su Ye.

·**CHANNELS ENTERED**：The foot greater yang and greater yin channels

·**Analysis of Formula**：(1) Fang Ji is great pungent, bitter, and cold. This moves to the twelve channels, opens orifice, and drains damp. This is main herb to treat wind swelling and water swelling.

(2) Huang Qi (raw) reaches exterior. This treats skin and flesh pain due to wind, warms seam of the flesh, and repletes the flesh.

(3) Bai Zhu fortifies the spleen and dries damp, with Huang Qi can check sweating, acting as minister.

(4) Fang Ji is harsh and rapid, therefore the sweet and neutral of Gan Cao is used to moderate it. And it can supplement earth and control water, acting as assistant.

(5) Sheng Jiang and Da Zao are pungent and sweet, and disperse. They regulate and harmonize the construction and defense, acts as courier.

·**RELATED FORMULA**：(1) When Bai Zhu, Sheng Jiang, and Da Zao are eliminated, and Fu Ling and Gui Zhi are added, this is called Fang Ji Fu Ling Tang, treats water in the skin, flesh, and limbs. This treats skin water.

(2) When Ren Shen, Sheng Jiang, Fang Ji, and Bai Zhu are added, this is called Fang Ji Tang, treats wind warmth, a pulse that is floating, profuse sweating, and generalized heaviness.

·**Original Source**：Jin Gui Yao Lue

7. 防己黃耆湯
　·總結：風水諸溼
　·組成：防己, 黃耆, 白朮, 甘草, 生薑, 大棗
　·主治：(1)治風水, 汗出惡風, 脈浮身重.
　　　　(2)及諸風諸溼, 麻木身痛.
　·加減：(1)腹痛加芍藥.
　　　　(2)喘加麻黃.
　　　　(3)有寒加細辛.
　　　　(4)氣上衝加桂枝.

275

(5)熱腫加黃芩.

(6)寒多掣痛加薑，桂.

(7)溼盛加茯苓，蒼朮.

(8)氣滿堅痛加陳皮，枳殼，蘇葉.

·歸經：足太陽太陰藥也

·方義：(1)防己大辛苦寒，通行十二經，開竅瀉溼，爲治風腫水腫之主藥.

(2)黃耆生用達表，治風注膚痛，溫分肉，實腠理.

(3)白朮健脾燥溼，與黃耆並能止汗爲臣.

(4)防己性險而捷，故用甘草甘平以緩之，又能補土制水爲佐.

(5)薑，棗辛甘發散，調和榮衛爲使也.

·變化方：(1)本方去白朮，薑，棗，加茯苓，桂枝，名防己茯苓湯，治水在皮膚四肢，聶聶而動，皮水爲病，四肢腫，水氣在皮膚中，聶聶而動者，名皮水.

(2)本方加人參，生薑，防己，白朮各增三倍，名防己湯，治風溫脈浮，多汗身重.

·來源：金匱

8. Shen Zhuo Tang. Kidney Fixity Decoction . 腎着湯

·**ACTIONS**：damp damaging the lumbus and kidney

·**COMPOSITION**：Gan Cao (mix fried), Gan Jiang, Fu Ling, Bai Zhu

·**INDICATIONS**：(1) treats damp damage, generalized heaviness, abdominal pain and cold lumbus without thirst, uninhibited urination, normal eating and drinking, and disease relating with the lower burner.

(2) Xuan Ming Lun Fang uses this formula to treat bladder impediment, heat pain of the bladder, rough voidings of urine, runny nose with clear snivel.

·**MODIFICATIONS**：for cold pattern, add Fu Zi.

·**CHANNELS ENTERED**：The lesser yin and greater yang channels

·**Analysis of Formula**：(1)①Gan Cao which is sweet and neutral, harmonizes the middle and supplements earth.

②Gan Jiang which is pungent and heat, dries damp.

(2) generally herbs for the spleen are used for kidney disease, boosting earth is to control water.

276

8. 腎着湯

　　·總結：溼傷腰腎

　　·組成：炙甘草, 炮乾薑, 茯苓, 白朮

　　·主治：(1)治傷溼身重, 腹痛腰冷不渴, 小便自利, 飲食如故, 病屬下焦.

　　　　　　(2)宣明用治胞痹, 膀胱熱痛, 濇於小便, 上爲清涕.

　　·加減：有寒者加附子.

　　·歸經：足少陰太陽藥也

　　·方義：(1)①甘草－甘平和中而補土.

　　　　　　　　②乾薑－辛熱以燥溼.

　　　　　　(2)此腎病而皆用脾藥, 益土正所以制水也.

9. Zhou Che Wan. Vessel and Vehicle Pill. 舟車丸

·**ACTIONS**：yang water with swelling and distention.

·**COMPOSITION**：Da Huang, Hei Qian Niu, Gan Sui, Da Ji, Yuan Hua, Ju Hong, Mu Xiang, Qing Pi, Jing Fen

·**INDICATIONS**：treats water swelling and water distention with replete physique and qi.

·**CHANNELS ENTERED**：The foot greater yang channel

·**Analysis of Formula**：(1) Da Huang, Qian Niu Zi, Gan Sui, Da Ji, and Yuan Hua, ; they are harsh herbs to move water, can move the water of the twelve channels.

　　　　　　Swelling is related with the spleen, distention is related with the liver, not moving of water is due to not moving of the spleen, not moving of the spleen is due to exuberant wood which rebels earth, these condition is unable to control water and causes overflowing.

　　　　　　(2) Qing Pi and Mu Xiang course the liver, drain the lung, and fortify the spleen, with Chen Pi summon qi and dry damp. When qi moves, water moves, and when the spleen moves and transforms, swelling disperses.

　　　　　　(3) Jing Fen enters every orifices and can eliminate accumulated phlegm, therefore use small dose. Only use it to replete pattern.

·**RELATED FORMULA**：When Yuan Hua, Da Ji, Qing Pi, Chen Pi, and Mu Xiang are reduced and Mang Xiao and Yu Li Ren are added, this is called Jun Chuan San.

·**Original Source**：Liu He Jian's formula

9. 舟車丸

　·總結：陽水腫脹

　·組成：大黃, 黑牽牛, 甘遂, 大戟, 芫花, 橘紅, 木香, 青皮, 輕粉

　·主治：治水腫水脹, 形氣俱實.

　·歸經：足太陽藥也

　·方義：(1)大黃, 牽牛, 甘遂, 大戟, 芫花, 皆行水之屬劑也, 能通行十二經之水.

　　　　　然腫屬於脾, 脹屬於肝, 水之不行, 由於脾之不運, 脾之不運, 由於木盛而來侮之, 是以不能防水而洋溢也.

　　　　　(2)青皮, 木香, 疏肝泄肺而健脾, 與陳皮均爲導氣燥溼之品, 使氣行則水行, 脾運則腫消也.

　　　　　(3)輕粉無竅不入, 能去積痰, 故少加之. 然非實證, 不可輕投.

　·變化方：本方減芫花, 大戟, 青皮, 陳皮, 木香, 加芒硝, 郁李仁, 名濬川散.

　·來源：河間

10. Shu Zao Yin Zi. Coursing and Piercing Drink. 疏鑿飲子

　·**ACTIONS**：yang water

　·**COMPOSITION**：Fu Ling Pi, Da Fu Pi, Qiang Huo, Qin Jiao, Shang Lu, Jiao Mu, Bing Lang, Chi Xiao Dou, Mu Tong, Ze Xie, Sheng Jiang Pi

　·**INDICATIONS**：treats generalized water swelling, panting with thirst, constipation and difficult urination.

　·**CHANNELS ENTERED**：The foot greater yang and hand and foot greater yin channels. [The bladder, lung, and spleen]

　·**Analysis of Formula**：(1) There is externally generalized swelling and internally thirst and constipation. There is disease in the interior, exterior, upper part and lower part.

　　　　　(2)① Da Fu Pi, Fu Ling Pi, and Sheng Jiang Pi have the character of acridity dissipating and bland percolation, therefor they move water in the skin and flesh.

　　　　　② Qiang Huo and Qin Jiao resolve exterior and course wind. They dissipate damp through wind, come out evil through sweating, and raise damp and evil to upward.

278

③Shang Lu, Bing Lang, Jiao Mu, and Chi Xiao Dou e
liminate distention and attack hardness, therefor they move water in the abdom
en and interior.

④ Mu Tong drains the water of the heart and the lung,
and frees to the small intestine.

⑤ Ze Xie drains the water of the spleen and kidney an
d frees to the bladder.

⑶ This formula disperses the water in the upper part, lower part,
interior, and exterior separately.

10. 疏鑿飲子
　·總結：陽水
　·組成：茯苓皮，大腹皮，羌活，秦艽，商陸，椒目，檳榔，赤小豆，木
通，澤瀉
　·主治：治遍身水腫，喘呼口渴，大小便秘.
　·歸經：足太陽手足太陰藥也
　·方義：⑴外而一身盡腫，內而口渴便秘，是上下表裡俱病也.
　　　　　⑵①腹皮，苓皮，薑皮—辛散淡滲，所以行水於皮膚.
　　　　　　②羌活，秦艽—解表疏風，使溼以風勝，邪由汗出，
而升於上.
　　　　　　③商陸，檳榔，椒目，赤豆—去脹攻堅，所以行水於
腹裡.
　　　　　　④木通—瀉心肺之水，達於小腸.
　　　　　　⑤澤瀉—瀉脾腎之水，通於膀胱.
　　　　　⑶上下內外分消其勢.

11. Shi Pi Yin. Bolster the Spleen Decoction. 實脾飲

·**ACTIONS**：yin water
·**COMPOSITION**：Da Fu Pi, Fu Ling, Bai Zhu, Gan Cao (mix fried), M
u Gua, Fu Zi, Hei Sheng Jiang, Cao Dou Kou, Mu Xiang, Hou Po
·**INDICATIONS**：treats edema of the limbs and body, emaciated comple
xion, low faint voice, absence of thirst, and uninhibited defecation and urinatio
n.
·**CHANNELS ENTERED**：The foot greater yin channel
·**Analysis of Formula**：⑴ for spleen damp, Da Fu Pi and Fu Ling are use

279

d to disinhibit damp.

    ⑵ for spleen vacuity, Bai Zhu, Fu Ling, and Gan Cao are used t
o supplement spleen qi.

    ⑶ for spleen cold, Sheng Jiang, Fu Zi, and Cao Dou Kou are us
ed to warm.

    ⑷ for spleen fullness, Mu Xiang and Hou Po are used to abduct.

    ⑸ Insufficient earth is due to superabundant wood, the sour and
warm of Mu Gua can drain wood in earth and move water. With Mu Xiang is t
he herb for pacifying the liver. When one makes wood not to overwhelm earth
and the liver to be in harmony, earth can control water and the spleen gets to re
plete. Nei Jing says that when damp overcomes, earth gets muddy, draining wat
er is right to repete earth.

11. 實脾飲
  ·總結：陰水
  ·組成：大腹皮, 茯苓, 白朮, 炙甘草, 木瓜, 附子, 黑薑, 草豆蔻, 木
香, 厚朴
  ·主治：治肢體浮腫, 色悴聲短, 口中不渴, 二便通利.
  ·歸經：足太陰藥也
  ·方義：⑴脾溼, 故以大腹, 茯苓利之.
      ⑵脾虛, 故以白朮, 苓, 草補之.
      ⑶脾寒, 故以薑, 附, 草蔻溫之.
      ⑷脾滿, 故以木香, 厚朴導之.
      ⑸然土之不足, 由於木之有餘, 木瓜酸溫, 能於土中瀉木,
兼能行水, 與木香同爲平肝之品, 使木不尅土而肝和, 則土能制水而脾實
矣. 經曰：「溼勝則地泥, 瀉水正所以實土也.」

12. Wu Pi Yin. Five-Peel Decoction. 五皮飲

  ·**ACTIONS**：water swelling of the skin and flesh
  ·**COMPOSITION**：Wu Jia Pi, Di Gu Pi, Fu Ling Pi, Da Fu Pi, Sheng Jia
ng Pi
  ·**INDICATIONS**：treats water disease with swelling and fullness, dyspne
a, panting, or swelling below the lumbus.
  ·**CHANNELS ENTERED**：The foot greater yang and yin channels
  ·**Analysis of Formula**：⑴① Wu Jia Pi eliminates wind and overcomes d

280

amp.

    ② Da Fu Pi descends qi and move water.

    ③ Fu Ling drains damp and fortifies the spleen. This regulates and supplements in the middle of draining the middle.

    ④ The dissipating acridity of Sheng Jiang disperses and assists yang.

    ⑤ Di Gu Pi abates heat and supplements vacuity.

    (2) The barks (skins) are used, water overflows in the skin and flesh, thus the skin part is treated with the barks.

·**Original Source**：Dan Liao

12. 五皮飲
  ·總結：皮膚水腫
  ·組成：五加皮, 地骨皮, 茯苓皮, 大腹皮, 生薑皮
  ·主治：治水病腫滿, 上氣喘急, 或腰以下腫.
  ·歸經：足太陽太陰藥也
  ·方義：(1)①五加祛風勝溼.
        ②大腹下氣行水.
        ③茯苓滲溼健脾, 於散瀉之中, 猶寓調補之意.
        ④生薑辛散助陽.
        ⑤地骨退熱補虛.
    (2)皆用皮者, 水溢皮膚, 以皮行皮也.
  ·又附方：(1)一方五加易陳皮.
       (2)羅氏五加易桑白皮, 治病後脾肺氣虛而致腫滿.
  ·來源：澹寮

13. Mai Men Dong Tang. Ophiopogonis Decoction. 麥門冬湯

·**ACTIONS**：The upper burner water

·**COMPOSITION**：Mai Men Dong, Ren Shen, Gan Cao (mix fried), Geng Mi, Da Zao, Ban Xia

·**INDICATIONS**：treats water overflowing to the upper burner, swelling of both the limbs and body..

·**CHANNELS ENTERED**：The hand greater yang channel

281

·**Analysis of Formula** : Wu He Gao says that, the lung is always concerne
d with swelling, food and drink enter the stomach, overflowing essence qi is tra
nsported upward to the spleen. The spleen qi spreads the essence, which turns u
pward to the lung. [The latter] frees and regulates the paths of the water, it trans
ports [the water] downward to the urinary bladder. If the lung is heat, this fails t
o descend qi, therefore water overflows to the upper burner and the skin and fle
sh, and this causes water swelling. A few doctors know this principle. Even tho
ugh one repletes the spleen and abducts water, it fails to recover. Therefore Mai
Men Dong is used to clear the lung and open the origin of descending. Geng Mi
boosts the spleen and banks up the mother of engendering of metal.

13. 麥門冬湯
　　·總結：上焦水
　　·組成：麥門冬, 人參, 炙甘草, 粳米, 大棗, 半夏
　　·主治：治水溢高原, 肢體皆腫.
　　·歸經：手太陽藥也
　　·方義：吳鶴皋曰：「肺非無為也, 飲食入胃, 游溢精氣, 上輸於脾,
脾氣散精, 上歸於肺, 通調水道, 下輸膀胱, 肺熱則失其下降之令, 以致水
溢高原, 淫於皮膚而為水腫. 醫罕明乎此, 實脾導水, 皆不能愈. 故用麥冬
清肺, 開其下降之源; 粳米益脾, 培乎生金之母.

14. Qiang Huo Sheng Shi Tang. Notopterygium Decoction t o Overcome Damp. 羌活勝濕湯

·**ACTIONS** : damp qi in the exterior
·**COMPOSITION** : Qiang Huo, Du Huo, Fang Feng, Gao Ben, Man Jing
Zi, Chuan Xiong, Gan Cao, Sheng Jiang
·**INDICATIONS** : treats damp qi in the exterior, headache, heavy-headedness, or
heavy pain in the lumbus, or generalized pain, mild heat effusion, and lassitude of e
ssence-sprit.
·**MODIFICATIONS** : for generalized and lumbar heaviness, and cold da
mp in the middle, add Fang Ji (washed with wine) and Fu Zi.
·**CHANNELS ENTERED** : The foot greater yang channel
·**Analysis of Formula** : (1) Nei Jing says that wind can overcome damp.
Qiang Huo, Du Huo, Fang Feng, Gao Ben, Man Jing Zi, and Chuan Xiong belo
ng to wind herb. When damp qi is the exterior, the pungent and warm of the six
herbs raise and disperse. All of them resolve exterior. If one makes damp come

282

out through sweating, then every evil get to disperse.

      (2) for water damp in the interior, the herbs which move and drain water should be used.

      (3) Gan Cao assists every herbs, pungent and sweet disperse and become yang, Gan Cao is sweet and neutral, this supplements during dispersing.

·**RELATED FORMULA**：(1) When Du Huo, Man Jing Zi, Chuan Xiong, and Gan Cao are eliminated, Sheng Ma and Cang Zhu are added, this is called Qiang Huo Chu Shi Tang, treats the contending of wind and damp, generalized pain.

      (2) When Chuan Xiong is eliminated and Huang Qi, Dang Gui, Cang Zhu, and Sheng Ma are added, this is called Sheng Yang Chu Shi Tang, treats water mounting(shan), large swelling, and incessant scrotal sweating. When again Mai Ya, Shen Qu, Zhu Ling, and Ze Xie are added, and Dang Gui and Huang Qi are eliminated, this is also called Sheng Yang Chu Shi Tang, treats spleen vacuity with diarrhea.

·**Original Source**：Ju Fang

14. 羌活勝濕湯

  ·總結：溼氣在表

  ·組成：羌活, 獨活, 防風, 藁本, 蔓荊子, 川芎, 甘草, 生薑

  ·主治：治溼氣在表, 頭痛頭重, 或腰脊重痛, 或一身盡痛, 微熱昏倦.

  ·加減：如身重腰中沈沈然, 中有寒溼也, 加酒洗防己, 附子.

  ·歸經：足太陽藥也

  ·方義：(1)經曰：「風能勝溼.」羌, 獨, 防, 藁, 芎, 蔓皆（風）藥也. 溼氣在表, 六者辛溫升散, 又皆解表之藥, 使溼從汗出, 則諸邪散矣.

      (2)若水溼在裡, 則當用行水滲洩之劑.

      (3)甘草助諸藥辛甘發散爲陽, 氣味甘平, 發中有補.

  ·變化方：(1)本方除獨活, 蔓荊, 川芎, 甘草, 加升麻, 蒼朮. 名羌活除溼湯, 治風溼相搏, 一身盡痛.

      (2)本方除川芎, 加黃耆, 當歸, 蒼朮, 升麻, 名升陽除溼湯, 治水疝腫大, 陰汗不絕. 再加麥芽, 神麯, 豬苓, 澤瀉, 除當歸, 黃耆, 亦名升陽除溼湯, 治脾虛瀉痢.

  ·來源：局方

15. Zhong Man Fen Xiao Wan. Center Fullness Separating

and Dispersing Pill.　中滿分消丸

·**ACTIONS**：center fullness and heat distention.

·**COMPOSITION**：Fu Ling, Ren Shen, Bai Zhu, Gan Cao (mix fried), S ha Ren, Jiang Huang, Gan Jiang, Hou Po, Zhi Shi, Zhi Mu, Huang Qin, Huang Lian, Ban Xia, Zhu Ling, Ze Xie, Chen Pi

·**INDICATIONS**：treats center fullness, timpanists, qi distention, water d istention, and heat distention.

·**CHANNELS ENTERED**：The foot greater yin and yang brightness cha nnels

·**Analysis of Formula**：(1) Ren Shen, Bai Zhu, and Gan Cao supplement t he spleen and stomach. If one makes qi move, distention gets to disperse.

(2) Gan Jiang boosts yang and dries damp.

(3) Hou Po and Zhi Shi move qi and disperse fullness.

(4) Zhi Mu clears the overwhelming fire of yang brightness, and moistens the kidney and nourishes yin.

(5) Huang Qin and Huang Lian drain heat and disperse glomus. J iang Huang and Sha Ren warm the stomach and fresh the spleen.

(6) Ban Xia moves water and disperses phlegm.

(7) Zhu Ling and Ze Xie drain the water of the spleen and kidney which moves frenetically. They raise clear and descend turbid.

(8) Chen Pi rectifies qi and harmonizes the middle.

15. 中滿分消丸

·總結：中滿熱脹

·組成：茯苓, 人參, 白朮, 炙甘草, 砂仁, 薑黃, 乾薑, 厚朴, 枳實, 知母, 黃芩, 黃連, 半夏, 豬苓, 澤瀉, 陳皮

·主治：治中滿鼓脹, 氣脹, 水脹, 熱脹.

·歸經：足太陰陽明藥也

·方義：(1)少加參, 朮, 苓, 草—以補脾胃, 使氣運則脹消也 .

(2)乾薑—益陽而燥溼.

(3)厚朴, 枳實—行氣而散滿.

(4)知母—治陽明獨勝之火潤腎滋陰.

(5)黃芩, 黃連—瀉熱而消痞. 薑黃, 砂仁—暖胃而快脾.

(6)半夏—行水而消痰.

(7)豬苓, 澤瀉—脾腎妄行之水, 升清降濁.

(8)陳皮—理氣而和中.

16. Zhong Man Fen Xiao Tang. Center Fullness Separating and Dispersing Decociton. 中滿分消湯

·ACTIONS：center fullness and cold distention.

·COMPOSITION：Gan Jiang, Sheng Jiang, Cao Kou Ren, Wu Zhu Yu, Bi Cheng Qie, Chuan Wu, Yi Zhi Ren, Huang Lian, Huang Bai, Fu Ling, Ze Xi e, Ban Xia, Mu Xiang, Chai Hu, Sheng Ma, Ren Shen, Huang Qi, Ma Huang, Dang Gui, Qing Pi, Hou Po

·INDICATIONS：treats center fullness, cold distention, cold abdominal colic, urinary and fecal stoppage, reverting cold of the limbs, immediate vomiti ng of ingested food, coldness in the abdomen, glomus below the heart, vacuity of the lower part, yin agitation, running piglet.

·CHANNELS ENTERED：The foot yang brightness and greater yin cha nnels

·Analysis of Formula：(1) Chuan Wu, Sheng Jiang, Gan Jiang, Wu Zhu Yu, Bi Cheng Qie, Yi Zhi Ren, and Cao Dou Kou eliminate damp, open depres sion, warm the stomach and kidney to eliminate the cold.

(2) Huang Lian and Huang Bai eliminate heat in the middle of da mp.

(3) Fu Ling and Ze Xie drain turbid.

(4) Ban Xia dries phlegm.

(5) Chen Pi regulates qi.

(6) Sheng Ma and Chai Hu raise the clear qi.

(7) Ren Shen and Huang Qi supplement the middle.

(8) Dang Gu harmonizes the blood.

(9) Ma Huang promotes sweating.

(10) Qing Pi and Hou Po disperse the fullness.

·Original Source：Li Dong Yuan

16. 中滿分消湯
·總結：中滿寒脹
·組成：乾薑, 生薑, 草蔻仁, 吳茱萸, 畢澄茄, 川烏, 益智仁, 黃連, 黃柏, 茯苓, 澤瀉, 半夏, 木香, 柴胡, 升麻, 人參, 黃耆, 麻黃, 當歸, 青皮, 厚朴

·主治：治中滿寒脹寒疝，二便不通，四肢厥冷，食入反出，腹中寒，心下痞，下虛陰躁，奔豚不收．

·歸經：足陽明太陰藥也

·方義：⑴川烏，二薑，吳茱，澄茄，益智，草蔻—除溼開鬱，暖胃溫腎，以袪其寒．

⑵黃連，黃柏—以去溼中之熱，又熱因寒用也．

⑶茯苓，澤瀉—以瀉其濁．

⑷半夏—以燥其痰．

⑸陳皮—以調其氣．

⑹升麻柴胡—以升其清．

⑺人參，黃耆—以補其中．

⑻當歸—以和其血．

⑼麻黃—以泄其汗．

⑽青皮，厚朴，以散其滿．

·來源：東垣

17. Da Ju Pi Tang. Major Tangerine Peel Decoction. 大橘皮湯

·**ACTIONS**：damp heat, distention and fullness

·**COMPOSITION**：Hua Shi, Gan Cao, Chi Fu Ling, Zhu Ling, Ze Xie, Bai Zhu, Rou Gui, Bing Lang, Chen Pi, Mu Xiang

·**INDICATIONS**：treats damp-heat attacking the interior, distention and fullness in the heart and abdomen, inhibited urination, efflux diarrhea, water swelling, and so on.

·**CHANNELS ENTERED**：The foot greater yang channel

·**Analysis of Formula**：(1) Chi Fu Ling, Zhu Ling, and Ze Xie drain fire and move water. Bai Zhu supplements the spleen. Rou Gui transforms qi. This is Wu Ling San.

(2) Hua Shi clears heat and inhibits damp, Gan Cao drains fire and regulates the middle. This is Liu Yi San.

(3) Damp-heat is severe in the interior, therefore Bing Lang which precipitates drastically, and Chen Pi and Mu Xiang which move qi are used. When qi moves, water moves. And when urine frees, stool gets harden.

17. 大橘皮湯

286

·總結：溼熱脹滿

·組成：滑石, 甘草, 赤茯苓, 豬苓, 澤瀉, 白朮, 桂, 檳榔, 陳皮, 木香

·主治：治溼熱內攻, 心腹脹滿, 小便不利, 大便滑瀉, 及水腫等證.

·歸經：足太陽藥也

·方義：(1)赤茯, 豬苓, 澤瀉瀉火行水；白朮補脾；　肉桂化氣. 此五苓散也.

(2)滑石清熱利溼, 甘草瀉火調中. 此六一散也.

(3)溼熱內甚, 故加檳榔峻下之藥, 陳皮, 木香行氣之品, 使氣行則水行, 以通小便而實大便也.

18. Yin Chen Hao Tang. Artemisia Scoparia Decoction. 茵陳蒿湯

·**ACTIONS**：damp heat and yang jaundice.

·**COMPOSITION**：Yin Chen Hao, Zhi Zi , Da Huang

·**INDICATIONS**：treats that when in cold damage yang brightness disease, there sweating only from the head, not from the body, and stopping at the neck, abdominal fullness, thirst, inhibited urination and defecation, damp heat with yellowing, and a pulse that is sunken and replete.

·**CHANNELS ENTERED**：The foot yang brightness channel

·**Analysis of Formula**：Cheng Wu Ji says that mild heat effusion should be harmonized with cool herb, great heat effusion should be dispersed with cold herb. Jaundice indicates that damp heat is severe, only very cold herb can control the heat, therefore Yin Chen acts as sovereign, Zhi Zi acts as minister, and Da Huang acts as assistant, they drain the heat separately through anterior and posterior(stool and urine), then abdominal distention resolves through urination and defecation.

·**RELATED FORMULA**：(1) When Da Huang is exchanged with Huang Lian, this is called Yin Chen San Wu Tang, treats same thing.

(2) When Hou Po, Zhi Shi, Huang Qin, Gan Cao, Sheng Jiang, and Deng Xin Cao are added, this is called Yin Chen Jiang Jun Tang, treats same thing.

(3) When Zhi Zi and Da Huang are eliminated and Fu Zi and Gan Jiang are added, treats cold damp with yin jaundice.

·**Original Source**：Zhong Jing

287

18. 茵陳蒿湯

　　·總結：溼熱陽黃

　　·組成：茵陳蒿, 梔子, 大黃

　　·主治：治傷寒陽明病, 但頭汗出, 腹滿口渴, 二便不利, 溼熱發黃, 脈沈實者.

　　·歸經：足陽明藥也

　　·方義：成無己曰：「小熱涼以和之, 大熱寒以散之. 發黃者, 溼熱甚也, 非大寒不能徹其熱. 故以茵陳爲君, 梔子爲臣, 大黃爲佐, 分泄前後, 則腹得利而解矣.」

　　·變化方：(1)本方大黃易黃連, 名茵陳三物湯, 治同.

　　　　　　(2)本方加厚朴, 枳實, 黃芩, 甘草, 入生薑, 燈草煎, 名茵陳將軍湯, 治同.

　　　　　　(3)本方去梔子, 大黃, 加附子, 乾薑, 治寒濕陰黃.

　　·來源：仲景

19. Ba Zheng San. Eight-Herb Powder for Rectification . 八正散

　·**ACTIONS**：damp heat with constipation

　·**COMPOSITION**：Qu Mai, Bian Xu, Che Qian Zi, Mu Tong, Hua Shi, shan Zhi Zi, Da Huang, Deng Xin, Gan Cao

　·**INDICATIONS**：treats damp-heat pouring down, dry throat, thirst, acute fullness in lower abdomen, urinary stoppage, or strangury and hematuria, or swelling in anterior yin due to heat.

　·**CHANNELS ENTERED**：The hand and foot greater yang, and foot lesser yang channels

　·**Analysis of Formula**：(1)① Zhi Zi and Da Huang are bitter and cold, move downward.

　　　　　② Hua Shi disinhibits orifice and disperses binds.

　　　　　③ they drain heat with disinhibiting damp.

　　　(2)① Che Qian Zi clears liver heat and frees the bladder. The liver channel connects to yin qi [anterior yin], and the bladder is the storehouse of the fluid and humor.

　　　　　② Mu Tong and Deng Xin Cao clear lung heat and descend heart fire. The lung is the source of qi transformation, and the heart is combined with the small intestine.

288

③ Qu Mai and Bian Xu descend fire and free strangur
y.

④ They disinhibit damp with draining heat.

⑶ Gan Cao with Hua Shi is Liu Yiu San. The tip of branch is us
ed to reach directly anterior part, and the sweet can moderate the pain.

⑷ Although this treats the lower burner but this does not only tr
eat the lower part, when triple burner free and is disinhibited, then water can m
ove downward.

19. 八正散

　·總結：濕熱便秘

　·組成：瞿麥, 扁蓄, 車前子, 木通, 滑石, 山梔子, 大黃, 燈芯, 甘草

　·主治：治濕熱下注, 咽乾口渴, 少腹急滿, 小便不通, 或淋痛尿血,
或因熱爲腫.

　·歸經：手足太陽足少陽藥也

　·方義：⑴①梔子, 大黃一苦寒下行.

　　　　　②滑石一利竅散結.

　　　　　③此皆瀉熱而兼利濕者也.

　　　⑵①車前一清肝熱而通膀胱, 肝脈絡於陰氣, 膀胱津液之府
也.

　　　　　②木通, 燈草一清肺熱而降心火, 肺爲氣化之源, 心
爲小腸之合也.

　　　　　③瞿麥, 扁蓄一降火通淋.

　　　　　④此皆利濕而兼瀉熱者也.

　　　⑶甘草合滑石爲六一散. 用梢者, 取其徑達莖中, 甘能緩痛
也.

　　　⑷雖治下焦而不專於治下, 必三焦通利, 水乃下行也.

20. Bi Xie Fen Qing Yin. Dioscorea Hypoglauca Decoction t
o Separate the Clear. 萆薢分清飲

·ACTIONS：damp heat and strangury-turbidity

·COMPOSITION：Bi Xie, Yi Zhi Ren, Shi Chang Pu, Wu Yao, Gan Ca
o, salt.

·INDICATIONS：treats yang vacuity with white turbidity, frequent urina

289

tion, something oily in urine, this is called unctuous strangury.

·**CHANNELS ENTERED**：The hand lesser yin. And foot reverting yin and yang brightness channels. [The heart, liver, and stomach]

·**Analysis of Formula**：(1)① Bi Xie can drain the damp heat of yang brightness and reverting yin, and eliminates turbidity and separates clear qi.

② Wu Yao can course all kinds of evil qi which counterfolws, expel cold, and warm the kidney.

③ Shi Chang Pu opens nine orifices and frees the heart.

④ Yi Zhi Ren belongs to spleen medicinal, and also enters the heart and kidney, secures kidney qi and disperses binds.

⑤ Gan Cao [tip] reaches directly yin part and relieves pain.

(2) when damp-heat removes, the heart and kidney free, then qi transforms and moves, and then strangury-turbid disappears. Therefore coursing treatment is contraindicated in unctuous strangury.

20. 萆薢分清飲
　　·總結：溼熱淋濁
　　·組成：萆薢, 益智仁, 石菖蒲, 烏藥, 甘草梢, 鹽
　　·主治：治陽虛白濁, 小便頻數, 漩白如油, 名曰膏淋.
　　·歸經：手足少陰足厥陰陽明藥也
　　·方義：(1)①萆薢－能泄陽明厥陰溼熱, 去濁而分清.
　　　　　　　②烏藥－能疏邪逆諸氣, 逐寒而溫腎.
　　　　　　　③石菖蒲－開九竅而通心.
　　　　　　　④益智－脾藥, 兼入心腎, 固腎氣而散結.
　　　　　　　⑤甘草梢－達莖中而止痛.
　　　　　(2)使溼熱去而心腎通, 則氣化行而淋濁止矣, 此以疏泄而爲
禁止者也.

21. Hou Po San. Magnolia Bark Powder. 琥珀散

·**ACTIONS**：damp heat with all kinds of strangury

·**COMPOSITION**：Hua Shi, Hu Po, Mu Tong, Bian Xu, Mu Xiang, Dang Gui, Yu Jin

·**INDICATIONS**：treats qi strangury, blood strangury, unctuous strangur y, and sand strangury.

    ·**CHANNELS ENTERED**：The hand lesser yin and greater yang channels.

    ·**Analysis of Formula**：(1) Hua Shi disinhibits orifice and moves water.

    (2) Bian Xu is bitter. This can descend. This disinhibits urination and frees strangury.

    (3) Hu Po can descend lung qi and free to the bladder.

    (4) Mu Tong can drain heart fire and enters the small intestine.

    (5) for blood strangury due to chaotic blood, Dang Gui can conduct blood to return channel.

    (6) for qi strangury due to qi stagnation, Mu Xiang can raise and descend every qi.

    (7) for all kinds of strangury due to the exuberant fire of the heart and liver, Yu Jin can cool the heart, disperse the liver, descend qi, and break blood.

21. 琥珀散
    ·總結：溼熱諸淋
    ·組成：滑石，琥珀，木通，扁蓄，木香，當歸，鬱金
    ·主治：治氣淋，血淋，膏淋，砂淋.
    ·歸經：手足少陰太陽藥
    ·方義：(1)滑石…滑可去着，利竅行水.
          (2)扁蓄…苦能下降，利便通淋.
          (3)琥珀…能降肺氣，通於膀胱.
          (4)木通…能瀉心火，入於小腸.
          (5)血淋由於血亂，當歸…能引血歸經.
          (6)氣淋由於氣滯，木香…能升降諸氣.
          (7)諸淋由心肝火盛，鬱金…能涼心散肝下氣而破血也.

22. Fang Ji Yin. Stephania Decoction. 防己飲

·**ACTIONS**：damp-heat with leg qi

·**COMPOSITION**：Fang Ji, Mu Tong, Bing Lang, Sheng Di Huang, Chuan Xiong, Bai Zhu, Cang Zhu, Huang Bai, Gan Cao, Xi Jiao

·**INDICATIONS**：treats leg qi with swollen pain in the foot and lower leg, abhorrence of cold and invigorating heat effusion.

291

·**MODIFICATIONS**：(1) for heat, add Huang Qin.

(2) for seasonal heat, add Shi Gao.

(3) for obese people with phlegm, add Zhu Li and Jiang Zhi (juice of ginger), or Nan Xing.

(4) for constipation, add Tao Ren and Hong Hua.

(5) for inhibited voiding of reddish urine, add Niu Xing, or Mu Gua and Yi Yi Ren.

·**CHANNELS ENTERED**：The foot greater yang channel.

·**Analysis of Formula**：(1) Fang Ji moves water and treats wind, and drains damp heat of the lower burner.

(2) Bing Lang attacks hardness, disinhibits water, and conducts every herbs to move downward.

(3) Mu Tong descends heart fire through urination.

(4) Gan Cao drains spleen fire and reaches directly anterior [yin] part.

(5) Huang Bai and Sheng Di Huang enrich kidney yin, cool blood, and resolve heat.

(6) Chang Zhu and Bai Zhu dry spleen damp and move the middle center.

(7) for swelling due to blood depression, Chuan Xiong is used to move qi in blood..

(8) for pain due to replete liver, Xi Jiao is used to cool the heart and clear the liver.

22. 防己飲

·總結：溼熱脚氣

·組成：防己，木通，檳榔，生地，川芎，白术，蒼术，黃柏，甘草梢，犀角

·主治：治脚氣足脛腫痛，憎寒壯熱

·加減：(1)熱…加黃芩.

(2)時令熱…加石膏.

(3)肥人有痰…加竹瀝.薑汁.或南星.

(4)大便秘…加桃仁.紅花.

(5)小便赤澀…加牛膝.或木瓜.薏苡.

·歸經：足太陽藥也.

·方義：(1)防己…行水療風，瀉下焦之濕熱.

292

(2)檳榔...攻堅利水, 墜諸藥使下行.

(3)木通...降心火由小便出.

(4)草梢...泄脾火徑達腎莖.

(5)黃柏.生地...滋腎陰而涼血解熱.

(6)蒼白二朮...燥脾濕而運動中樞.

(7)腫由血鬱, 川芎...行血中之氣.

(8)痛由肝實, 犀角...涼心而清肝

23. Dang Gui Nian Tong Tang. Tangkuei Decoction to Lift the Pain. 當歸拈痛湯

·**ACTIONS**：all kinds of damp heat disease.

·**COMPOSITION**：Yin Chen, Qiang Huo, Fang Feng, Sheng Ma, Ge Gen, Bai Zhu, Gan Cao, Huang Qin, Ku Shen, Zhi Mu, Dang Gui, Zhu Ling, Ze Xie

·**INDICATIONS**：(1) treats contending of damp and heat, vexed pain in the limbs and joints, heaviness in the shoulder and back, or generalized pain, or leg qi with swelling and pain, sore in the lumbus and knee, incessant pus and water.

(2) and damp heat with jaundice, a pulse that is sunken, replete, tight, rapid, stirring, and slippery.

·**CHANNELS ENTERED**：The foot greater yang and yang brightness channels.

·**Analysis of Formula**：(1) Qiang Huo outthrusts joints. Fang Feng disperses wind damp. They act as sovereign.

(2) The light of Sheng Ma and Ge Gen conduct other herbs to move upward and the bitter effuses [qi].

(3) Bai Zhu is sweet, warm, harmonious, and neutral. Cang Zhu is pungent, warm, and strong. They fortify the spleen and dry damp, acting as minister.

(4) When warm and heath combine together, vexed pain in the limbs and joints occurs. Therefore the bitter and cold of Ku Shen, Huang Qin, Zhi Mu, Yin Chen are used to drain warn and heat.

(5) Congested blood is hard to flow and causes pain, Dang Gui is pungent and warm, this disperses it.

(6) Ren Shen and Gan Cao are sweet and warm, they supplement

293

and nourish the right qi, and let bitter and cold not to damage the spleen and sto mach.

(7) When treating damp, if disinhibiting of urination is not used, this is not right treatment. Zhu Ling and Ze Xie are sweet, bland, salty, and neu tral, they abduct the lodged rheum, acting as assistant.

·**Original Source**：Li Dong Yuan

23. 當歸拈痛湯

·總結：溼熱諸病

·組成：茵陳，羌活，防風，升麻，葛根，白朮，甘草，黃芩，苦參，知母，當歸，豬苓，澤瀉

·主治：(1)治溼熱相搏，肢節煩痛，肩背沉重，或徧身疼痛，或脚氣腫痛，脚膝生瘡，膿水不絕.

(2)及溼熱發黃，脈沉實緊數動滑者.

·歸經：足太陽陽明藥

·方義：(1)羌活...透關節.防風...散風濕；爲君.

(2)升葛...味薄引而上行，苦以發之.

(3)白朮...甘溫和平.蒼朮...辛溫雄壯；健脾燥濕爲臣.

(4)溫熱和合，肢節煩痛...苦參，黃芩，知母，茵陳...苦寒以泄之，酒炒以爲因用.

(5)血壅不流則爲痛，當歸...辛溫以散之.

(6)人參.甘草...甘溫，補養正氣，使苦寒不傷脾胃.

(7)治濕不利小便，非其治也，豬苓.澤瀉...甘淡鹹平，導其留飲爲佐

·來源：東垣

24. Yu Gong San. Water Controller Yu Powder. 禹功散

·**ACTIONS**：cold damp and water mounting(shan)

·**COMPOSITION**：Hei Qian Niu, Xiao Hui Xiang

·**INDICATIONS**：treats cold damp, water mounting(shan), scrotal swelli ng and distention, and inhibited defecation and urination.

·**MODIFICATIONS**：or add Mu Xiang (one liang)

·**CHANNELS ENTERED**：The lesser yin greater yang channel.

·**Analysis of Formula**：(1) Qian Niu Zi is pungent and harsh. This can rea ch the kidney (life gate), enters essence track. This moves water and drains dam

294

p, and also frees wind or qi constipation.

(2) Xiao Hui Xiang is pungent and heat, warms and disperses. This can warms cinnabar field, eliminate cold qi of the small intestine, and enters the lower burner to drain yin evil.

·**Original Source**：Zhang Zi He

24. 禹功散

·總結：寒溼水疝

·組成：黑牽牛, 茴香

·主治：治寒濕水疝, 陰囊腫脹, 大小便不利.

·加減：或加木香一兩

·歸經：足少陰太陽藥.

·方義：(1)牽牛辛烈…能達右腎命門, 走精隧, 行水泄濕, 兼通大腸風秘氣秘

(2)茴香辛熱溫散…能暖丹田, 祛小腸冷氣, 同入下焦以泄陰邪也.

·來源：子和

25. Sheng Yang Chu Shi Fang Feng Tang. Yang–Upbearing Damp-Eliminting Decoction with Saposhnikovia. 升陽除濕防風湯

·**ACTIONS**：eliminates damp and raises yang

·**COMPOSITION**：Cang Zhu, Fang Feng, Fu Ling, Bai Zhu, Shao Yao

·**INDICATIONS**：(1) treats constipation, or tenesmus, or stool with white pus or blood.

(2) Do not use precipitation thoughtlessly, this causes severe disease or depression.

(3) This formula raises yang, then yin spontaneously descends.

·**MODIFICATIONS**：for stomach cold with diarrhea and borborigmus, add Yi Zhi Ren, Ban Xia (respectively five fen), Sheng jiang, and Da Zao.

·**CHANNELS ENTERED**：The foot greater yang and yang brightness channels.

·**Analysis of Formula**：(1) Cang Zhu is pungent, warm, dry, and harsh. This raises clear yang and opens all kinds of depression, therefore this acts as sovereign.

295

(2) Bai Zhu is sweet and warm. Fu Ling is sweet and bland. They fortify the spleen and disinhibit damp, acting as assistant.

(3) Fang Feng is pungent and warm. It overcomes damp and raises yang.

(4) Bai Shao Yao is sour and cold. This restrains yin and harmonizes the spleen.

·**Original Source**：Li Dong Yuan

25. 升陽除濕防風湯
　·總結：除溼升陽
　·組成：蒼朮, 防風, 茯苓, 白朮, 芍藥
　·主治：⑴治大便閉塞, 或裏急後重, 數至圊而不能便, 或有白膿, 或血.

　　　　　⑵慎勿利之, 利之則必至重病, 反鬱結而不通矣.

　　　　　⑶以此湯升舉其陽, 則陰自降矣.

　·加減：如胃寒泄瀉腸鳴…加益智仁.半夏各五分, 薑.棗煎.

　·歸經：足太陽陽明藥也.

　·方義：⑴蒼朮辛溫燥烈…升清陽而開諸鬱, 故以爲君.

　　　　　⑵白朮…甘溫；茯苓…甘淡；佐之以健脾利濕.

　　　　　⑶防風辛溫…勝濕而升陽.

　　　　　⑷白芍酸寒…斂陰而和脾也.

　·來源：東垣

Chapter 13. Dryness-Moistening Formulas. 潤燥之劑

1. Qiong Yu Gao. Beautiful Jade Paste. 瓊玉膏

·**ACTIONS**：dry cough
·**COMPOSITION**：Di Huang, Fu Ling, Ren Shen, Honey
·**INDICATIONS**：treats dry cough.
·**CHANNELS ENTERED**：The hand greater yin channel.
·**Analysis of Formula**：(1) Di Huang nourishes yin and engenders water, water can restrain fire.

(2) Honey is sweet, cool, and moisture. Moisture can eliminate dryness.

(3) Metal is the mother of water, earth is the mother of metal, therefore Ren Shen and Fu Ling are used to supplement earth and engender metal. Generally Ren Shen boosts lung qi and drains fire, Fu Ling clears lung heat and generates the fluids.

1. 瓊玉膏
　·總結：乾欬
　·組成：地黃, 茯苓, 人參, 白蜜
　·主治：治乾咳嗽.
　·加減：決瞿仙加琥珀.沉香各五錢, 自云奇妙.
　·歸經：手太陰藥也.
　·方義：(1)地黃…滋陰生水, 水能制火.
　　　　　(2)白蜜…甘涼性潤, 潤能去燥.
　　　　　(3)金爲水母, 土爲金母, 故用參, 苓…補土生金. 蓋人參益肺氣而瀉火, 茯苓清肺熱而生津也.

2. Zhi Gan Cao Tang. Honey-Fried Licorice Decoction. 炙甘草湯

·**ACTIONS**：boosts blood and engenders the fluid.
·**COMPOSITION**：Gan Cao (mix fried), Ren Shen, Da Zao, Gui Zhi, Sh

eng Jiang, Di Huang, E Jiao, Mai Men Dong, Ma Zi Ren

·**INDICATIONS**：(1) cold damage with a pulse that is bound and intermit tent, and stirring, heart palpitations, and lung wilting with copious cough, seethi ng in the heart with desire to vomit.

(2) Wei Sheng Bao Jian use this formula to treat hiccup.

·**CHANNELS ENTERED**：The hand and foot greater yin channels.

·**Analysis of Formula**：(1) Ren Shen, Mai Men Dong, Gan Cao, and Da Z a boost qi and restore pulse.

(2) Sheng Di Huang and E Jiao assist construction and blood and quiet the heart.

(3) Ma Zi Ren is moisture and lubricative. This moderates the sp leen and stomach.

(4) Sheng Jiang and Gui Zhi are pungent and warm. They disper se residual evil.

(5) The sweet of Ma Zi Ren, E Jiao, Mai Men Dong, and Di Hua ng moistens the channels, boosts blood, restores pulse, and frees the heart.

·**Original Source**：Zhong Jing

2. 炙甘草湯

　·總結：益血生津

　·組成：炙甘草, 人參, 大棗, 桂枝, 生薑, 地黃, 阿膠, 麥門冬, 麻子仁

　·主治：(1)治傷寒脈結代, 心動悸, 及肺痿咳唾多, 心中溫溫液液者.

　　　　(2)寶鑑用治呃逆.

　·歸經：手足太陰（肺, 脾）藥也.

　·方義：(1)人參, 麥冬, 甘草, 大棗…益中氣而復脈.

　　　　(2)生地, 阿膠…助營血而寧心.

　　　　(3)麻仁潤滑…以緩脾胃.

　　　　(4)薑, 桂辛溫…以散餘邪.

　　　　(5)麻仁, 阿膠, 麥冬, 地黃之甘…潤經益血, 復脈通心也.

　·來源：仲景

3. Mai Men Dong Tang, Opohiopogon Decoction. 麥門冬湯

·ACTIONS：descends fire and disinhibits throat.

·COMPOSITION：Mai Men Dong, Ban Xia, Ren Shen, Gan Cao, Da Zao, Geng Mi

·INDICATIONS：treats fire counterfolw with dyspnea, discomfort in the throat.

·CHANNELS ENTERED：The hand greater yin and foot yang brightness channels.

·Analysis of Formula：(1) In Zhong Jing, Mai Men Dong, Ren Shen, Geng Mi, Gan Cao, and Da Zao greatly supplement the middle qi and engender the fluid and humor. The one flavor of Ban Xia's pungent are used to disinhibit throat and descend qi.

·Original Source：Jin Gui Yao Lue

3. 麥門冬湯

·總結：降火利咽

·組成：麥門冬, 半夏, 人參, 甘草, 大棗, 粳米

·主治：治火逆上氣, 咽喉不利.

·歸經：手太陰足陽明藥也.

·方義：(1)仲景於麥冬, 人參, 粳米, 甘草, 大棗…大補中氣, 大生津液隊中, 增入半夏之辛溫一味 → 用以利咽下氣.

·來源：金匱

4. Huo Xue Run Zao Sheng Jin Tang. Blood-Quickening Dryness-Moistening Liquid-Engendering Decoction. 活血潤燥生津湯

·ACTIONS：internal dryness.

·COMPOSITION：Dang Gui, Bai Shao Yao, Shu Di Huang, Tian Men Dong, Mai Men Dong, Gua Lou, Tao Ren, Hong Hua

·INDICATIONS：treats internal dryness and desiccated and scant fluid and humor.

·CHANNELS ENTERED：The hand greater yin and foot reverting yin channels.

299

·**Analysis of Formula**：⑴ Dang Gui, Shao Yao, and Di Huang nourish yin and engender blood.

⑵ Gua Lou, Tian Men Dong, and Mai Men Dong moisten dryness and can engender the fluid.

⑶ Tao Ren and Hong Hua activate blood and moisten dryness

·**Original Source**：Dan Xi

4. 活血潤燥生津湯
·總結：內燥
·組成：當歸，白芍，熟地黃，天冬，麥冬，栝簍，桃仁，紅花
·主治：治內燥津液枯少.
·歸經：手太陰足厥陰藥也.
·方義：⑴歸.芍.地黃…滋陰可以生血.
⑵栝簍.二冬…潤燥兼能生津.
⑶桃仁.紅花…活血又可潤燥
·來源：丹溪

5. Qing Zao Tang. Eliminate Dryness Decoction. 清燥湯

·**ACTIONS**：clears metal and moistens dryness

·**COMPOSITION**：Huang Qi, Cang Zhu, Bai Zhu, Chen Pi, Ze Xie, Ren Shen, Fu Ling, Sheng Ma, Dang Gui, sheng Di Huang, Mai Men Dong, Gan Cao, Shen Qu, Huang Bai, Zhu Ling, Chai Hu, Huang Lian, Wu Wei Zi

·**INDICATIONS**：treats lung metal contracting the evil of damp heat, leg flaccidity, panting, thoracic fullness with light eating, whitish complexion and lusterless hair, dizziness, generalized heaviness, generalized pain, fatigued cumbersome limbs, thirst, and constipation.

·**CHANNELS ENTERED**：The hand and foot greater yin and yang brightness channels. [The lung, spleen, large intestine, and stomach]

·**Analysis of Formula**：⑴ The lung is related with pungent metal and controls qi. Large intestine is related with Geng metal and controls the fluid. If dry metal contracts the evil of damp heat, the source which engenders and transforms cold water generates expires. If the source expires, kidney water gets depleted.

⑵ Metal is the mother of water, qi is the source of water.

⑶ Huang Qi boosts source qi and replenishes the skin and fur, t

300

herefore this acts as sovereign.

(4) Bai Zhu, Chang Zhu, Ren Shen, Fu Ling, Gan Cao, Ju Pi, and Shen Qu fortify the spleen, dry damp, rectify qi, and transform stagnation. This makes earth move, because earth is the mother of metal.

(5) Mai Men Dong and Wu Wei Zi preserve the lung and engender the fluid.

(6) Dang Gui and Sheng Di Huang nourish yin and tonify blood.

(7) Huang Bai and Huang Lian dry damp and clear heat.

(8) Sheng Ma Chai Hu raise clear qi.

(9) Zhu Ling and Ze Xie descend turbidity.

·**Original Source**：Li Dong Yuan

5. 清燥湯

·總結：清金潤燥

·組成：黃耆，蒼朮，白朮，陳皮，澤瀉，人參，茯苓，升麻，當歸，生地黃，麥冬，甘草，神曲，黃柏，豬苓，柴胡，黃連，五味子

·主治：治肺金受濕熱之邪，痿躄喘促，胸滿少食，色白毛敗，頭眩體重，身痛肢倦，口渴便秘.

·歸經：手足太陰陽明藥也.

·方義：(1)肺屬辛金而主氣；大腸屬庚金而主津. 燥金受濕熱之邪，則寒水生化之源絕，源絕則腎水虧.

(2)金者水之母也，氣者水之源也.

(3)黃耆...益元氣而實皮毛，故以爲君.

(4)二朮，參，苓，甘，橘，神麴...健脾燥濕，理氣化滯...所以運動其土，土者金之母也.

(5)麥冬，五味...保肺以生津.

(6)當歸，生地...滋陰而養血.

(7)黃柏，黃連...燥濕而清熱.

(8)升麻，柴胡...所以升清.

(9)豬苓，澤瀉...所以降濁.

·來源：東垣

6. Zi Zao Yang Ying Tang. Dryness-Enriching Constructio n-Nourishing Decoction. 滋燥養榮湯

·**ACTIONS**：blood vacuity and wind-dryness.

·**COMPOSITION**：Dang Gui, Sheng Di Huang, Shu Di Huang, Shao Ya o, Huang Qin, Qin Jiao, Fang Feng, Gan Cao

·**INDICATIONS**：treats fire scorching metal, blood vacuity with external dryness, dry cracked skin, sinew hypertonicity, desiccated nail, or constipation.

·**CHANNELS ENTERED**：The hand greater yin and foot reverting yin c hannels.

·**Analysis of Formula**：(1) Dang Gui moistens dryness and tonifies blood, acting as sovereign.

(2) Sheng Di Huang and Shu Di Huang enrich kidney water and supplement the liver.

(3) Shao Yao drains liver fire and boosts blood, acting as ministe r.

(4) Huang Qin clears lung heat, and can nourish yin and abate ya ng.

(5) Qin Jiao and Fang Feng disperse liver wind. They are moistu re medicinal in wind medicinal.

(6) also Qin Jiao can tonify blood and flourish sinew. Fang Feng conducts other herbs to blood part.

(7) Gan Cao is sweet and neutral, drains fire, with moisture herb supplements yin blood, acting as assistant and courier.

6. 滋燥養榮湯

   ·總結：血虛風燥

   ·組成：當歸, 生地黃, 熟地黃, 芍藥, 黃芩, 秦艽, 防風, 甘草

   ·主治：治火爍金, 血虛外燥, 皮膚皴揭, 筋急爪枯, 或大便風秘.

   ·歸經：手太陰足厥陰藥也.

   ·方義：(1)當歸…潤燥養血爲君.

        (2)二地…滋腎水而補肝.

        (3)芍藥…瀉肝火而益血爲臣.

        (4)黃芩…清肺熱, 能養陰退陽.

        (5)艽.防…散肝風, 爲風藥潤劑.

        (6)又秦艽能養血榮筋, 防風…乃血藥之使.

(7)甘草...甘平瀉火, 入潤劑則補陰血...爲佐使也.

7. Sou Feng Shun Qi Wan. Wind-Tracking Qi Normalizing Pill. 搜風順氣丸

·**ACTIONS**：wind constipation, qi constipation.

·**COMPOSITION**：Da Huang, Ma Zi Ren, Yu Li Ren, Shan Yao, Shan Zhu Yu, Che Qian Zi, Niu Xi, Tu Si Zi, Du Huo, Fang Feng, Bing Lang, Zhi Ke

·**INDICATIONS**：(1) treats wind or qi constipation caused by wind stoke, inhibited urination and defecation, generalized vacuous itch, a pulse that is floating and rapid when coming.

(2) also treats intestinal wind with precipitation of blood, wind stroke with paralysis.

·**CHANNELS ENTERED**：The hand and foot yang brightness channels.

·**Analysis of Formula**：(1) Da Huang is bitter, cold, and drastic. This can precipitate dry bound stool and eliminate stasis heat, acting as sovereign.

(2) Ma Zi Ren is lubricant, Yu Li Ren is sweet and moisture. They can enter the large intestine, moisten dryness, and free dark gate.

(3) Che Qian Zi disinhibits water. Niu Xi moves downward. They can boost the liver kidney.

(4) Dryness is originated from wind, the pungent of Du Huo and Fang Feng moistens the kidney and tracks wind.

(5) Stagnation is causes by qi, the bitter of Zhi Ke and Bing Lang breaks stagnation and normalizes qi.

(6) A few herbs attack and disperse [qi], therefore Shan Yao is used to boost qi and secure the spleen. Shan Zhu Yu is used to warm the liver and supplement the kidney. Tu Si Zi is used to boost yang and strengthen yin. They supplement and assist the right qi.

7. 搜風順氣丸

·總結：風秘氣秘

·組成：大黃, 大麻仁, 郁李仁, 山藥, 山茱肉, 車前子, 牛膝, 菟絲子, 獨活, 防風, 檳榔, 枳殼

·主治：(1)治中風, 風秘氣秘, 便溺阻隔, 遍身虛癢, 脈來浮數.

(2)亦治腸風下血, 中風癱瘓.

303

·歸經：手足陽明藥也.

·方義：(1)大黃苦寒峻猛…能下燥結而袪瘀熱.

(2)麻仁滑利，李仁甘潤…並能入大腸而潤燥通幽.

(3)車前利水，牛膝下行…又能益肝腎而不走元氣.

(4)燥本於風，獨活，防風之辛…以潤腎而搜風.

(5)滯由於氣，枳殼，檳榔之苦…以破滯而順氣.

(6)數藥未免攻散，故又用…山藥益氣固脾；山茱溫肝補腎；

菟絲益陽強陰…以補助之也.

8. Run Chang Wan. Moisten the Intestines Pill. 潤腸丸

·**ACTIONS**：wind constipation, blood constipation.

·**COMPOSITION**：Qiang Huo, Dang Gui Wei, Tao Ren, Da Huang, Ma Zi Ren

·**INDICATIONS**：treats latent fire in the intestines and stomach, constipation, no thought of food, wind binds, blood binds.

·**MODIFICATIONS**：for wind damp, add Qin Jiao and Zao Jiao.

·**CHANNELS ENTERED**：The hand and foot yang brightness channels.

·**Analysis of Formula**：(1) Dang Gui Wei and Tao Ren moisten dryness and activate blood.

(2) Qiang Huo tracks wind and disperses evil.

(3) Da Huang breaks binds and frees stool.

(4) Ma Zi Ren lubricates the intestines and disinhibits orifice.

·**RELATED FORMULA**：(1) When Fang Feng, Zao Jiao Ren, and Honey are added, this is called Huo Xue Run Chang Wan, treats same things..

(2) When Qiang Huo is eliminated and Sheng Ma, Hong Hua, Sheng Di Huang, and Shu Di Huang are added, this is called Run Chang Tang, treats same things.

·**Original Source**：Li Dong Yuan

8. 潤腸丸

·總結：風秘血秘

·組成：羌活，當歸尾，桃仁，大黃，麻仁

·主治：治腸胃有伏火，大便秘澀，全不思食，風結血結.

·加減：風濕加…秦艽；皂角子.

·歸經：手足陽明藥也.
·方義：⑴歸尾.桃仁...潤燥活血.
　　　　⑵羌活...搜風散邪.
　　　　⑶大黃...破結通幽.
　　　　⑷麻仁...滑腸利竅.
·變化方：⑴本方加防風, 皂角仁, 蜜丸...名活血潤燥丸⇒治同.
　　　　　⑵本方去羌活, 加升麻, 紅花, 生熟二地...名潤燥湯⇒治同
·來源：東垣

9. Tong You Tang. Dark-Gate-Freeing Decoction. 通幽湯

·**ACTIONS**：dysphagia. Constipation

·**COMPOSITION**：Dang Gui Shen, Sheng Ma, Tao Ren, Hong Hua, Gan Cao, sheng Di Huang, Shu Di Huang, or Bing Lang (powder, five fen)

·**INDICATIONS**：treats dark gate stoppage, surging upward to breath gate, dysphagia, inability of qi descending, constipation, this is called lower stomach stoppage, the place where to treat is in dark gate.

·**CHANNELS ENTERED**：The hand and foot yang brightness channels.

·**Analysis of Formula**：(1) Dang Gui, Shu Di Huang, and Sheng Di Huang nourish yin and tonifys blood.

⑵ Tao Ren and Hong Hua moisten dryness and move blood.

⑶ Bing Lang expels downward and breaks qi stagnation.

⑷ Sheng Ma is added. Descending after ascending is the principle of nature. If clear yang does not ascend, then turbid yin is unable to descend. Nei Jing says that earth qi ascends to be cloud and heaven qi descends to be rain.

·**RELATED FORMULA**：When Da Huang and Ma Zi Ren are added, this is called Dang Gui Run Chang Tang, treats same things..

·**Original Source**：Li Dong Yuan

9. 通幽湯
　·總結：噎塞便秘
　·組成：當歸身, 升麻, 桃仁, 紅花, 甘草, 生地黃, 熟地黃, 或加檳榔
末五分
　·主治：治幽門不通, 上攻吸門, 噎塞不開, 氣不得下, 大便艱難, 名
曰下脘不通, 治在幽門.

·歸經：手足陽明藥也.
·方義：(1)當歸.二地...滋陰以養血.
　　　　(2)桃仁.紅花...潤燥而行血.
　　　　(3)檳榔...下墜而破氣滯.
　　　　(4)加升麻者...天地之道...能升而後能降，清陽不升，則濁陰
不降...經所謂：地氣上爲雲，天氣下爲雨也.
·變化方：本方加大黃，麻仁...名當歸潤腸湯⇒治同.
·來源：東垣

10. Jiu Zhi Niu Ru Yin. Chinese Leek [Leaf] Juice and Milk Beverage. 韭汁牛乳飲

·**ACTIONS**：stomach reflux and dry blood.

·**COMPOSITION**： Jiu Zhi and Niu Ru

·**INDICATIONS**：treats dead blood in stomach duct, dryness and desiccation, pain after eating, stomach reflux, and constipation.

·**MODIFICATIONS**：(1) for phlegm, add Jiang Zhi (juice of ginger).

(2) When milk is eliminated and Chen Jiu is added, this treats blood diaphragm [Xue Ge].

·**CHANNELS ENTERED**：The foot yang brightness channel.

·**Analysis of Formula**：(1) Jiu Zhi is pungent and warm. This boosts the stomach and disperses stasis.

(2) Niu Ru is sweet and warm. This moistens dryness and tonifies blood. If stasis is eliminated, there is no obstruction in the stomach, and if blood is moisture, the large intestine frees and food is able to descend.

·**Original Source**：Dan Xi

10. 韭汁牛乳飲
·總結：翻胃血燥
·組成：韭菜汁，牛乳
·主治：治胃脘有死血，乾燥枯槁，食下作痛，翻胃便秘.
·加減：(1)有痰汁者...加薑汁.(2)本方去牛乳，加陳酒...>治血膈.
·歸經：足陽明藥也.
·方義：(1)韭汁辛溫...益胃消瘀.
　　　　(2)牛乳甘溫...潤燥養血；瘀去則胃無阻，血潤則大腸通而食

306

得下矣.

　·來源：丹溪

11. Huang Qi Tang. Astragalus Decoction. 黃耆湯

　·**ACTIONS**：engenders the fluid and eliminates dryness.

　·**COMPOSITION**：Huang Qi, Shu Di Huang, Shao Yao, Wu Wei Zi, Mai Men Dong, Tian Men Dong, Ren Shen, Gan Cao, Fu Ling

　·**INDICATIONS**：treats vexation in the heart, inability to engender the fluid and humor, no though of food and drink.

　·**CHANNELS ENTERED**：The hand and foot greater yin channels.

　·**Analysis of Formula**：(1) Huang Qi and Ren Shen supplement qi.

　　　　(2) Shu Di Huang and Shao Yao supplement blood.

　　　　(3) Wu Mei and Wu Wei Zi restrain exhaustion and engender the fluid.

　　　　(4) Tian Men Dong and Mai Men Dong drain fire and supplement water.

　　　　(5) Fu Ling is bland. This disinhibits damp.

　　　　(6) Gan Cao is sweet. This harmonizes the middle. When damp is eliminated and qi moves, the spleen gets harmonious, one gets to think of food, the fluid is engendered, and dryness retreats.

　·**Original Source**：Ben Shi Fang

11. 黃耆湯
　·總結：生津去燥
　·組成：黃耆, 熟地黃, 芍藥, 五味子, 麥冬, 天冬, 人參, 甘草, 茯苓
　·主治：治心中煩燥, 不生津液, 不思飲食.
　·歸經：手足太陰藥也.
　·方義：(1)黃耆, 人參...補氣.
　　　　(2)熟地, 芍藥...補血.
　　　　(3)烏梅, 五味...斂耗生津.
　　　　(4)天冬, 麥冬...瀉火補水.
　　　　(5)茯苓...淡以利濕.
　　　　(6)甘草...甘以和中；濕去氣運, 則脾和而思食, 津生而燥退矣.

·來源：本事

12. Xioa Ke Fang. Wasting Thirst Formula. 消渴方

·ACTIONS：wasting-thirst

·COMPOSITION：Huang Lian, Tian Hua Fen, Sheng Di Huang (juice), Ou Jie (juice), Niu Ru

·INDICATIONS：treats thirst pattern with stomach heat, swift digestion.

·CHANNELS ENTERED：The hand and foot greater yin and yang brightness channels. [The lung, spleen, large intestine, and stomach]

·Analysis of Formula： Nei Jing says that when heart heat spreads to the lung, this causes diaphragm wasting-thirst. Exuberant fire scorches metal, this metal is unable to engender water, therefore vexation and thirst occur.

(1) Huang Lian is bitter cold. This drains heart fire.

(2) Sheng Di Huang is great cold. This engenders kidney water.

(3) Tian Hua Fen and Ou Jie (juice) descend fire and engender the fluid.

(4) Niu Ru supplements blood. Moisture eliminates dryness. When fire retreats, dryness eliminates, when the fluid engenders, blood is effulgent, then thirst spontaneously allays.

·Original Source：Dan Xi

12. 消渴方

·總結：消渴

·組成：黃連, 天花粉, 生地汁, 藕汁, 牛乳

·主治：治渴證胃熱, 善消水穀.

·歸經：手足太陰陽明藥也.

·方義：經曰：心移熱於肺, 傳爲鬲消.火盛灼金, 不能生水, 故令燥渴.

(1)黃連苦寒...以瀉心火.

(2)生地大寒...以生腎水.

(3)花粉, 藕汁...降火生津.

(4)牛乳...補血, 潤以去燥；火退燥除, 津生血旺, 則渴自止矣.

·煎服法：(1)將黃連, 花粉, 爲末調服.

(2)或加薑汁, 蜂蜜爲膏, 噙化.

·來源：丹溪

13. Di Huang Yin Zi. Rehmannia Decoction. 地黃飲子

·**ACTIONS**：wasting-thirst, vexation and agitation

·**COMPOSITION**：Ren Shen, Huang Qi, Gan Cao, sheng Di Huang, Shu Di Huang, Tian Men Dong, Mai Men Dong, Pi Pa Ye, Shi Hu, Ze Xie, Zhi Ke

·**INDICATIONS**：treats wasting-thirst, vexation and agitation, dry throat, and reddish complexion.

·**CHANNELS ENTERED**：The hand and foot greater yin and yang brig htness channels.

·**Analysis of Formula**：喻嘉言 says that this formula engenders essence, supplements blood, moistens dryness, and allays thirst. Ze Xie and Zhi Ke cour se and abduct the small and large intestine, acting as assistant. When small inte stine is clear and disinhibited, heart fire gets to descend. When the large intestin e frees and is uninhibited, the lung channel becomes moisture. Abiding heat is e liminated, and then the thirst spontaneously allays.

·**Original Source**：Yi Jian

13. 地黃飲子

·總結：消渴煩躁

·組成：人參, 黃耆, 甘草, 生地黃, 熟地黃, 天冬, 麥冬, 枇杷葉, 石斛, 澤瀉, 枳殼

·主治：治消渴煩躁, 咽乾面赤.

·歸經：手足太[陰陽明藥也.

·方義：喻嘉言曰：此方生精補血, 潤燥止渴. 佐以澤瀉, 枳殼疏導二腑, 使小腑清利則心火下降；大腑流暢則肺經潤澤. 宿熱既除, 其渴自止矣.

·來源：易簡

14. Bai Fu Ling Wan. White Poria Pill. 白茯苓丸

·**ACTIONS**：kidney wasting-thirst.

·**COMPOSITION**：Fu Ling, Huang Lian, Tian Hua Fen, Bi Xie, Shu Di Huang, Fu Pen Zi, Ren Shen, Xuan Shen, Shi Hu, She Chuang Zi, Ji Zhun Pi.

·**INDICATIONS**：treats kidney wasting-thirst, both legs which gradually get weak and thin, the forceless of the lumbus and leg.

·**CHANNELS ENTERED**：The lesser yin channel.

·**Analysis of Formula**：(1) Fu Ling descends heart fire and interacts with the kidney.

(2) Huang Lian clears spleen fire and drains the heart.

(3) Shu Di Huang and Xuan Shen engender kidney water.

(4) Shi Hu pacifies stomach heat and astringes the kidney.

(5) Fu Pen Zi and She Chuang Zi secure kidney essence.

(6) Ren Shen supplements qi.

(7) Tian Hua Fen engenders the fluid.

(8) Bi Xie clears heat and disinhibits damp.

(9) Ji Zhun Pi is the spleen of the fowls. This can digest grain, frees the small intestine and bladder, checks frequent urination, and treats well wasting-thirst.

(10) The color of Ci Shi is black which enter the kidney to supplement Kidney and boost essence, therefore this acts as courier.

14. 白茯苓丸

·總結：腎消

·組成：茯苓，黃連，花粉，萆解，熟地黃，覆盆子，人參，玄參，石斛，蛇床子，鷄肫皮

·主治：治腎消兩腿漸細，腰脚無力.

·歸經：足少陰藥也.

·方義：(1)茯苓…降心火而交腎.

(2)黃連…清脾火而瀉心.

(3)熟地，玄參…生腎水.

(4)石斛…平胃熱而濇腎.

(5)覆盆，蛇床…固腎精.

(6)人參…補氣.

(7)花粉…生津.

(8)萆解…清熱利濕.

(9)鷄肫皮鷄之脾也…能消水穀，通小腸膀胱而止便數，善治膈消.

(10)磁石色黑入腎…補腎益精，故 假之爲使也.

15. Zhi Jiu Sou Fang. Enduring Cough Treating Formula.

310

治久嗽方

·**ACTIONS**：enduring cough
·**COMPOSITION**：Honey, Sheng Jiang
·**CHANNELS ENTERED**：The hand greater yin channel.
·**Analysis of Formula**：(1) Honey is lubricative. This can moisten the lun
g.

  (2) Sheng Jiang is pungent. This can disperse cold.
·**Original Source**：Tian Jin Yao Fang

15. 治久嗽方
  ·總結：久嗽
  ·組成：白蜜，生薑
  ·歸經：手太陰藥也.
  ·方義：(1)白蜜…滑能潤肺.
      (2)生薑…辛能散寒.
  ·來源：千金

16. Zhu Gao Jiu. Pork Lard Wine. 豬膏酒

·**ACTIONS**：extreme of the sinew.
·**COMPOSITION**：Zhu Zhi (pork lard), Jiang Zhi (juice of ginger), Win
e
·**INDICATIONS**：treats overexertion of the limbs, exhaustion of sinew h
umor, frequent cramp, pain in the all of nails, inability to stand for long time, th
is is called extreme of the sinew.
·**CHANNELS ENTERED**：The foot reverting yin channel.
·**Analysis of Formula**：Exhausted fluid and desiccated sinew cannot be tr
eated with only herbs.

  (1) Zhu Gao (pork lard) is moisture, this can nourish the sinew.

  (2) Jiang Zhi (juice of ginger) is pungent, this can moisten dryne
ss.

  (3) Wine harmonizes blood and the character moves well and rea
ches easily the limbs.
·**RELATED FORMULA**：(1) When Jiang Zhi (juice of ginger)is elimina
ted and Hair Decoction is added, hair has the character of dispersing, this is call

311

ed Zhu Gao Fa Jian, treats all kinds of jaundice, this makes jaundice come out t
hrough urination.

(2) When Jiang Zhi (juice of ginger) is eliminated and Jin Yin H
ua is added, this treats sore and scabies.

16. 豬膏酒

　·總結：筋極

　·組成：豬脂，薑汁，酒

　·主治：治過勞四肢筋液耗竭，數數轉筋，爪甲皆痛，不能久立，名曰
筋極.

　·歸經：足厥陰藥也.

　·方義：津竭筋枯，非草木之藥卒能責效…

　　　　　(1)豬膏…潤能養筋.

　　　　　(2)薑汁…辛能潤燥.

　　　　　(3)酒和血…而性善行，取易達於四肢也.

　·變化方：(1)本方除薑汁，加亂髮煎，髮消藥成…名豬膏髮煎⇒治諸黃，
令病從小便出.

　　　　　(2)本方除薑汁，加金銀花，煮酒飲⇒治瘡疥最良.

　·煎服法：分三服.

17. Ma Ren Su Zi Zhou. Hemp Seed and Perilla Fruit Grue
l. 麻仁蘇子粥

·ACTIONS：constipation of women after childbirth and old people.

·COMPOSITION：Da Ma Ren, Zi Su Zi

·INDICATIONS：treats defecation stoppage after childbirth, and wind c
onstipation of old people.

·CHANNELS ENTERED：The hand yang brightness channel.

·Analysis of Formula：(1) Ma Ren is the medicinal of yang brightness. T
his lubricates intestines and moistens dryness, and disinhibits defecation and eli
minates wind.

(2) Su Zi enters greater yin with large intestine. This moistens the lung and
frees intestines, harmonizes blood and descends qi, moves downward but is not dra
stic, is moderate but can free. The qi and blood of woman after childbirth and old p
eople is insufficient, therefore this is appropriate to use.

·Original Source：Ben Shi Fang

312

17. 麻仁蘇子粥

　　·總結：產婦老人便秘

　　·組成：大麻仁，紫蘇子

　　·主治：治產後大便不通，及老人風秘.

　　·歸經：手陽明藥也.

　　·方義：(1)麻仁陽明正藥...滑腸潤燥，利便除風.

　　　　　　(2)蘇子兼走太陰...潤肺通腸，和血下氣，行而不峻，緩而能

通.

　　　　　...故老人產婦氣血不足者所宜用之.

·來源：本事方

Chapter 14. Fire-Draining Formulas. 瀉火之劑

1. Huang Lian Jie Du Tang. Coptis Decoction to Relieve Toxicity. 黃連解毒湯

·**ACTIONS**：replete fire of triple burner

·**COMPOSITION**：Huang Qin, Huang Lian, Huang Bai, Zhi Zi

·**INDICATIONS**：treats all kinds of fire and heat, exuberance of both exterior and interior, mania with agitation, vexation in the heart, dry mouth, dry throat, great heat with, dry retching, disordered speech, insomnia, hematemesis, epistaxis, severe heat with macula.

·**CHANNELS ENTERED**：The hand and foot yang brightness, and the hand lesser yang channels [the large intestine, stomach, and triple burner]

·**Analysis of Formula**：(1) Heat is accumulated in the triple burner and evil fire moves frenetically, therefor Huang Qin is used to drain lung fire in the upper burner, Huang Lian is used to drain spleen fire in the middle burner, Huang Bai is used to drain kidney fire in the lower burner. Zhi Zi is used to free and drain the fire of the triple burner and make it out through the bladder.

(2) Generally when yang is exuberant, yin gets debilitated, when fire is exuberant, water gets debilitated, therefore medicinal which are great bitter and cold are used to retrain yang and support yin, and drain hyperactive fire and rescue water which is about to expire.

·**RELATED FORMULA**：(1) When Zhi Zi is eliminated, this is called Bai Pi Tang, treats triple burner's replete heat. When this is made with gruel into pill, this is called San Bu Wan, treats triple burner with fire, dry pharynx and throat, blocked urine and stool, damp phlegm, and heat effusion at night.

(2) When Huang Qin and Huang Lian are eliminated and Gan Cao is added, this is called Zhi Zi Bai Pi Tang, treats that when in cold damage, there is jaundice, and generalized heat effusion.

(3) When Huang Bai and Zhi Zi in this formula are added with Da Huang (soaked in wine), this is called San Huang Xie Xin Tang, treats glomus and heat below the heart, insufficiency of heart qi, hematemesis, and epistaxis.

(4) When Shi Gao, Dan Dou Chi, and Ma Huang are added, this is called San Huang Shi Gao Tang.

1. 黃連解毒湯

·總結：三焦實火

·組成：黃芩, 黃連, 黃柏, 梔子

·主治：治一切火熱, 表裏俱盛, 狂躁煩心, 口燥咽乾, 大熱乾嘔, 錯語不眠, 吐血衄血, 熱甚發斑.

·歸經：此手足陽明手少陽藥也(大腸, 胃, 三焦)

·方義：(1)三焦積熱, 邪火妄行, 故用黃芩瀉肺火於上焦, 黃連瀉脾火於中焦, 黃柏瀉腎火於下焦, 梔子通瀉三焦之火, 從膀胱出.

(2)蓋陽盛則陰衰, 火盛則水衰, 故用大苦大寒之藥, 抑陽而扶陰, 瀉其亢甚之火, 而救其欲絕之水也.

·變化方：(1)本方去梔子, 名柏皮湯, 治三焦實熱. 用粥丸, 名三補丸, 治三焦有火, 嗌燥喉乾, 二便閉結, 及淫瘀夜熱.

(2)本方去芩, 連, 加甘草, 名梔子柏皮湯, 治傷寒發黃身熱.

(3)本方黃柏, 梔子, 加酒浸大黃, 名三黃瀉心湯, 治心下痞熱, 心氣不足, 吐血衄血.

(4)本方加石膏, 淡豉, 麻黃, 名三黃石膏湯.

2. Fu Zi Xie Xin Tang. Aconite Heart-Draining Decoction. 附子瀉心湯

·**ACTIONS**：glomus and fullness in cold damage

·**COMPOSITION**：Fu Zi, Da Huang, Huang Lian, Huang Qin

·**INDICATIONS**：treats when in cold damage there is glomus below the heart, aversion to cold, and sweating.

·**CHANNELS ENTERED**：The foot greater yang and hand lesser yin channels [the bladder and heart]

·**Analysis of Formula**：Wu He Gao says that owing to glomus below the heart, the three Huang are used to drain glomus, owing to aversion to cold and sweating, Fu Zi is used to secure yang. Without three huang, it is unable to eliminate glomus and glomus heat, and Fu Zi is used, because there is worry that three huang damage yang, cold and heat medicinal are used together.

RELATED FORMULA：When Fu Zi is eliminated, this is called San Huang Xie Xin Tang, again when Huang Qin is eliminate, this is called Da Huang Huang Liand Xie Xin Tang, treats that when there is a glomus below the heart that is soft when pressure is applied, and the pulse is floating on the bar.   ·**Original Source**：Zhong Jing

315

2. 附子瀉心湯

　　·總結：傷寒痞滿

　　·組成：附子，大黃，黃連，黃芩

　　·主治：治傷寒心下痞，而復惡寒汗出者.

　　·歸經：此足太陽手少陰藥也(膀胱，心)

　　·方義：吳鶴臯：「心下痞，故用三黃以瀉痞，惡寒汗出，故用附子以固陽. 非三黃不能痞去痞熱，無附子恐三黃益損其陽，寒熱並用，斯爲有制之兵矣.」

　　·變化方：本方去附子名三黃瀉心湯，再去黃芩，名大黃黃連瀉心湯，治傷心下痞，按之濡，關上脈浮.

　　·來源：仲景

3. Ban Xia Xie Xin Tang. Pinellia Heart-Draining Decoction. 半夏瀉心湯

·**ACTIONS**： vacuous glomus in cold damage

·**COMPOSITION**：Huang Lian, Huang Qin, Ban Xia, Gan Jiang, Ren Shen, Gan Cao, Da Zao

·**INDICATIONS**：treats that when in cold damage, precipitation is used too early, thoracic fullness without pain is glomus, if there is generalized cold, retching, and inability to descend food and drink, this is not Chai Hu pattern.

·**CHANNELS ENTERED**：The hand lesser yin and the foot greater yin channels. [The heart and spleen]

·**Analysis of Formula**：Cheng Wu Ji says that bitter first enter the heart. Bitter should be used to drain the heart. Therefore Huang Lian acts as sovereign, Huang Qin acts as minister, they descend yang and raise yin. Pungent runs to qi, pungent should be used to disperse glomus. Therefore Ban Xia and Gan Jiang act as assistant to separate yin and move yang. To make the upper and lower free and interact, one should harmonize the middle, therefore Ren Shen, Gan Cao, and Da Zao act as courier to supplement the spleen and harmonize the middle. Then glomus heat disperses and profuse sweating resolves.

·**RELATED FORMULA**：⑴ When Ren Shen is eliminated and Gan Cao is added again, this is called Gan Cao Xie Xin Tang, treats that when in cold damage or wind strike, the physician has used precipitation, the person will have diarrhea ten times per day containing food that has not been transformed, with thunderous rumbling in the abdomen, fullness and a hard glomus below the heart, dry retching, and vexation that cannot be quieted. When the physician sees

316

a glomus below the heart, suggesting the illness has not finished, and again use s precipitation, yet as a result the glomus increase in severity, it is because heat bind is absent; only stomach vacuity is present with counterflow ascent of visiti ng qi, causing hardness.

(2) When Sheng Jiang (four liang) are added, this is called Sheng Jiang Xie Xin Tang, treats that when in cold damage after sweat has issued and brought resolution of the exterior, the stomach is in disharmony, there is a hard glomus below the heart, dry retching with malodor of food, water qi under the r ib-side, thunderous rumbling in the abdomen, and diarrhea.

(3) When Huang Qin and Da Zao are eliminated and Zhi Shi, Ho u Po, Mai Ya, Bai Zhu, and Fu Ling are added, this is called Zhi Shi Xiao Pi W an.

·**Original Source**：Zhong Jing

3. 半夏瀉心湯

　·總結：傷寒虛痞

　·組成：黃連, 黃芩, 半夏, 乾薑, 人參, 甘草, 大棗

　·主治：治傷寒下之早, 胸滿而不痛者爲痞, 身寒而嘔, 飲食不下, 非柴胡證.

　·歸經：此手少陰足太陰藥也(心脾)

　·方義：成氏曰：「否而不泰爲痞. 苦先入心, 瀉心者必以苦, 故以黃連爲君, 黃芩爲臣, 以降陽而升陰也. 辛走氣, 散痞者必以辛, 故以半夏, 乾薑爲佐, 以分陰而行陽也. 欲通上下交陰陽者, 必和其中, 故以人參, 甘草, 大棗爲使, 以補脾而和中. 則痞熱消而大汗以解矣.」

　·變化方：(1)本方除人參, 再加甘草, 名甘草瀉心湯, 治傷中風, 醫反下之, 下利穀不化, 腹中雷鳴, 心下痞硬而滿, 乾嘔心煩, 醫復下之, 其痞益甚, 此非結熱, 但以胃虛客氣上逆, 故使經也.

　　　(2)本方加生薑四兩, 名生薑瀉心湯, 治傷寒汗解後胃中不和, 心中痞硬, 乾噫嗳食臭, 完穀不化, 脅下有水氣, 腹中雷鳴下利.

　　　(3)本除黃芩, 大棗, 加枳實, 厚朴, 麥芽, 白朮, 茯苓, 蒸餅糊丸, 名枳實消痞丸.

　·來源：仲景

4. Bai Hu Tang. White Tiger Decoction. 白虎湯

·**ACTIONS**： replete heat of the lung and stomach.

317

·**COMPOSITION**：Zhi Mu, Shi Gao, Gan Cao (mix fried), Geng Mi

·**INDICATIONS**：(1) treats that when in cold damage, the pulse is floatin g and slippery. This means there is heat in the exterior and cold in the interior

(2) and in combination disease of the three yang, there is abdomi nal fullness, generalized heaviness, difficulty turning sides, insensitivity of the mouth, grimy face, delirious speech, and enuresis. If sweating is promoted, ther e will be delirious speech, and if precipitation is used, sweat will arise on the fo rehead and there will be reversal cold of the extremities. If sweat spontaneously issues, this formula governs.

(3) treats the combination disease of three yang, a pulse that is su rging, large, and long, there is absence of aversion to cold, instead, aversion to heat, headache, spontaneous sweating, thirst, eye pain, dry nose, inability to sle ep, vexation and agitation in the heart, late afternoon tidal heat effusion.

(4) or yang toxin with macula, all kinds of stomach heat disease.

·**CHANNELS ENTERED**： The foot yang brightness and the hand great er yin channels. [The stomach and heart]

·**Analysis of Formula**：(1) Excessive heat should be effused with bitter an d cold, therefore Zhi Mu which is bitter and cold, acts as sovereign.

(2) Heat tends to damage qi, the qi should be assisted by sweet a nd cold, therefore Shi Gao acts as minister.

(3) The fluid and humor is scorched in the interior, Gan Cao and Geng Mi are sweet and neutral, they boost and moderate qi and act as courier in order not to damage the stomach.

(4) Vexation is generated from the lung and the agitation is from the kidney, Shi Gao clears the lung and drains stomach fire, Zhi Mu clears the l ung and drains kidney fire, Gan Cao harmonizes the middle and drains the fire of the heart and spleen. This formula drains the son of the stomach, or drains th e mother of the stomach, this does not only treat the heat in qi part of yang brig htness.

·**RELATED FORMULA**：(1) When Ren Shen (three liang) is added, this is called Ren Shen Bai Hu Tang, treats that when in cold damage there is thirst with a desire to drink water, absence of exterior pattern, and dry tongue. And al so treats when in cold damage there is no great heat effusion, dry mouth, thirst, heart vexation, and mild aversion to cold in the back. Also treats that when in g reater yang summerheat stroke, there is generalized heat effusion, sweating, the cold of the feet, a pulse that is faint, and thirst. Also treats that when fire damag es the lung and stomach, this becomes diaphragm wasting-thirst.

(2) When Cang Zhu is added, this is called Bai Hu Jia Cang Zhu

318

Tang, treats damp warmth and a pulse that is sunken and fine.

(3) When Gui Zhi is added, this is called Gui Zhi Bai Hu Tang, t reats warm malaria, only heat effusion without aversion to cold, pain in bone an d joint, and periodic retching.

(4) When Chai Hu, Huang Qin, and Ban Xia are added, this is ca lled Chai Hu Shi Gao Tang, treats summerheat with cough, panting, and thirst.

(5) When Geng Mi is eliminated and Ren Shen is added, this is called Hua Ban Tang, treats stomach heat with macula and a pulse that is vacuous.

·**Original Source**：Zhong Jing

4. 白虎湯
·總結：肺胃實熱
·組成：知母, 石膏, 炙甘草, 粳米
·主治：(1)治傷寒脈浮滑, 表有熱, 裏有寒.

(2)及三陽合病, 脈浮大, 腹滿身重, 難以轉側, 口不仁而面垢, 譫語遺尿, 發汗則譫語, 下之則頭上生汗, 手足逆冷, 汗出者.

(3)通治陽明病脈洪大而長, 不惡寒, 反惡熱, 頭痛自汗, 口渴舌胎, 目痛鼻乾, 不得臥, 心煩躁亂, 日晡潮熱.

(4)或陽毒發斑, 胃熱諸病.
·歸經：此足陽明手太陰藥也(胃, 心)
·方義：(1)熱淫於內, 以苦寒發之, 故以知母苦寒爲君.

(2)熱則傷氣, 必以甘寒爲助, 故以石膏爲臣.

(3)津液內爍, 故以甘草, 粳米甘平益氣緩之爲使, 不致傷胃也.

(4)又煩出於肺, 躁出於腎, 石膏清肺而瀉胃火, 知母清肺而瀉腎火, 甘草和中而瀉心脾之火. 或瀉其子, 或瀉其母, 不專治陽明氣分熱也.

·變化方：(1)本方加人參三兩, 名人參白虎湯, 治傷寒渴欲飲水, 無表證者, 口乾舌燥者. 亦治傷寒無大熱, 口燥渴, 心煩背微惡寒者. 亦治太陽中暍, 身熱, 汗出, 足冷, 脈微而渴. 亦治火傷肺胃, 傳爲膈消.

(2)本方加蒼朮, 名白虎加蒼朮湯, 濕溫脈沈細者.

(3)本方加桂枝, 名桂枝白虎湯, 治溫瘧, 但熱無寒, 骨節疼痛, 時嘔.

(4)本方加柴胡, 黃芩, 半夏, 名柴胡石膏湯, 治暑嗽喘渴.

(5)本方除粳米, 加人參, 名化斑湯治胃熱發斑脈虛者.
·來源：仲景

319

5. Zhu Ye Shi Gao Tang. Lophatherum and Gypsum Decoction. 竹葉石膏湯

·**ACTIONS**： vacuous heat of the lung and stomach

·**COMPOSITION**： Zhu Ye, Shi Gao, Ban Xia, Gan Cao (mix fried), Geng Mi, Mai Men Dong, Ren Shen

·**INDICATIONS**： (1) treats that after cold damage has resolved, there is vacuous emaciation, shortage of qi, qi counterflow, and a desire to vomit.

(2) also treats summerheat damage with thirst and a pulse that is vacuous.

·**CHANNELS ENTERED**： The hand greater yin and foot yang brightness channels [the heart and the stomach]

·**Analysis of Formula**： (1) Zhu Ye and Shi Gao are pungent and cool, they disperse residual heat.

(2) Ren Shen, Gan Cao, Mai Men Dong, and Geng Mi are sweet and neutral. They boost the lung, quiet the stomach, supplement vacuity, and engender the fluid.

(3) Ban Xia is pungent and warm, this sweeps phlegm and checks retching.

Therefore this formula eliminates heat and does not damage the true yin, and conduct counterflow qi and can boosts qi.

·**Another Side Formula**： Zhu Ye, Shi Gao, Mu Tong, Bo He, Jie Geng, Gan Cao, this is also called Zhu Ye Shi GaoTang, treats replete stomach and exuberant fire with thirst.

·**Original Source**： Zhong Jing

5. 竹葉石膏湯

·總結：肺胃虛熱

·組成：竹葉，石膏，半夏，炙甘草，粳米，麥冬，人參

·主治：(1)治傷寒解後，虛贏少氣，氣逆欲吐.

(2)亦治傷暑發渴脈虛.

·歸經：手太陰足陽明藥也(心，胃)

·方義：(1)竹葉石膏之辛涼，以散餘熱.

(2)人參，甘草，麥冬，粳米之甘平，以益肺安胃，補虛生津.

(3)半夏之辛溫，以谿痰止嘔.

故去熱而不損其眞，導逆而能益其氣也.

·又附方：竹葉，石膏，木通，薄荷，桔梗，甘草，亦名竹葉石膏湯，治

胃實火盛而作渴.

·來源：仲景

6. Sheng Yang San Huo Tang. Raise the Yang and Disperse the Fire Decoction. 升陽散火湯

·**ACTIONS**：fire depression

·**COMPOSITION**：Chai Hu, Sheng Ma, Ge Gen, Qiang Huo, Fang Feng, Du Huo, Gan Cao (mix fried), Sheng Gan Cao, Ren Shen, Bai Shao Yao

·**INDICATIONS**：(1) treats flesh heat, exterior heat, heat effusion in the l imbs, heat in the bone marrow, heat effusion as burning, when rubbing, it feels like an iron. .

(2) this disease occurs due to blood vacuity, and also stomach va cuity with overeating of cold food and drink causes yang qi to be depressed in s pleen earth, both case should be treated with this formula.

·**CHANNELS ENTERED**：The hand and foot lesser yang channels. [Th e triple burner and gall bladder]

·**Analysis of Formula**：(1) Chai Hu effuse the fire of lesser yang, acting a s sovereign.

(2) Sheng Ma and Ge Gen effuse the fire of yang brightness, Qia ng Huo and Fang Feng effuse the fire of greater yang, Du Huo effuses the fire o f lesser yin, acting as minister. They are thin in flavor and light in qi, and move upward. Therefore this formula raises the yang and makes the triple burner to b e uninhibited, then all of fire evils get to disperse.

(3) Ren Shen and Gan Cao boost spleen earth and drain heat, Sha o Yao drains spleen fire and restrains yin. The sour is astringent and the sweet moderates, therefore this formula disperses in the middle of contracting, and m akes yin qi not to reach detriment, acting as assistant and courier.

·**Original Source**：Li Dong Yuan

6. 升陽散火湯

·總結：火鬱

·組成：柴胡，升麻，葛根，羌活，防風，獨活，炙甘草，生甘草，人參，白芍

·主治：(1)治肌熱表熱，四肢發熱，骨髓中熱，熱如火燎，捫之烙手.

(2)此病多因血虛得之，及胃虛過食冷物，抑遏陽氣於脾土，

並宜服此.

　·歸經：此手足少陽藥也(三焦，膽)

　·方義：(1)柴胡以發少陽之火爲君.

　　　　　(2)升，葛以發陽明之火，羌，防以發太陽之火，獨活以發少陰之火爲臣. 此皆味薄氣輕，上行之藥，所以升擧其陽，使三焦暢遂，而火邪皆散矣.

　　　　　(3)人參，甘草益脾土而瀉熱，芍藥瀉脾火而斂陰，且酸斂甘緩，散中有收，不致有損陰氣而佐使也.

　·來源：東垣

7. Liang Ge San. Cool the Diaphragm Powder. 涼膈散

　·ACTIONS：fire in the upper and middle burner.

　·COMPOSITION：Da Huang, Mang Xiao, Bo He, Huang Qin, Zhi Zi, Lian Qiao, Gan Cao

　·INDICATIONS：(1) treats exuberant heart fire, dryness and repletion in the middle burner, vexation and agitation, thirst, reddish eye, dizziness, mouth sore, cracked lips, hematemesis, epistaxis, inhibited urination, constipation, wind convulsions, stomach heat with macula and mania.

　　　　　(2) and child fright, pox sore.

·CHANNELS ENTERED：this formula drains the fire of the upper and middle burner.

·Analysis of Formula：(1) Excessive heat in the interior should be treated with salty and cold and is assisted with bitter and sweet, therefore Lian Qiao, Huang Qin, Zhu Ye, and Bo He raise and disperse heat to upward. Da Huang and Mang Xiao precipitate harshly and flush the middle. They make fire evil ascend upward and move downward, and then the diaphragm spontaneously clears.

　　　　　(2) Gan Cao and raw Honey are used, because disease is in the diaphragm, the sweet moderate it.

　·Original Source：Ju Fang

7. 涼膈散

　·總結：上中二焦火

　·組成：大黃，芒硝，薄荷，黃芩，梔子，連翹，甘草

　·主治：(1)治心火上盛，中焦燥實，煩燥口渴，目赤頭眩，口瘡脣裂，吐血衄血，大小便祕，諸風瘛瘲，胃熱發斑發狂.

(2)及小兒驚急, 痘瘡黑陷.

·歸經：此上中二焦瀉火藥

·方義：(1)熱淫於內, 治以鹹寒, 佐以苦甘, 故以連翹, 黃芩, 竹葉, 薄荷升散於上；而以大黃, 芒硝之猛利推蕩其中, 使上升下行, 而膈自清矣.

(2)用甘草, 生蜜者, 病在膈, 甘以緩之也.

·來源：局方

8. Dang Gui Long Hui Wan. Tangkuei, Gentiana and Aloe Pills. 當歸龍薈丸

·ACTIONS：The fire of the liver and gall bladder

·COMPOSITION：Dang Gui, Lu Hui, Mu Xiang, She Xiang, Long Dan Cao, Qing Dai, Huang Qin, Huang Lian, Huang Bai, Zhi Zi, Da Huang

·INDICATIONS：(1) treats all kinds of the fire of the liver and gall bladder, unquiet spirit-mind, fright and palpitations, convulsion, agitated mania, dizziness, dizzy vision, tinnitus, deafness, glomus blockage in the chest and diaphragm.

(2) inhibited throat, dry intestines and stomach, both rib side pain stretched to lesser abdomen, liver heat spreading to the lung with cough.

(3) also treats night sweating.

·CHANNELS ENTERED：The foot reverting yin and the hand and foot lesser yang channels. [The liver, triple burner, and gall bladder]

·Analysis of Formula：(1) Liver wood is the root of engendering fire, when liver fire is exuberant, the fire of all of the channels keep uprising, the disease caused by this condition is not one kind. Therefore Long Dan Cao and Qing Dai directly enter the original channel to break it and Da Huang, Huang Qin, Huang Lian, Zhi Zi, and Huang Bai free and pacify the fire of triple burner.

(2) Lu Hui is great bitter and cold, the qi is animal order, and enter the liver, this can conduct every herbs to enter the reverting yin. This first calms exuberant liver fire and then fire of all of the channels get calm.

(3) The above herbs are bitter and cold. Dang Gui is pungent and warm, can enter the reverting yin, harmonizes blood and supplements yin, therefore acting as sovereign.

(4) Small dose of Mu Xiang and She Xiang move qi and free orifice.

·Original Source：Gao Ming

323

8. 當歸龍薈丸

　·總結：肝膽火

　·組成：當歸，蘆薈，木香，麝香，龍膽草，青黛，黃芩，黃連，黃柏，
梔子，大黃

　·主治：(1)治一切肝膽之火，神志不寧，驚悸搐搦，躁擾狂越，頭運目
眩，耳鳴耳聾，胸膈痞塞．

　　　　(2)咽嗌不利，腸胃燥澀，兩脇痛引少腹，肝移熱於肺而欬嗽．

　　　　(3)亦治盜汗．

　·歸經：足厥陰手足少陽藥也．

　·方義：(1)肝木為生火之本，肝火盛則諸經之火相因而起，為病不止一
端矣．故以龍膽，青黛直入本經而折之，而以大黃，芩，連，梔，柏：通平
上下三焦之火也．

　　　　(2)蘆薈大苦大寒，氣躁入肝，能引諸藥同入厥陰，先平其甚
者，而諸經之火無不漸平矣．

　　　　(3)諸藥苦寒已甚，當歸辛溫，能入厥陰，和血而補陰，故以
為君．

　　　　(4)少加木香，麝香者，取其行氣通竅也．

　·來源：高明

9. Long Dan Xie Gan Tang. Gentiana Decoction to Drain the Liver. 龍膽瀉肝湯

·ACTIONS：The fire of the liver and gall bladder

·COMPOSITION：Long Dan Cao, Huang Qin, Zhi Zi, Chai Hu, Sheng Di Huang, Dang Gui, Gan Cao, Mu Tong, Che Qian Zi, Ze Xie

·INDICATIONS：(1) treats replete fire and damp heat in the liver and gall bladder channels, rib side pain, deafness, overflowing gall with bitter taste in the mouth

(2) sinew wilting, genital sweating, genital swelling, genital pain, white turbidity, and hematuria.

·CHANNELS ENTERED：The foot reverting yin and lesser yang channels.

·Analysis of Formula：(1) Long Dan Cao drains the heat of the reverting yin.

(2) Chai Hu pacifies the heat of the lesser yang.

(3) Huang Qin and Zhi Zi clear the heat of the lung and triple burner, acting as assistant.

324

(4) Ze Xie drains the damp of the kidney channel.

(5) Mu Tong and Che Qian Zi drain the damp of the small intestine and bladder, acting as assistant.

(6) Dang Gui and Sheng Di Huang are used to tonify blood and supplement the liver.

(7) Gan Cao is used to moderate the middle and not to damage the stomach, acting as minister and courier.

·Another Side Formula：(1) Li Dong Yuan eliminates Huang Qin, Zhi Zi, and Gan Cao, this is also called Long Dan Xie Gan Tang, treats heat, itch, and urine odor in genitals.

(2) In the other formula, Dang Gui, Sheng Di Huang, Mu Tong, Ze Xie, and Che Qian Zi are eliminated and Ren Shen, Wu Wei Zi, Tian Men Dong, Mai Men Dong, Huang Lian, and Zhi Mu are added, this is also called Long Dan Cao Xie Gan Tang, treats sinew wilting, hypertonicity, bitter taste in the mouth, desiccated nails, and also the above pattern.

·**Original Source**：Ju Fang

9. 龍膽瀉肝湯

·總結：肝膽火

·組成：龍膽草, 黃芩, 栀子, 柴胡, 生地黃, 當歸, 甘草, 木通, 車前子, 澤瀉

·主治：(1)治肝膽經實火濕熱, 脇痛耳聾, 膽溢口苦

(2)筋痿陰汗, 陰腫陰痛, 白濁溲血.

·歸經：此足厥陰少陽藥也.

·方義：(1)龍膽：瀉厥陰之熱.

(2)柴胡：平少陽之熱.

(3)黃芩, 栀子：清肺與三焦之熱以佐之.

(4)澤瀉：瀉腎經之濕.

(5)木通, 車前：瀉小腸膀胱之濕以佐之.

(6)用歸地：以養血而補肝.

(7)用甘草：以緩中而不使腸胃爲臣使也.

·又附方：(1)東垣無黃芩, 栀子, 甘草, 亦名龍膽瀉肝湯. 治前陰熱癢臊臭.

(2)一方除當歸, 生地, 木通, 澤瀉, 車前, 加人參, 五味, 天冬, 麥冬, 黃連, 知母, 亦名龍膽瀉肝湯. 治筋痿攣急, 口苦爪枯, 亦治前證.

325

·來源：局方

10. Zuo Jin Wan. Left Metal Pill. 左金丸

·**ACTIONS**：liver fire

·**COMPOSITION**：Huang Lian, Wu Zhu Yu.

·**INDICATIONS**：(1) treats exuberant fire and dryness of the liver, pain in the l eft rib side, acid regurgitation, acid vomiting, sinew mounting(shan), glomus and binds.

(2) also treats food-denying dysentery, immediate vomiting as so on as a decoction enters the mouth.

·**CHANNELS ENTERED**：The foot reverting yin channel.

·**Analysis of Formula**：(1) Replete liver causes pain, the heart is the son o f the liver, when the liver is replete, one should drain the son.

(2) Therefore Huang Lian is used to drain the heart and clear fire, acting as sovereign. This makes fire not to restrain metal, metal can restrain wo od, and then the liver gets calm.

(3) Wu Zhu Yu is pungent and heat, this can enter the reverting y in, moves qi and resolves depression, this also can conduct heat to move down ward, therefore this acts as counteracting assistant. In this formula, one herb is cold and the other herb is heat, draining heat with cold is right treatment, count eracting assistant with heat herb is following treatment, heat pattern treated wit h heat herb is counteracting treatment. Therefore they can help each other to m ake treat effect. The liver resides in the left and moves upward, the lung resides in the right and moves downward. The name of this formula is Zuo Jin (Left M etal), this means that this formula make metal qi to move in the left side and pa cifies the liver.

·**RELATED FORMULA**：(1) Zhu Lian Wan：Huang Qin (stir-baked), Cang Zhu, and Chen Pi are added, treats same things..

(2) Wu Ji Wan is this formula with Shao Yao, treats heat dysente ry and heat diarrhea.

(3) Lian Fu Liu Yi Tang：When Wu Zhu Yu is eliminated and F u Zi (one liang) is added, this is Lian Fu Liu Yi Tang, treats stomach duct pain, this treats heat disease with heat herbs.

(4) Xie Xin Tang. : only huang lian, this treats heart heat.

10. 左金丸

·總結：肝火

·組成：黃連, 吳茱萸.

·主治：(1)治肝火燥盛, 左脇作痛, 吞酸吐酸, 筋疝痞結.

　　　　(2)亦治噤口痢, 湯藥入口即吐.

·歸經：此足厥陰藥也.

·方義：(1)肝實則作痛, 心者肝之子, 實則瀉其子.

　　　　(2)故用黃連：瀉心清火爲君, 使火不剋金, 金能制木, 則肝平矣.

　　　　(3)吳茱萸：辛熱, 能入厥陰, 行氣解郁, 又能引熱下行, 故以爲反佐. 一寒一熱, 寒者正治, 熱者從治, 以熱治熱, 從其性而治之, 亦曰反治. 故能相濟以立功, 肝居於左, 肺處於右. 左金者：謂使金令得行於左而平肝也.

·變化方：(1)茱連丸：本方加炒芩, 蒼朮, 陳皮. 治同.

　　　　(2)戊己丸：本方和芍藥等分爲丸. 治熱痢熱瀉.

　　　　(3)連附六一湯：本方除吳茱萸加附子一兩, 治胃脘痛, 寒因熱用也.

　　　　(4)瀉心湯：單黃連煎服. 治心熱.

11. Xie Qing Wan. Drain the Green Pill. 瀉青丸

·ACTIONS：liver fire

·COMPOSITION：Long Dan Cao, Da Huang, Fang Feng, Qiang Huo, Chuan Xiong, Dang Gui, Shan Zhi Zi.

·INDICATIONS：treats liver fire, congested heat, inability to lay down, often fright and anger, sinew wilting, reddish, swollen, and aching eyes.

·CHANNELS ENTERED：The foot reverting yin and lesser yang channels. [The liver and gall bladder]

·Analysis of Formula：(1) The liver holds the office of general. Excessive wind and intense fire are not easy to come down.

(2) Long Dan Cao and Da Huang are bitter, cold, and thick flavor, deep yin tends to move downward. They directly enter reverting yin and disperse and drain wind fire, they break the anger fire and move this downward.

(3) The qi of Qiang Huo is strong and Fang Feng is good at dispersing, therefore they can track liver wind down and disperse liver fire.

(4) Fire repletion of lesser yang causes headache and reddish eyes. Chuan Xiong can move upward to the head and eyes, and expels wind evil.

327

(5) The congested fire of lesser yang causes vexation and agitati
on, Zhi Zi can disperse the congested fire of the triple burner and make evil hea
t to move downward through urination.

(6) And Chuan Xiong and Dang Gui belong to blood part herbs.
They can nourish liver blood and moisten dry liver. And they are qi medicinal i
n blood, pungent can disperse and warm can harmonize.

·**Original Source**：Qian Yi

11. 瀉青丸

·總結：肝火

·組成：龍膽草，大黃，防風，羌活，川芎，當歸，山梔.

·主治：治肝火郁熱，不能安臥，多驚多怒，筋痿不起，目赤腫痛.

·歸經：此足厥陰少陽藥也.

·方義：(1)肝者將軍之官，風淫火熾，不易平也.

(2)龍膽，大黃：苦寒厚味，沉陰下行，直入厥陰而散瀉之，
所以抑其怒而折之於下也.

(3)羌活：氣雄，防風：善散，故能搜肝風而散肝火.

(4)少陽火實，多頭痛目赤，川芎能上行頭目而逐風邪.

(5)少陽火郁，多煩燥，梔子能散三焦郁火而使邪熱從小便下
行.

(6)且川芎，當歸乃血分之藥，能養肝血而潤肝燥，又皆血中
氣藥，辛能散而溫能和兼以培之也.

·來源：錢乙

12. Xie Huang San. Drain the Yellow Powder. 瀉黃散

·**ACTIONS**：spleen fire

·**COMPOSITION**：Shan Zhi Zi, Huo Xiang, Shi Gao, Gan Cao, Fang Fe
ng.

·**INDICATIONS**：treats latent fire of the spleen and stomach, dry mouth,
dry lip, mouth sore, fetid mouth odor, vexation, thirst, rapid hungering, and hea
t in the flesh.

·**CHANNELS ENTERED**：The foot greater yin and yang brightness cha
nnels. [The spleen and stomach]

·**Analysis of Formula**：(1) Shan Zhi Zi clears the fire of the heart and lun
g. This makes heat fire to move downward and come out through urination.

328

(2) Huo Xiang rectifies the qi of the spleen and lung, eliminates congested heat in the upper burner, repels malign, and regulates the middle.

(3) Shi Gao is great cold. This drains heat with resolving the flesh.

(4) Gan Cao is sweet and neutral. This harmonizes the middle and also can drain fire.

(5) Lots of Fang Feng is used. This raises yang and can disperse latent fire in the spleen and drain wood in earth.

12. 瀉黃散
　·總結：脾火
　·組成：山梔子，藿香，石膏，甘草，防風.
　·主治：治脾胃伏火，口燥唇乾，口瘡口臭，煩渴易飢，熱在肌肉.
　·歸經：此足太陰陽明藥也.
　·方義：(1)山梔：清心肺之火，使屈曲下行，從小便出.
　　　　　(2)藿香：理脾肺之氣，去上焦壅熱，辟惡調中.
　　　　　(3)石膏：大寒瀉熱，兼能解肌.
　　　　　(4)甘草：甘平和中，又能瀉火.
　　　　　(5)重用防風者：取其升陽，能發脾中伏火，又能於土中瀉木也.

13. Qing Wei San. Clear the Stomach Powder. 清胃散

·ACTIONS：stomach fire with toothache

·COMPOSITION：Sheng Ma, sheng Di Huang, Dang Gui, Huang Lian, Mu Dan Pi, Shi Gao

·INDICATIONS：(1) treats the accumulated heat in the stomach, toothache stretching to the head and brain, heat effusion in whole face.

(2) the tooth liking something cold and disliking something heat, or gingivitis, or often gingival bleeding, or mumps.

·CHANNELS ENTERED：The foot yang brightness channel. [The stomach]

·Analysis of Formula：(1) Huang Lian drains heart fire and also drains spleen fire. The spleen is the son of the heart and has interior exterior relationship with the stomach.

(2) Dang Gui harmonizes blood, Sheng Di Huang and Mu Dan P

329

i cool blood. They nourish yin and retreat yang.

    (3) Shi Gao drains great heat of yang brightness.

    (4) Sheng Ma raises clear yang of yang brightness. When clear a
scends and heat descends, swelling disperses and pain stops.

 ·Original Source：Li Dong Yuan

13. 清胃散
 ·總結：胃火牙痛
 ·組成：升麻, 生地黃, 當歸, 川黃連, 牡丹皮, 石膏
 ·主治：(1)治胃有積熱, 上下牙痛, 牽引頭腦, 滿面發熱.
    (2)其牙喜寒惡熱, 或牙齦潰爛, 或牙宣出血, 或唇口頰腮腫
痛.
 ·歸經：此足陽明藥也.
 ·方義：(1)黃連：瀉心火, 亦瀉脾火, 脾爲心子, 而與胃相表裏.
    (2)當歸：和血, 生地, 丹皮：涼血, 以養陰而退陽.
    (3)石膏：瀉陽明之大熱.
    (4)升麻：升陽明之清陽, 清升熱降, 則腫消而痛止.
 ·來源：東垣

14. Gan Lu Yin. Sweet Dew Decoction. 甘露飲

 ·ACTIONS：damp heat in the stomach.

 ·COMPOSITION：Shu Di Huang, Sheng Di Huang, Tian Men Dong, M
ai Men Dong, Shi Hu, Huang Qin, Pi Pa Ye, Yin Chen, Zhi Ke, Gan Cao

 ·INDICATIONS：treats damp heat in the stomach, fetid mouth odor, sor
e throat, exposed gums, and hematemesis, epistaxis, and gingival bleeding.

 ·MODIFICATIONS：When Gui Zhi and Fu Ling are added, this is calle
d Gui Ling Gan Lu Yin. In Ben Shi Fang, Xi Jiao is added.

 ·CHANNELS ENTERED：The foot yang brightness and lesser yin chan
nels. [The stomach and kidney]

 ·Analysis of Formula：(1) Vexing heat is mainly related with vacuity. Th
e sweet of Shu Di Huang and Sheng Di Huang, Mai Men Doing, Tian Men Don
g, Gan Cao, and Shi Hu treats vacuous heat in the kidney and stomach, they dra
ins vacuous heat with supplementing yin.

    (2) The bitter and cold of Yin Chen Huang Qin breaks heat and e
liminates damp.

(3) When fire heat moves upward, this causes disease, therefore Zhi Ke, and Pi Pa Ye repress and descend fire heat.

·Another Side Formula：Liu He Jian's Gui Ling Gan Lu Yin.：Hua Shi, Shi Gao, Han Shui Shi, Gan Cao, Bai Zhu, Fu Ling, Ze Xie, Zhu Ling, and Rou Gui. This treats summerheat with damp, copious drinking of water, headache, v exation, thirst, damp heat with constipation.

·**Original Source**：Ju Fang

14. 甘露飲

·總結：胃中溼熱

·組成：熟地黃, 生地黃, 天門冬, 麥門冬, 石斛, 黃芩, 枇杷葉, 茵陳, 枳殼, 甘草

·主治：治胃中濕熱, 口臭喉瘡, 齒齦宣露, 及吐衄齒血.

·加減：一方加桂苓, 名桂苓甘露飲, 本事方加犀角.

·歸經：此足陽明少陰藥也.

·方義：(1)煩熱多屬於虛, 二地, 二冬, 甘草, 石斛之甘：治腎胃之虛熱, 瀉而兼補.

(2)茵陳黃芩之苦寒：折熱而去濕.

(3)火熱上行爲患, 故又以枳殼, 枇杷葉抑而降之也.

·又附方：河間桂苓甘露飲：滑石, 石膏, 寒水石, 甘草, 白朮, 茯苓, 澤瀉, 豬苓, 肉桂. 治中暑受濕, 引飲過多, 頭痛煩渴, 濕熱便秘.

·來源：局方

15. Xie Bai San. Drain the White Powder. 瀉白散

·**ACTIONS**：lung fire

·**COMPOSITION**：Sang Bai Pi, Di Gu Pi, Gan Cao, Geng Mi.

·**INDICATIONS**：treats lung fire, steaming heat in the skin, aversion to c old and heat effusion, getting severe in late afternoon, panting, cough, and rapi d breathing.

·**CHANNELS ENTERED**：The hand greater yin channel. [The lung]

·**Analysis of Formula**：(1) The sweet of Sang Bai Pi boosts insufficient s ource qi, the pungent drains surplus lung qi, eliminates phlegm, and allays coug h.

(2) The cold of Di Gu Pi drains latent fire in the lung and vacuou s heat of the liver and kidney, and cools blood and treats steaming heat.

331

(3) Gan Cao drains fire and boosts the spleen.

(4) Geng Mi clears the lung and supplements the stomach. This can drain heat through urination.

(5) The lung controls west side, therefore this is called Xie Bai.

·**RELATED FORMULA**：(1) **Jia Jian Xie Bai San**.：When Ren Shen, Wu Wei Zi, Fu Ling, Qing Pi, and Chen Pi are added, this treats cough, panting, and acute vomiting.（Li Dong Yuan Fang）

(2) **Jia Jian Xie Bai San.**：When Zhi Mu, Huang Qin, Jie Geng, Qing Pi, and Chen Pi are added, this treats cough, vexing heat, thirst, inhibited chest diaphragm.(Bao Jian Fang)

(3) **Jia Jian Xie Bai San.**：When Gan Cao and Geng Mi are eliminated and Huang Qin, Zhi Mu, Mai Men Dong, Wu Wei Zi, and Jie Geng are added, this treats excessive drinking damaging the lung, fishy smell form mouth, spittle of sticky snivel, inhibited throat, bitter taste in the mouth, and dry mouth.(Luo Qian Fu Fang)

·**Original Source**：Qian Yi

15. 瀉白散

·總結：肺火

·組成：桑白皮, 地骨皮, 甘草, 粳米.

·主治：治肺火皮膚蒸熱, 灑淅寒熱, 日晡尤甚, 喘嗽氣急.

·歸經：此手太陰藥也.

·方義：(1)桑白皮：甘益元氣之不足, 辛瀉肺氣之有餘, 除痰止嗽.

(2)地骨皮：寒瀉肺中伏火, 淡泄肝腎虛熱, 涼血退蒸.

(3)甘草：瀉火而益脾.

(4)粳米：清肺而補胃, 能瀉熱從小便出.

(5)肺主西方, 故曰瀉白.

·變化方：(1)加減瀉白散：本方加人參, 五味, 茯苓, 青皮, 陳皮. 皮治欬嗽喘急嘔吐.（東垣方）

(2)加減瀉白散：本方加知母, 黃芩, 桔梗, 青皮, 陳皮. 治欬而氣喘, 煩熱口渴, 胸膈不利.(寶鑑方)

(3)加減瀉白散：本方除甘草, 粳米, 加黃芩, 知母, 麥冬, 五味, 桔梗治過飲傷肺, 氣出腥臭, 唾涕稠黏, 嗌喉不利, 口苦乾燥.(羅謙甫方)

·來源：錢乙

16. Dao Chi San. Guide Out the Red Powder. 導赤散

·**ACTIONS**： the fire of the heart and small intestine.

·**COMPOSITION**：Sheng Di Huang, Mu Tong, Gan Cao, Dan Zhu Ye.

·**INDICATIONS**：treats the small intestine with fire, reddish urine, stran gury, reddish complexion, mania, agitation, oral erosion, tongue sore, grinding of the teeth, and thirst.

·**CHANNELS ENTERED**：The hand lesser yin and greater yang channel s. [The heart and small intestine]

·**Analysis of Formula**：(1) Sheng Di Huang cools heart blood.

(2) Zhu Ye clears heart qi.

(3) Mu Tong descends heart fire and enters the small intestine.

(4) Gan Cao reaches the middle and relieves pain. All of them ab duct the fire of Bing Ding, and the fire comes out through urination. The small i ntestine is related with Bing Fire, the heart is Ding Fire.

Heart heat should be treated with draining the small intestine.

·**Original Source**：Qian Yi

16. 導赤散
·總結：心小腸火
·組成：生地, 木通, 甘草梢, 淡竹葉.
·主治：治小腸有火, 便赤淋痛, 面赤狂躁, 口糜舌瘡, 咬牙口渴.
·歸經：此手少陰太陽藥也.
·方義：(1)生地：涼心血.
(2)竹葉：清心氣.
(3)木通：降心火, 入小腸.
(4)草梢：達中而止痛, 以共導丙丁之火, 由小水而出也. 小腸爲丙火, 心爲丁火.
心熱泄小腸.
·來源：錢乙

17. Lian Zi Qing Xin Yin. Lotus Seed Decoction to Clear th e Heart. 蓮子清心飲

·**ACTIONS**：heart fire with strangury and turbid

·**COMPOSITION**：Shi Lian Rou, Gan Cao, Huang Qi, Ren Shen, Di Gu

Pi, Chai Hu, Huang Qin, Mai Men Dong, Fu Ling, Che Qian Zi.

·**INDICATIONS**：(1) treats depression due to anxiety and thought, heat e ffusion, and vexation and agitation.

(2) or excessive drinking of alcohol and eating, exuberant fire res training metal, bitter taste in the mouth, dry throat, wasting-thirst, seminal emis sion, strangury and turbid, fatigued cumbersome limbs, vexing heat in the five hearts, stable at night and severe at day.

(2) and metrorrhagia and leukorrhargia in woman.

·**CHANNELS ENTERED**：The hand and foot lesser yin and foot lesser yang and greater yin channels. [The heart, kidney, gall bladder, and spleen]

·**Analysis of Formula**：(1) Ren Shen, Huang Qi, and Gan Cao supplemen t yang vacuity and drain fire, and assist qi to transform and to reach bladder.

(2) Di Gu Pi retreats vacuous heat of the liver and kidney.

(3) Chai Hu disperses fire evil of the liver and gall bladder.

(4) Huang Qin and Mai Men Dong clear heat in the heart, lung, a nd upper burner.

(5) Fu Ling and Che Qian Zi disinhibit damp in the bladder and l ower part.

(6) Shi Lian Rou clears the heart fire and make the heart and the kidney interact, then every pattern disappear.

·**Original Source**：Ju Fang

17. 蓮子清心飲

·總結：心火淋濁

·組成：石蓮肉，甘草，黃耆，人參，地骨皮，柴胡，黃芩，麥冬，茯苓，車前子.

·主治：(1)治憂思抑郁，發熱煩躁.

(2)或酒食過度，火盛剋金，口苦咽乾，漸成消渴，遺精淋濁，遇勞即發，四肢倦怠，五煩熱，夜靜晝甚.

(2)及女人崩帶.

·歸經：此手足少陰足少陽太陰藥也.

·方義：(1)參，耆，甘草：所以補陽虛而瀉火，助氣化而達州都.

(2)地骨：退肝腎之虛熱.

(3)柴胡：散肝膽之火邪.

(4)黃芩，麥冬：清熱於心肺上焦.

(5)茯苓，車前：利濕於膀胱下部.

(6)用以石蓮：清心火而交心腎，則諸證悉退也.
　·來源：局方

18. Dao Chu Ge Ban Tang. 導赤各半湯

·**ACTIONS**：cold damage with heart heat

·**COMPOSITION**：Huang Lian, Xi Jiao, Zhi Zi, Hua Shi, Gan Cao, Mai Men Dong, Huang Qin, Ren Shen, Fu Shen, Zhi Mu, Deng Xin, Da Zao, Sheng Jiang.

·**INDICATIONS**：(1) treats that after cold damage, there is absence of hardness below the heart, absence of abdominal fullness, normal urination and defecation, absence of generalized heat effusion, gradual change of loss of consciousness with inability to speak.

(2) or a soliloquy in sleep, reddish eyes, dry mouth, non-drinking of water, if one gives gruel to patient, the patient eats, but if one does not, there is no thought of gruel, and looking like lush. This is called Yue Jing (skipping channels) pattern.

·**CHANNELS ENTERED**：The hand lesser and greater yin and greater yang channels. [The heart, lung, and large intestine]

·**Analysis of Formula**：(1) Chen Lai Zhang says that when heat enters heart channel, cool the heat with Huang Lian, Xi Jiao, and Zhi Zi.

(2) When heart heat passed into the small intestine, drain Hua Shi, Gan Cao, and Deng Xin.

(3) When heart heat pressures upward to the lung, clear the heat with Huang Qin, Zhi Zi, and Mai Men Dong.

(4) If evil which skips channels, passes into the heart, this indicates that heart spirit is originally insufficient, therefore Ren Shen and Fu Shen are added to supplement the heart.

·**Original Source**：Jie An

18. 導赤各半湯

　·總結：傷寒心熱

　·組成：黃連, 犀角, 梔子, 滑石, 甘草, 麥冬, 黃芩, 人參, 茯神, 知母, 燈心, 大棗, 生薑.

　·主治：(1)治傷寒後心下不硬, 腹中不滿, 二便如常, 身無熱, 漸變神昏不語.

335

(2)或睡中獨語, 目赤口乾, 不飲水, 與粥則嚥, 不與勿思, 形如醉人, 名越經證.

·歸經：此手少陰太陰太陽藥也.

·方義：(1)陳來章曰：熱入心經, 涼之以黃連, 犀角, 梔子.

(2)心移熱於小腸, 泄之以滑石, 甘草, 燈心.

(3)心熱上逼於肺, 清之以黃芩, 梔子, 麥冬.

(4)然邪之越經而傳於心者, 以心神本不足也, 故又加人參, 茯神以補之.

·來源：節庵

19. Pu Ji Xiao Du Yin. Universal Benefit Decoction to Eliminate Toxin. 普濟消毒飲

·**ACTIONS**：massive head scourge

·**COMPOSITION**：Huang Qin, Huang Lian, Lian Qiao, Ban Lan Gen, Sheng Ma, Bo He, Shu Nian Zi, Jiang Can, Chai Hu, Jie Geng, Xuan Shen, Ma Bo, Gan Cao, Chen Pi

·**INDICATIONS**：treats massive head scourge, feeling of abhorrence of cold and generalized heaviness at first, and then swelling in the head and face, inability of opening of eyes, panting, discomfort in the throat, thirst, and dry tongue.

·**MODIFICATIONS**：for constipation, add Da Huang.

·**CHANNELS ENTERED**：The hand greater and lesser yin and foot lesser yang and yang brightness channels. [The lung, heart, gall bladder, and stomach]

·**Analysis of Formula**：(1) Huang Qin and Huang Lian are bitter and cold. They drain the heat of the heart and lung, acting as sovereign.

(2) Xuan Shen is bitter and cold. Ju Hong is bitter and pungent. Gan Cao is sweet and cold. They drain fire and supplement qi, acting as minister.

(3) Lian Qiao, Bo He, and Shu Nian Zi are pungent, bitter, and neutral. Ban Lan Gen is sweet and cold. Ma Bo and Jiang Can are bitter and neutral. They disperse swelling, dissipate toxin, and stabilize panting, acting as assistant.

(4) Sheng Ma and Chai Hu are bitter and neutral. They move yang qi of lesser yang and yang brightness.

(5) Jie Geng is pungent and warm. This makes every herb to move upward.

·**Original Source**：Li Dong Yuan

19. 普濟消毒飲

·總結：大頭天行

·組成：黃芩, 黃連, 連翹, 板藍根, 升麻, 薄荷, 鼠黏子, 殭蠶, 柴胡, 桔梗, 玄參, 馬勃, 甘草, 陳皮

·主治：治大頭天行, 初覺憎寒體重, 次傳頭面腫盛, 目不能開, 上喘, 咽喉不利, 口渴舌燥.

·加減：便秘者：加大黃.

·歸經：此手太陰少陰足少陽陽明藥也.

·方義：(1)芩連：苦寒, 瀉心肺之熱爲君.

(2)玄參：苦寒, 橘紅：苦辛, 甘草：甘寒, 瀉火補氣爲臣.

(3)連翹, 薄荷, 鼠粘：辛苦而平, 藍根：甘寒, 馬勃, 殭蠶：苦平, 散腫消毒定喘爲佐.

(4)升麻, 柴胡：苦平, 行少陽陽明二經之陽氣不得伸.

(5)桔梗；辛溫, 爲舟楫, 不令下行, 爲載也.

·來源：東垣

20. Qing Zhen Tang. Clearing Invigoration Decocotion. 清震湯

·**ACTIONS**：thunder head wind

·**COMPOSITION**：Cang Zhu, Sheng Ma, He Ye.

·**INDICATIONS**：treats thunder head wind, pimple, swelling, and pain in the head and face, abhorrence of cold and invigorating heat, looking like cold damage.

·**CHANNELS ENTERED**：The foot yang brightness channel. [The stomach]

·**Analysis of Formula**：(1) The qi (charater) of Sheng Ma is related with yang, the flavor is sweet. The qi rises. This can resolve one hundred toxins.

(2) Cang Zhu is pungent and harsh. This dries damp and strengthens the spleen. This can expel miasmic toxin.

(3) He Ye is blue, the qi is aromatic. The form looks like thunder.

This can assist clear yang in the stomach to move upward.

(4) The sweet, warm, and pungent herbs are used to disperse mia smic toxin and make the evil come out upward. And also those herbs secure sto mach to make evil not to pass the interior.

·**Original Source**：Liu He Jian's formula

20. 清震湯

　·總結：雷頭風

　·組成：蒼朮，升麻，荷葉．

　·主治：治雷頭風，頭面疙瘩腫痛，憎寒壯熱，狀如傷寒．

　·歸經：此足陽明藥也．

　·方義：(1)升麻：性陽，味甘，氣升，能解百毒．

　　　　　(2)蒼朮：辛烈，燥濕強脾，能辟瘴癘．

　　　　　(3)荷葉：色青氣香，形仰象震，能助胃中清陽上行．

　　　　　(4)用甘溫辛散藥以升發之，使其邪從上越，且固胃氣，使邪

不傳裏．

　·來源：河間

21. Zi Xue Dan. Purple Snow Elixir. 紫雪丹

·**ACTIONS**：all kinds of fire and heat

·**COMPOSITION**： Huang Jin, Han Shui Shi, Shi Gao, Hua Shi, Ci Shi, Sheng Ma, Yuan Shen, Gan Cao, Xi Jiao, Ling Yang Jiao, Chen Xiang, Mu Xia ng, Ding Xiang, Mang Xiao, Xiao Shi, Chen Sha, She Xiang.

·**INDICATIONS**：(1) treats unresolved vexed heat in the interior and exte rior, mania, running with shouting, macular eruption, jaundice, mouth sore, leg qi, miasmic toxin, parasitic toxin, heat toxin, and drug toxin.

(2) and fright epilepsy of child.

·**CHANNELS ENTERED**： The hand and foot lesser yin and foot revert ing yin and yang brightness channels. [The heart, kidney, liver, and stomach]

·**Analysis of Formula**：(1) Han Shui Shi, Shi Gao, Hua Shi, and Xiao Shi drain fire of every channels and disinhibit water, acting as sovereign.

(2) Ci Shi and Xuan Shen enrich kidney water and supplement yi n, acting as minister.

(3) Xi Jiao and Ling Yang Jiao clear the heart and quiet the liver.

(4) Sheng Ma and Gan Cao raise yang and resolve toxin.

338

(5) Chen Xiang, Mu Xiang, and Ding Xiang warm the stomach and regulate qi.

(6) She Xiang outthrusts bone and frees orifices.

(7) Dan Sha and Huang Jin settle fright, quiet ethereal soul, drains the heat of the heart and liver, acting as assistant and courier.

·**Original Source**：Ju Fang

21. 紫雪丹

·總結：一切火熱

·組成：黃金, 寒水石, 石膏, 滑石, 磁石, 升麻, 元參, 甘草, 犀角, 羚羊角, 沉香, 木香, 丁香, 朴硝, 硝石, 辰砂, 麝香當門子.

·主治：(1)治內外煩熱不解, 狂易叫走, 發斑發黃, 口瘡脚氣, 瘴毒蠱毒, 熱毒藥毒.

(2)及小兒驚癇.

·歸經：此手足少陰足厥陰陽明藥也.

·方義：(1)寒水石, 石膏, 滑石, 硝石：以瀉諸經之火, 而兼利水爲君.

(2)磁石, 玄參：以滋腎水, 而兼補陰爲臣.

(3)犀角, 羚角：以清心寧肝.

(4)升麻, 甘草：以升陽解毒

(5)沉香木香, 丁香：以溫胃調氣.

(6)麝香：以透骨通竅.

(7)丹砂, 黃金：以鎮驚安魂, 瀉心肝之熱爲佐使.

·來源：局方

22. Ren Shen Qing Qi San. Jinseng Clearing Qi Powder. 人參清肌散

·**ACTIONS**：vacuous heat in the forenoon.

·**COMPOSITION**：Ren Shen, Bai Zhu, Fu Ling, Gan Cao, Ban Xia, Dang Gui, Chi Shao, Chai Hu, Ge Gen.

·**INDICATIONS**：treats tidal heat effusion in the forenoon and qi vacuity with absence of sweating.

·**CHANNELS ENTERED**：The foot lesser yang and yang brightness channels. [The gall bladder and stomach]

·**Analysis of Formula**：(1) Si Jun Zi Tang supplements yang vacuity.

339

(2) Dang Gui and Shao Yao regulate yin and blood.

(3) Ban Xia harmonizes the stomach and moves phlegm.

(4) Chai Hu and Ge Gen raise yang and abate heat.

(5) The sweet and warm drains fire, the sour and cold activate blood, and the pungent and sweet resolves the flesh. The absence of sweating here is different with one in cold damage, therefore this formula just resolves flesh heat and there is no need to promote sweating.

·**RELATED FORMULA**：Ren Shen San: This adds Huang Qin and Sheng Jiang to this formula. This treats evil heat visiting the channels and networks, phlegm with cough, vexed heat, headache, blurred vision, night sweating, fatigue, and all kinds of blood heat and vacuous taxation.

22. 人參清肌散
　·總結：午前虛熱
　·組成：人參, 白朮, 茯苓, 甘草, 半夏麴, 當歸, 赤芍藥, 柴胡, 乾葛.
　·主治：治午前潮熱, 氣虛無汗.
　·歸經：此足少陽陽明藥也.
　·方義：(1)四君：以補陽虛.
　　　　　(2)歸, 芍：以調陰血.
　　　　　(3)半夏：和胃而行痰.
　　　　　(4)柴葛：升陽而退熱.
　　　　　(5)而以甘溫瀉火, 酸寒活血, 辛甘解肌, 此之無汗, 與傷寒無汗不同, 故但解其肌熱, 而不必發出其汗.
　·變化方：人參散：本方加黃芩, 加薑棗煎. 治邪熱客於經絡, 痰嗽煩熱, 頭痛目昏, 盜汗倦息, 一切血熱虛勞.

23. Bai Zhu Chu Shi Tang. Ovate Atractylodes Eliminating Damp Decoction. 白朮除濕湯

·**ACTIONS**：heat effusion in the afternoon.

·**COMPOSITION**：Bai Zhu, Ren Shen, Gan Cao, Chi Fu Ling, Ze Xie, Zhi Mu, Di Gu Pi, Chai Hu, sheng Di Huang.

·**INDICATIONS**：(1) treats heat effusion in the afternoon, aversion to wind in the back, fatigued limbs and yellow urine.

(2) also treats heat effusion after promotion of sweating.

·**MODIFICATIONS**：for stabbing pain, add Dang Gui, for uninhibited u

340

rination, reduce the dose of Fu Ling and Ze Xie to the half.

·**CHANNELS ENTERED**：The foot greater and lesser yin and lesser yang channels. [The spleen, kidney, and gall bladder]

·**Analysis of Formula**：(1) Yang falls into the yin and heat is in the blood part, therefore Sheng Di Huang enriches lesser yin and Zhi Mu and Di Gu Pi drain latent fire in the blood.

(2) Chai Hu raises yang to resolve the flesh.

(3) Fu Ling and Ze Xie disinhibit damp with clearing heat.

(4) Ren Shen, Bai Zhu, and Gan Cao boost qi and assist the spleen.

(5) When qi is sufficient and yang rises, vacuous heat spontaneously retreats, and when the spleen moves, damp is also eliminated.

·**Original Source**：Li Dong Yuan

23. 白朮除濕湯

·總結：午後發熱

·組成：白朮, 人參, 甘草, 赤茯苓, 澤瀉, 知母, 地骨皮, 柴胡, 生地黃.

·主治：(1)治午後發熱, 背惡風, 四肢沉困, 小便色黃.

(2)又治汗後發熱.

·加減：如有刺痛加當歸, 小便利減苓瀉一半.

·歸經：此足太陰少陰少陽藥也.

·方義：(1)陽陷陰中, 熱在血分, 故以生地滋其少陰, 而以知母, 地骨瀉血中伏火也.

(2)柴胡：升陽以解其肌.

(3)苓澤：利濕兼清其熱.

(4)參朮, 甘草：益氣助脾.

(5)氣足陽升, 虛熱自退, 脾運而濕亦除矣.

·來源：東垣

24. Qing Gu San. Cool the Bones Powder. 清骨散

·**ACTIONS**：steaming bone

·**COMPOSITION**：Di Gu Pi, Hu Huang Lian, Zhi Mu, Bie Jia, Qing Hao, Qin Jiao, Yin Chai Hu, Gan Cao

·**INDICATIONS**：treats steaming bone and taxation fever.

·**CHANNELS ENTERED**：The foot lesser yang and reverting yin channels. [The gall bladder and liver]

341

·**Analysis of Formula**：(1) Di Gu Pi, Huang Lian, and Zhi Mu are bitter and cold. They can eliminate heat in the yin part and pacify in the interior.

(2) Chai Hu, Qing Hao, and Qin Jiao are pungent and cold. They can eliminate the heat of the liver and gall bladder and disperses in the exterior.

(3) Bie Jia belongs to yin family and the shell belongs to bone. This can conduct every herbs to enter bone and supplement yin.

(4) Gan Cao is sweet and neutral. This can harmonize every herbs and retreat vacuous heat.

24. 清骨散
　·總結：骨蒸
　·組成：地骨皮, 胡黃連, 知母, 鱉甲, 青蒿, 秦艽, 銀柴胡, 甘草
　·主治：治骨蒸勞熱.
　·歸經：此足少陽厥陰藥也.
　·方義：(1)地骨皮, 黃連, 知母：苦寒, 能除陰分之熱, 而平之於內.
　　　　　(2)柴胡, 青蒿, 秦艽：辛寒, 能除肝膽之熱, 而散之於表.
　　　　　(3)鱉：陰類而甲屬骨, 能引諸藥入骨而補陰.
　　　　　(4)甘草：甘平, 能和諸藥而退虛熱也.

25. Shi Gao San. Gypsum Powder. 石膏散

·**COMPOSITION**：Shi Gao.

·**INDICATIONS**：treats taxation fever, steaming bone, mild weak limbs, sweating, and a pulse that is long.

·**CHANNELS ENTERED**：The foot yang brightness channel. [The stomach]

·**Analysis of Formula**：(1) Shi Gao is great cold and heavy. This can enter the interior and descend fire.

(2) The flavor is pungent and the qi is light, this can penetrate the exterior and resolve the flesh.

(3) Although this is cold and sweet, this can moderate the spleen and boost qi

(4) Taxation fever belongs to replete heat, therefore the other formula cannot treat this.

·**Original Source**：Wai Tai Mi Yao

25. 石膏散

　　·組成：石膏.

　　·主治：治勞熱骨蒸, 四肢微瘦, 有汗, 脈長者.

　　·歸經：此足陽明藥也.

　　·方義：(1)石膏：大寒質重, 能入裏降火.

　　　　　　(2)味辛氣輕, 能透表解肌.

　　　　　　(3)雖寒而甘, 能緩脾益氣

　　　　　　(4)火勞實熱者, 非此不爲功.

　　　　　·來源：外臺

26. Er Mu San. Anemarrhena and Fritillaria Powder. 二母散

·COMPOSITION：Zhi Mu, Bei Mu.

·INDICATIONS：treats lung taxation with heat. This formula is used when qi cannot be supplemented.

·CHANNELS ENTERED：The hand greater yin channel. [The Lung]

·Analysis of Formula：(1) Effulgent fire melts metal, therefore lung vacuity and taxation heat occur. If this pattern can be treated with warming and supplementing method, this is easy case, but if this cannot be treated with, that case is difficult. Therefore this method of nourishing yin is made.

(2) Bei Mu transforms phlegm and drains lung fire.

(3) Zhi Mu enriches the kidney and clears lung metal

(4) The bitter can drain heat, the cold can overcome heat, and the moisture can eliminate dry.

26. 二母散

　　·組成：知母, 貝母.

　　·主治：治肺勞有熱, 不能服補氣之劑者.

　　·歸經：此手太陰藥也.

　　·方義：(1)火旺鑠金, 肺虛勞熱, 能受溫補者易治, 不能受溫補者難治, 故又設此法以滋陰.

　　　　　　(2)用貝母：化痰瀉肺火.

　　　　　　(3)知母：滋腎清肺金

　　　　　　(4)取其苦能泄熱, 寒能勝熱, 潤能去燥.

343

27. Li Ge Tang. Benefit the Diaphragm Decoction. 利膈湯

·**ACTIONS**：diaphragm heat and sore throat

·**COMPOSITION**：Bo He, Jing Jie, Fang Feng, Jie Geng, Gan Cao, Niu Bang Zi, Ren Shen.

·**INDICATIONS**：treat the fire-heat of the spleen and lung, vacuous vexation, congestion in the upper, sore throat with sores.

·**MODIFICATIONS**：or add Jiang Can.

·**CHANNELS ENTERED**：The hand greater and lesser yin channels. [The lung and heart]

·**Analysis of Formula**：(1) Sore throat and dry throat are due to fire depression. The composition of Jie Geng and Gan Cao is Gan Jie Tang. The pungent and bitter disperse cold, the sweet and neutral eliminates heat to clear diaphragm and disinhibit throat.

(2) Bo He, Jing Jie, and Fang Feng disperse fire and eliminate wind.

(3) Niu Bang Zi moistens the intestines and resolves toxin.

(4) Fire is the enemy of source qi. When the right qi is vacuous, evil fire gets to intense, therefore Ren Shen is added to supplement vacuity and abate heat.

·**Original Source**：Ben Shi Fang

27. 利膈湯

·總結：膈熱咽痛

·組成：薄荷，荊芥，防風，桔梗，甘草，牛蒡子，人參.

·主治：治脾肺火熱，虛煩上壅，咽痛生瘡.

·加減：或加殭蠶.

·歸經：此手太陰少陰藥也.

·方義：(1)咽痛咽乾，由於火郁，桔梗，甘草，甘桔湯也：辛苦散寒，甘平除熱爲清膈利咽之要藥.

(2)加薄荷，荊芥，防風：以散火除風.

(3)加牛蒡子：以潤腸解毒

(4)火者元氣之賊，正氣虛則邪火熾，故又加人參：以補虛退熱.

·來源：本事

344

28. Gan Jie Tang. Licorice and Platycodon Decoction.甘桔湯

·**COMPOSITION**：Gan Cao, Jie Geng.

·**INDICATIONS**：(1) treats lesser yin sore throat, throat impediment, lung welling abscess with vomiting of pus, dry cough without phlegm, and fire depressed in the lung.

(2) also treats cough originated form the heart, cough causing heart pain, the sensation of obstruction in the throat.

·**MODIFICATIONS**：Wang Hao Gu's variant method.

(1) for loss of voice, add He Zi.

(2) for aphonia, add Ban Xia.

(3) for dyspnea, add Chen Pi.

(4) for drool and cough, add Zhi Mu and Bei Mu.

(5) for cough and thirst, add Wu Wei Zi.

(6) for alcoholic toxin, add Ge Gen.

(7) for shortage of qi, add Ren Shen

(8) for retching, add Ban Xia and Sheng Jiang.

(9) for vomiting of pus and blood, add Zi Wan.

(10) for lung disease, add E Jiao.

(11) for inhibited chest and diaphragm, add Zhi Ke.

(12) for glomus and fullness, add Zhi Shi.

(13) for reddish eyes, add Zhi Zi and Da Huang.

(14) for face edema, add Fu Ling.

(15) for skin pain, add Huang Qi

(16) for macular eruption, add Jing Jie and Fang Feng.

(17) for phlegm fire, add Niu Bang Zi and Da Huang.

(18) for insomnia, add Zhi Zi.

·**CHANNELS ENTERED**：The hand greater and lesser yin channels. [The spleen and lung]

·**Analysis of Formula**：(1) Gan Cao is sweet and neutral, resolves toxin and drains fire.

(2) Jie Geng is bitter and pungent, clears the lung and disinhibits diaphragm, and also can open and raise blood and qi, disperses cold evil in the exterior, expels pus and blood, and supplements the lung.

(3) Therefore this formula treats sore throat, throat impediment, lung welling abscess with cough. The pungent and bitter disperses cold and the sweet and neutral eliminates heat.

·**RELATED FORMULA**：(1) Gan Cao Tang.：This eliminates Jie Geng from this formula. This treats same things.

(2) Gan Jie Fang Feng Tang.：This adds Fang Feng in this formula. This treats same things.

(3) Ru Sheng Tang.：This adds Fang Feng, Jing Jie, and Lian Qiao in this formula. This treats wind heat in the upper burner.

(4) Jie Geng Tang.：This adds Lian QiaoBo He, Zhu Ye, Zhi Zi, and Huang Qin in this formula. This treats wind heat in the upper burner.

(6) He Zi Qing Yin Tang.：This adds He Zi and child's urine. This treats wind stroke.

(7) Zhi Jie Tang.：This eliminates Gan Cao and adds Zhi Ke. This treats glomus and oppression in the chest, belching qi, acid vomiting, or cough.

·Another Side Formula：Jie Geng, Sang Pi, Bei Mu, Gua Lou, Dang Gui, Zhi Ke, Yi Yi Ren, Fang Ji, Huang Qi, Xing Ren, Bai He, Gan Cao, and Sheng Jiang, this is also called Jie GengTang. (Ji Sheng Fang). This treats lung welling abscess, vomiting of pus, dry throat, thirst. For fecal block, add Da Huang, for reddish urine, add Mu Tong.

28. 甘桔湯
·組成：甘草, 桔梗.
·主治：(1)治少陰咽痛喉痺, 肺癰吐膿, 乾欬無痰, 火郁在肺.
(2)亦治心臟發欬, 欬則心痛, 喉中介介如梗狀.
·加減：王好古加減法：
(1)失音；加訶子.
(2)聲不出：加半夏.
(3)上氣：加陳皮.
(4)涎嗽：加知母, 貝母.
(5)欬渴；加五味.
(6)酒毒：加葛根.
(7)少氣；加人參
(8)嘔：加半夏, 生薑.
(9)吐膿血：加紫菀.

(10)肺病；加阿膠.

(11)胸膈不利：加枳殼.

(12)痞滿：加枳實.

(13)目赤：加梔子，大黃.

(14)面腫；加茯苓.

(15)膚痛；加黃耆

(16)發斑：加荊芥，防風.

(17)痰火：加牛蒡大黃.

(18)不能睡眠加梔子.

·歸經：此手太陰少陰葯也.

·方義：(1)甘草；甘平解毒而瀉火.

(2)桔梗；苦辛清肺而利膈，又能開提血氣，表散寒邪，排膿血而補內漏.

(3)故治咽痛喉痺，肺癰欬嗽，取其辛苦散寒，甘平除熱也.

·變化方：(1)甘草湯：本方除桔梗治同.(金匱方)

(2)甘桔防風湯：本方加防風.治同.

(3)如聖湯：本方加防風，荊芥，連翹.治上焦風熱.(宋仁宗方)

(4)桔梗湯：本方加連翹薄荷，竹葉，梔子，黃芩.治上焦風熱.

(6)訶子清音湯：本方加訶子.加童便服.治中風不譔.

(7)枳桔湯：本方除甘草，加枳殼.治胸中痞塞，噫氣吐酸或欬.

·又附方：桔梗，桑皮，貝母，栝樓，當歸，枳殼，苡仁，防己，黃耆，杏仁，百合，甘草，加薑煎，亦名桔梗湯.(濟生方)治肺癰吐膿，嗌乾多渴.如大便閉，加大黃；小便赤加大通.

29. Yuan Shen Sheng Ma San. Scrophularia and Cimicifaga Powder. 元參升麻散

·**ACTIONS**：clears throat and disperses macule.

·**COMPOSITION**：Yuan Shen, Sheng Ma, Gan Cao.

·**INDICATIONS**：treats macular eruption and sore throat.

·**CHANNELS ENTERED**：The foot yang brightness and lesser yin channels. [The stomach and kidney.

·**Analysis of Formula**：(1) Sheng Ma can enter yang brightness, and raise s yang and resolves toxin.

(2) Yuan Shen can enter lesser yin, and invigorates water to restrain fire.

(3) Gan Cao is sweet and neutral. This can disperse and harmonize, therefore this can disinhibit throat in the upper and disperse macule in the interior.

·**RELATED FORMULA**：When Yuan Shen is eliminated and Xi Jiao, She Gan, Huang Qin, and Ren Shen are added, this is called Yang Du Sheng Ma Tang, treats yang toxin with macular eruption, pain in the head, nape, and back, manic agitation with bad language, swollen throat, and hematemesis. Take this warmly and make one to sweat.

·**Original Source**：Huo Ren

29. 元參升麻散
   ·總結：清咽散斑
   ·組成：元參，升麻，甘草.
   ·主治：治發斑咽痛.
   ·歸經：此足陽明少陰藥也.
   ·方義：(1)升麻：能入陽明，升陽而解毒.
          (2)元參：能入少陰，壯水以制火.
          (3)甘草：甘平，能散能和，故上可利咽，而內可以散斑.
   ·變化方：本方除元參，加犀角，射干，黃芩，人參，名陽毒升麻湯，治陽毒發斑，頭項背痛，狂躁罵詈，咽腫吐血溫服取汗.
   ·來源：活人

30. Xiao Ban Qing Dai Yin. Macule-Dispersing Indigo Beverage. 消斑青黛飲

·**ACTIONS**：stomach heat and dissipated macule.

·**COMPOSITION**：Huang Lian, Qing Dai, Xi Jiao, Shi Gao, Zhi Mu, Yuan Shen, Sheng Di Huang, Zhi Zi, Ren Shen, Chai Hu, Gan Cao, Sheng Jiang, Da Zao

·**INDICATIONS**：treats that when in cold damage, heat evil passes into the interior, the interior gets replete and the exterior becomes vacuous, there is yang toxin with macule.

·**MODIFICATIONS**：for solid stool, eliminate Ren Shen and add Da Huang.

·**CHANNELS ENTERED**：The foot yang brightness channel. [The stomach]

·**Analysis of Formula**：(1) Macular eruption is due to stomach heat and the fire of every channels assists the stomach heat.

(2) Qing Dai and Huang Lian clear liver fire.

(3) Zhi Zi clears the fire of the heart and lung.

(4) Yuan Shen, Zhi Mu, and Sheng Di Huang clear kidney fire.

(5) Xi Jiao and Shi Gao clear stomach fire.

(6) Chai Hu is used as channel conductor, this makes herbs to reach the flesh exterior.

(7) Sheng Jiang and Da Zao harmonize the construction and defense

(8) Ren Shen and Gan Cao harmonize the stomach. Owing to stomach vacuity, heat toxin exploits vacuity, enters the interior, and then erupts in the flesh occurs.

·**Original Source**：Jie An

30. 消斑青黛飲
　·總結：胃熱散斑
　·組成：黃連, 青黛, 犀角, 石膏, 知母, 元參, 生地, 栀子, 人參, 柴胡, 甘草
　·主治：治傷寒熱邪傳裏, 裏實表虛, 陽毒發斑.
　·加減：大便實：去人參, 加大黃.
　·歸經：此足陽明藥也.
　·方義：(1)發斑雖出胃熱, 亦諸經之火有以助之.
　　　　(2)青黛, 黃連：以清肝火.
　　　　(3)栀子：以清心肺之火.
　　　　(4)元參, 知母, 生地：以清腎火.
　　　　(5)犀角, 石膏：以清胃火.
　　　　(6)引以柴胡：使達肌表.
　　　　(7)使以薑棗：以和營衛
　　　　(8)其用人參, 甘草者：以和胃也, 胃虛故熱毒乘虛入裏, 而發於肌肉.
　·來源：節庵

31. Yu Xie Wu You San. Jade Scraps Non Anxiety Powder. 玉屑無憂

·**ACTIONS**：throat–entwining wind

·**COMPOSITION**：Yuan Shen, Han Shui Shi, Huang Lian, Guan Zhong, Shan Dou Gen, Fu Ling, Hua Shi, Jing Jie, Gan Cao, Peng Sha, Sha Ren

·**INDICATIONS**：(1) treats throat–entwining wind and impediment, swel ling and pain in the throat, and some obstacle in the throat.

(2) or stagnated wind and drool, mouth and tongue sores, alcohol ic pattern of adult, mammary aggregation of child, bone fragment blocking the throat.

(3) this can eliminate San Shi, remove eight evil, expel scourge e pidemic, and treat thirst.

·**CHANNELS ENTERED**：The foot yang brightness and lesser yin chan nel. [The stomach and kidney]

·**Analysis of Formula**：(1) Yuan Shen, Huang Lian, and Han Shui Shi cle ar fire.

(2) Guan Zhong and Shan Dou Gen resolve toxin.

(3) Hua Shi and Fu Ling disinhibit water.

(4) Sha Ren softens hardness.

(5) Jing Jie disperses binds.

(6) Gan Cao harmonizes the middle.

·**Original Source**：Chen Wu Ze

31. 玉屑無憂散

·總結：風纏咽喉

·組成：元參, 寒水石, 黃連, 貫衆, 山豆根, 茯苓, 滑石, 荊芥, 甘草, 硼砂, 砂仁

·主治：(1)治纏喉風痹, 咽喉腫痛, 咽物有礙.

(2)或風涎壅滯, 口舌生瘡, 大人酒癥, 小兒媚癖, 及骨屑哽 塞.

(3)能除三尸, 去八邪, 辟瘟療渴.

·歸經：此足陽明少陰藥也.

·方義：(1)元參, 黃連, 寒水石：清火

(2)貫衆, 山豆根：解毒.

(3)滑石, 茯苓：利水.

(4)砂仁砂：軟堅.

(5)荊芥：散結.

(6)甘草：和中.

·來源：陳無擇

32. Xiang Lian Wan. Aucklandia and Coptis Pills. 香連丸

·**ACTIONS**：heat diarrhea.

·**COMPOSITION**：Huang Lian, Mu Xiang.

·**INDICATIONS**：treats red or white diarrhea mixed with pus and blood, interior tenesmus.

·**MODIFICATIONS**：(1) for food-denying dysentery, add Shi Lian Rou.

(2) for heat dysentery and accumulation, double Da Huang.

·**CHANNELS ENTERED**：The hand and foot yang brightness channel. [The large intestine and stomach]

·**Analysis of Formula**：(1) Dysentery is due to irregularities of food and drink, cold and summerheat damage, and stagnation of damp-heat.

(2) The bitter of Huang Lian dries damp, the cold overcomes heat. This directly breaks the fire of the heart and spleen, therefore acts as sovereign.

(3) Wu Zhu Yu can disinhibit stagnated qi of the large intestine and kills the great cold character of Huang Lian.

(4) Interior tenesmus is due to qi stagnation. The pungent of Mu Xiang moves qi and the warm harmonizes the spleen. This can free and disinhibit the triple burner, drain the lung to pacify the lung. When one makes wood evil not to restrain spleen earth, qi gets to move and stagnation is eliminated.

·**RELATED FORMULA**：(1) When Wu Zhu Yu, Rou Dou Kou, and Wu Mei Tang are added, this treats diarrhea.

(2) Huang Lian Wan.：When He Zi and Long Gu are added, this treats dysentery.

·**Original Source**：Zhi Zhi

32. 香連丸

·總結：熱痢

·組成：黃連, 木香.

·主治：治下痢赤白, 膿血相雜, 裏急後重.

351

·加減：⑴噤口痢：加石蓮肉.

　　　　⑵熱痢積滯：倍大黃.

·歸經：此手足陽明藥也.

·方義：⑴痢爲飲食不節, 寒暑所傷, 濕熱蒸郁而成.

　　　　⑵黃連：苦燥濕, 寒勝熱, 直折心脾之火, 故以爲君.

　　　　⑶用吳茱萸, 同炒者：取其能利大腸壅氣, 且以殺大寒之性.

　　　　⑷裏急由於氣滯, 木香辛行氣, 溫和脾, 能通利三焦, 泄肺
以平肺, 使木邪不剋脾土, 氣行而滯去也.

·變化方：⑴本方加吳茱萸, 肉豆蔻, 烏梅湯丸. 治痢疾斷下.

　　　　⑵黃連丸：本方加訶子, 龍骨. 並治痢疾斷下.

·來源：直指

33. Bai Tou Weng Tang. Pulsatilla Decoction.　白頭翁湯

·**ACTIONS**：heat diarrhea.

·**COMPOSITION**：Bai Tou Weng, Qin Pi , Huang Lian, Huang Bai.

·**INDICATIONS**：treats when in cold damage there is diarrhea with rectal heaviness, and a desire to drink water.

·**CHANNELS ENTERED**：The foot yang brightness and lesser and reverting yin channels. [The stomach, kidney, and liver]

·**Analysis of Formula**：(1) Bai Tou Weng is bitter and cold. This can enter blood part of yang brightness, cool blood, and relieve diarrhea.

　　　　(2) Qin Pi is bitter, cold, and astringent. This can cool the liver, boost the kidney, and secure the lower burner.

　　　　(3) Huang Lian cools the heart and clears the liver.

　　　　(4) Huang Bai drains fire and supplements water. This also can dry damp, relieves diarrhea, and riches the intestines.

　　　　(5) The cold can overcome heat, bitter can consolidate the kidney, the astringent can stop diarrhea.

·**Original Source**：Zhong Jing

33. 白頭翁湯

·總結：熱痢

·組成：白頭翁, 秦皮, 黃連, 黃柏.

·主治：治傷寒痢下重, 欲飲水者.

·歸經：此足陽明少陰厥陰藥也.
·方義：(1)白頭翁：苦寒，能入陽明血分，而涼血止澼.
　　　　(2)秦皮：苦寒，性濇，能涼肝益腎而固下焦.
　　　　(3)黃連：涼心清肝.
　　　　(4)黃柏：瀉火補水，並能燥濕止利而厚腸.
　　　　(5)取其寒能勝熱，苦能堅腎，濇能斷下.
·來源：仲景

34. Shen Re Tang. Kidney Heat Decoction. 腎熱湯

·**ACTIONS**：kidney heat with deafness

·**COMPOSITION**：Ci Shi, Mu Li, sheng Di Huang, Shao Yao, Gan Cao, Mai Men Dong, Cong Bai, Da Zao, Bai Zhu.

·**INDICATIONS**：treats kidney heat, pus and blood flowing from the ear, loss of hear.

·**CHANNELS ENTERED**：The lesser yin channel. [The kidney]

·**Analysis of Formula**：(1) Ci Shi is heavy, pungent, salty, and black. This supplements the kidney, eliminates heat, frees the ear, and improves vision, therefore acts as sovereign.

(2) Mu Li is salty and cold. This softens phlegm and breaks binds.

(3) Sheng Di Huang is greatly cold. This drains fire and enriches the kidney.

(4) Mai Men Dong and Gan Cao supplements the lung and clears metal.

(5) Bai Shao Yao is sour and cold. This pacifies the liver and harmonizes blood.

(6) Bai Zhu, Gan Cao, and Da Zao supplements the spleen, boosts earth qi to restrain kidney evil.

(7) Cong Bai is added to conduct kidney qi to free upward to the ear.

·**Original Source**：Tian Jin Yao Fang

34. 腎熱湯
　·總結：腎熱耳聾
　·組成：磁石，牡蠣，生地黃汁，芍藥，甘草，麥冬，蔥白，大棗，白朮.

·主治：治腎熱耳流膿血，不聞人聲.

·歸經：此足少陰藥也.

·方義：(1)磁石：体重辛鹹，色黑補腎袪熱，通耳明目，故以爲君.

　　　(2)牡蠣：鹹寒，軟痰破結.

　　　(3)生地：大寒，瀉火滋腎.

　　　(4)麥冬，甘草：補肺清金.

　　　(5)白芍：酸寒平肝和血.

　　　(6)白朮，甘草，大棗：補脾之品，益土氣以制腎邪也.

　　　(7)加蔥白者：以引腎氣上通於耳也.

·來源：千金

35. Xin Yi San. Magnolia Flower Powder. 辛夷散

·**COMPOSITION**：Xin Yi, Bai Zhi, Sheng Ma, Mu Tong, Gan Cao, Gao Ben, Fang Feng, Chuan Xiong, Xi Xin.

·**INDICATIONS**：treats nose engendering polyp, breathing stoppage, and loss of smell.

·**CHANNELS ENTERED**：The hand greater yin and foot yang brightness channels. [The lung and stomach]

·**Analysis of Formula**：(1) Nei Jing says that heaven qi frees to the lung. If there is not phlegm fire and accumulated heat in the stomach, something rising upward normally in body becomes clear qi. If dry fire blazes internally, wind-cold fetters externally, blood and qi are congested, therefore nose generates polyp and is blocked.

(2) Xin Yi, Sheng Ma, and Bai Zhi are pungent, warm, light, and floating. They can conduct clear qi in the stomach to move upward to the head and brain.

(3) Fang Feng and Gao Ben are pungent. They can ascend to enter vertex, overcome damp, and eliminate wind.

(4) Xi Xin disperses heat, breaks binds, frees essence qi, and disinhibits nine orifices.

(5) Chuan Xiong supplements the liver, moistens dry, disperses every stagnation, and assists clear yang.

(6) Mu Tong frees the middle. .

(7) herbs with clear, cold, and bitter can move downward to drain fire.

354

·**Original Source**：Yan Shi

35. 辛夷散

   ·組成：辛夷, 白芷, 升麻, 木通, 甘草, 藁本, 防風, 川芎, 細辛.

   ·主治：治鼻生瘜肉, 氣息不通, 不聞香臭.

   ·歸經：此手太陰足陽明藥也.

   ·方義：(1)經曰：天氣通於肺, 若腸胃無痰火積熱, 則平常上升, 皆清氣也. 由燥火內焚, 風寒外束, 血氣壅滯故鼻生瘜肉而窒塞不通也.

        (2)辛夷, 升麻, 白芷：辛溫輕浮, 能引胃中清氣上行頭腦.

        (3)防風, 藁本：辛溫雄壯, 亦能上入巔頂, 勝濕祛風.

        (4)細辛：散熱破結, 通精氣而利九竅.

        (5)芎藭：補肝潤燥, 散諸郁而助清陽.

        (6)木通：通中.

        (7)茶清寒苦：以下行瀉火.

        ·來源：嚴氏

36. Cang Er San. Xanthium Powder. 蒼耳散

·**ACTIONS**：wind heat with sinusitis

·**COMPOSITION**：Cang Er Zi, Xin Yi, Bai Zhi, Bo He.

·**INDICATIONS**：treats sinusitis.

·**CHANNELS ENTERED**：The hand greater yin and foot yang brightness channels. [The lung and stomach]

·**Analysis of Formula**：(1) general the disease of the head and face occurs when clear yang does not ascend and turbid yin counterfolw upward.

      (2) Bai Zhi controls the hand and foot yang brightness, moves upward to the head and face, frees orifices and effuses exterior sweat, eliminates damp, and disperses wind.

      (3) Xin Yi frees nine orifices and disperses wind heat. This can assist clear yang in the stomach to move upward to the head and brain.

      (4) Cang Er Zi courses wind, disperses damp, frees upward to brain and vertex, and reaches the skin and flesh.

      (5) Bo He drains the lung, courses the liver, and clears and disinhibits the head and eye.

      (6) Cong Bai raises yang and frees qi.

(7) When clear yang raises and turbid yin descends, wind-heat di
sperses and brain humor spontaneously gets secured.

·**Original Source**：Wu Ze

36. 蒼耳散

    ·總結：風熱鼻淵

    ·組成：蒼耳子, 辛夷, 白芷, 薄荷.

    ·主治：治鼻淵.

    ·歸經：此手太陰足陽明藥也.

    ·方義：(1)凡頭面之疾，皆由清陽不升，濁陰逆上所致.

           (2)白芷：主手足陽明, 上行頭面, 通竅表汗, 除濕散風.

           (3)辛夷：通九竅, 散風熱, 能助胃中清陽上行頭腦.

           (4)蒼耳：疏風散濕, 上通腦頂, 外達皮膚

           (5)薄荷：泄肺疏肝, 清利頭目.

           (6)葱白：升陽通氣.

           (7)使清升濁降, 風熱散而腦液自固矣.

    ·來源：無擇

Chapter 15. Phlegm-Eliminating Formulas. 除痰之劑

1. Er Chen Tang. Two-Cured Decoction. 二陳湯

·**ACTIONS**：damp phlegm

·**COMPOSITION**：Ban Xia, Chen Pi, Fu Ling, Gan Cao.

·**INDICATIONS**：treats all kinds of phlegm disease, cough, distention and fullness, vomiting, nausea, dizziness, and palpitations.

·**MODIFICATIONS**：(1) for wind phlegm, add Nan Xing, Bai Fu, Zao Jiao, Zhu Li.

(2) for cold phlegm, add Ban Xia, Jiang Zhi (juice of ginger).

(3) for fire phlegm, add Shi Gao, Qing Dai.

(4) for damp phlegm, add Cang Zhu, Bai Zhu.

(5) for dry phlegm, add Gua Lou, Xing Ren

(6) for food phlegm, add Shan Zha, Mai Ya, Shen Qu.

(7) for old phlegm, add Zhi Shi, Hai Shi, Mang Xiao.

(8) for qi phlegm, add Xiang Fu, Zhi Ke.

(9) for phlegm in rib sides, add Bai Jie Zi.

(10) for phlegm in the limbs, add Zhu Li.

·**CHANNELS ENTERED**：The foot greater yin and yang brightness channels. [The spleen and stomach]

·**Analysis of Formula**：(1) Ban Xia is pungent and warm. The body is lubricative but the character is dry. This moves water and disinhibits phlegm, acting as sovereign.

(2) In case of phlegm due to qi stagnation, when qi normalizes, phlegm descends, therefore Ju Hong is used to disinhibit qi.

(3) In case of phlegm engendered by damp, when damp eliminates, then phlegm disappears, therefore Fu Ling is used to drain damp, acting as minister.

(4) When the middle is not harmonious, phlegm and drool gather, Gan Cao harmonizes the middle and supplements earth, acting as assistant.

·**RELATED FORMULA**：(1) Liu Jun Zi Tang.：Ren Shen and Bai Zhu are added, this treats qi vacuity with phlegm.

(2) Chen Pi Ban Xia Tang.：Fu Ling and Gan Cao are eliminate

357

d.

(3) Jie Geng Ban Xia Tang. : Jie Geng is added to Chen Pi Ban Xia Tang.

(4) Ban Xia Fu Ling Tang. : Chen Pi and Gan Cao are eliminated.

(5) Xiao Ban Xia Jia Fu Ling Tang. : Sheng Jiang is added to Ban Xia Fu Ling Tang. This treats water qi, retching, and nausea.

(6) Fu Ling Ban Xia Tang. : Huang Qin is added. This treats heat phlegm.

(7) Er Chen Jia Zhi Lian Sheng JiangTang. : Huang Lian, Zhi Zi, and Sheng Jiang are added. This treats heat phlegm over the diaphragm. This makes one to vomit.

(8) Sha Zhi Er Chen Tang. : Sha Ren and Zhi Ke are added. This moves phlegm and disinhibits qi.

(9) Dao Tan Tang. : Dan Nan Xing and Zhi Shi are added. This treats stubborn phlegm.

(10) Shun Qi Dao Tan Yin. : Dao Tan Tang with Mu Xiang and Xiang Fu. This treats phlegm binds, thoracic fullness, panting, cough, and dyspnea.

(11) When Zhi Shi, Lai Fu Zi, Shan Zha, Shen Qu, and Gua Lou are added, this treats food accumulation, phlegm cough, and heat effusion.

(12) Jia Wei Er Chen Tang. : Cang Zhu, Zhi Ke, and Jiang Huang are added, this treats phlegm attack, eye swelling, drinker with heaviness, pain, and numbness of the hand and arms.

(13) Wen Zhong Hua Tan Wan. : When Gan Cao is eliminated and Gan Jiang, and Jiang Zhi (juice of ginger) are added, this treats cold phlegm in the chest and diaphragm.

(14) San Sheng Wan. : When Fu Ling and Gan Cao are eliminated and Huang Lian are added, this treats phlegm fire with gastric upset.

(15) Ju Pi Tang. : only using of Chen Pi and Sheng Jiang. This treats dry retching, hiccup, the reverse of the limbs.

(16) Sheng Jiang Ban Xia Tang. : only using of Ban Xia and Jiang Zhi (juice of ginger). This treats condition like panting but not panting, condition like retching but not retching, condition like hiccup but not hiccup.

·**Original Source** : Ju Fang

1. 二陳湯

358

·總結：溼痰

·組成：半夏，陳皮，茯苓，甘草.

·主治：治一切痰飲爲病，欬嗽脹滿，嘔吐惡心，頭眩心悸.

·加減：(1)風痰：加南星，白附，皂角，竹瀝.

(2)寒痰：加半夏，薑汁.

(3)火痰：加石膏，青黛.

(4)溼痰：加蒼朮，白朮.

(5)燥痰：加栝蔞，杏仁

(6)食痰：加山查，麥芽，神麴.

(7)老痰：加枳實，海石，芒硝.

(8)氣痰：加香附，枳殼.

(9)脇痰在皮裏膜外：加白芥子.

(10)四肢痰：加竹瀝.

·歸經：此足太陰陽明藥也.

·方義：(1)半夏：辛溫体滑，性燥，行水利痰爲君.

(2)痰因氣滯，氣順則痰降，故以橘紅利氣.

(3)痰由溼生，溼去則痰消，故以茯苓滲溼爲臣.

(4)中不和則痰涎聚，又以甘草和中補土爲佐.

·變化方：(1)六君子湯：本方加人參，白朮. 治氣虛有痰.

(2)陳皮半夏湯：本方去茯苓，甘草.

(3)桔梗半夏湯：上方加桔梗.

(4)半夏茯苓湯：本方去陳皮，甘草.

(5)小半夏加茯苓湯：上方加生薑. 並治水氣嘔惡.

(6)茯苓半夏湯：本方加黃芩. 治熱痰.

(7)二陳加梔連生薑湯：本方加黃連，梔子，生薑. 治膈上熱痰，令人嘔吐.

(8)砂枳二陳湯：本方加砂仁，枳殼. 行痰利氣.

(9)導痰湯：本方加膽星，枳實. 治頑痰膠固.

(10)順氣導痰飲：導痰湯加木香，香附. 治痰結胸滿，喘欬上氣.

(11)本方加枳實，菔子，山查，神麴，栝蔞. 治食積痰嗽發熱.

(12)加味二陳湯：本方加蒼朮，枳殼，片子薑黃. 治痰攻眼腫，併酒家手臂重痛麻木.

(13)溫中化痰丸：本方除甘草，加乾薑，薑汁糊丸. 治胸膈寒痰不快.

(14)三聖丸：本方除茯苓，甘草，加黃連，麴糊丸，薑湯下治痰火嘈雜.

(15)橘皮湯：單用陳皮生薑. 治乾嘔噦，及手足厥者.

(16)生薑半夏湯：單用半夏，薑汁治似喘不喘，似嘔不嘔，似噦不噦.

·來源：局方

2. Run Xia Wan. Moist Precipitation Pills. 潤下丸

·**ACTIONS**：phlegm in the diaphragm

·**COMPOSITION**：Guang Chen Pi, Gan Cao

·**INDICATIONS**：treats phlegm in the diaphragm.

·**MODIFICATIONS**：(1) for excessive damp, add Dan Nan Xing and Ban Xia.

(2) for exuberant fire, add Huang Qin and Huang Lian.

·**CHANNELS ENTERED**：The foot greater yin and yang brightness channels. [The spleen and stomach]

·**Analysis of Formula**：(1) Chen Pi dries damp and disinhibits qi. When damp removes, phlegm dries, and when qi normalizes, phlegm moves.

(2) eating of salt precipitates with moistness and softens hardness. Precipitation with moistness descends phlegm, softening of hardness disperses hardness.

(3) Phlegm is in the diaphragm, therefore Gan Cao is used as channel conductor, this enters the stomach, this can fortify the spleen and regulates the stomach. When the spleen and stomach fortify, phlegm spontaneously moves.

·**Contraindication**：weak constitution.

2. 潤下丸

·總結：膈痰

·組成：廣陳皮，甘草

·主治：治膈中痰飲.

·加減：(1)濕勝加星，夏.

(2)火盛加芩，連.

·歸經：足太陰陽明藥.

·方義：(1)陳皮燥濕而利氣，濕去而痰涸，氣順而痰行.

(2)食鹽潤下而軟堅, 潤下則痰降, 軟堅則痰消.

(3)痰在膈中, 故用甘草引之入胃, 甘草經蜜炙能健脾調胃, 脾胃健則痰自行矣.

·禁 忌：虛弱人慎用.

3. Gui Ling Gan Zhu Tang. Cinnamon Twig, Poria, Licorice, and Ovate Atractylodes Decoction. 桂苓甘朮湯

·**ACTIONS**：phlegm

·**COMPOSITION**：Fu Ling, Gui Zhi, Bai Zhu, Gan Cao

·**INDICATIONS**：treats phlegm below the heart, propping fullness in the chest and rib-side, and dizzy vision.

·**CHANNELS ENTERED**：The foot greater yin channel. [The spleen]

·**Analysis of Formula**：喻嘉言 says that Fu Ling treats phlegm, quells kidney evil, and drains water way. Gui Zhi frees yang qi, opens the channels and networks, and harmonizes the construction and defense.

Bai Zhu dries phlegm water, eliminates distention and fullness, and treats wind dizziness. Gan Cao with Fu Ling does not support fullness and instead drains fullness, therefore Ben Cao says that Gan Cao can descend qi, eliminate vexation and fullness. This pattern is phlegm restraining yang, therefore this formula raises yang and transforms qi.

·**Original Source**：Jin Gui Yao Lue

3. 桂苓甘朮湯

·總結：痰飲

·組成：茯苓, 桂枝, 白朮, 甘草

·主治：治心下有痰飲, 胸脅支滿, 目眩.

·歸經：足太陰藥.

·方義： 喻嘉言曰：「茯苓治痰飲, 伐腎邪, 滲水道. 桂枝通陽氣, 開經絡, 和營衛.

白朮燥痰水, 除脹滿, 治風眩. 甘草得茯苓, 則不資滿而反泄滿, 故本草曰：『甘草能下氣, 除煩滿.』此證爲痰飲阻抑其陽, 故用陽藥以升陽而化氣也.」

·來源：金匱

4. Qing Qi Hua Tan Wan. Clear the Qi and Transform Phl egm Pill. 清氣化痰丸

·**ACTIONS**：heat phlegm

·**COMPOSITION**：Ban Xia, Ju Hong, Fu Ling, Huang Qin, Gua Lou Ren, Zhi Shi, Dan Nan Xing, Ku Xing Ren

·**INDICATIONS**：treats heat phlegm.

·**CHANNELS ENTERED**：The hand and foot greater yin channels. [The lung and spleen]

·**Analysis of Formula**：(1) This is general formula for phlegm fire. Qi can effuse fire, fire can eliminate phlegm.

(2) Ban Xia and Nan Xing dry damp qi, Gua Lou and Huang Qin pacify damp qi, Chen Pi normalizes interior qi, Xing Ren descends counterfolw qi, Zhi Shi breaks accumulated qi, and Fu Ling moves water qi.

(3) Water, damp, fire, and heat, they are the root of engendering of phlegm.

4. 清氣化痰丸
    ·總結：熱痰
    ·組成：半夏, 橘紅, 茯苓, 黃芩, 栝蔞仁, 枳實, 膽星, 苦杏仁
    ·主治：治熱痰.
    ·歸經：手足太陰藥.
    ·方義：(1)治痰火之通劑也. 氣能發火, 火能役痰.
        (2)半夏, 南星以燥濕氣, 瓜蔞, 黃芩以平濕氣, 陳皮以順裏氣, 杏仁以降逆氣, 枳實以破積氣, 茯苓以行水氣.
        (3)水濕火熱, 皆生痰之本也.

5. Shun Qi Xiao Shi Hua Tan Wan. Qi-Normalizing Food-d ispersing Phlegm-Transforming Pills. 順氣消食化痰丸

·**ACTIONS**：food phlegm

·**COMPOSITION**：Ban Xia, Dan Nan Xing, Xing Ren, Su Zi, Lai Fu Zi, Qing Pi, Chen Pi (without the white part), Xiang Fu, Ge Gen, Shen Qu, Shan Zha, Mai Ya

·**INDICATIONS**：treats phlegm engendered by wind and food, distensio

362

n and oppression in the chest and diaphragm, fifth-watch cough.

·**CHANNELS ENTERED**：The hand and foot greater yin channels. [The spleen and lung]

·**Analysis of Formula**：(1) for phlegm originated from damp, Ban Xia and Nan Xing dry damp.

(2) for phlegm due to qi rising, Su Zi, Lai Fu Zi, and Xing Ren descend qi.

(3) for phlegm due to qi stagnation, Qing Pi, Chen Pi, and Xiang Fu abduct stagnation.

(4) for phlegm due to wine and food, Ge Gen and Shen Qu resolve wind, and Shan Zha and Mai Ya transform food.

(5) When damp eliminates and food disperses, then phlegm is not generated. When qi normalizes, then cough stops, phlegm stagnation is already eliminated, fullness and oppression spontaneously disappear.

·**Original Source**：Tang Zhu Rui

5. 順氣消食化痰丸

·總結：食痰

·組成：半夏, 膽星, 杏仁, 蘇子, 萊菔子, 青皮, 陳皮去白, 香附, 葛根, 神麴, 山楂, 麥芽

·主治：治酒食生痰, 胸膈膨悶, 五更咳嗽.

·歸經：手足太陰藥.

·方義：(1)痰由溼生, 半夏, 南星, 所以燥溼.

(2)痰由氣升, 蘇子, 菔子, 杏仁, 所以降氣.

(3)痰由氣滯, 青皮, 陳皮, 香附, 所以導滯.

(4)痰因於酒食, 葛根, 神麴, 所以解酒；山楂, 麥芽, 所以化食.

(5)溼去食消, 則痰不生. 氣順則咳嗽止, 痰滯既去, 滿悶自除也.

·來源：瑞竹堂

6. Qing Fei Yin. Clear the Lung Drink. 清肺飲

·**ACTIONS**：phlegm cough

·**COMPOSITION**：Wu Wei Zi, Jie Geng, Ju Hong, Fu Ling, Bei Mu, Xing Ren, Gan Cao

·**INDICATIONS** : treats phlegm and damp, qi counterflow, and cough.

·**MODIFICATIONS** : (1) In spring, if there is wind damage, cough, runn y nose with clear snivel, one should treat with clearing and resolving. Add Bo He, Fang Feng, Zi Su Ye, and Huang Qing.

(2) In summer, the weather is fire heat, one should treat with clea ring and descending, add Sang Pi, Mai Men Dong, Huang Qin, Zhi Mu, Shi Ga o.

(3) In fall, the weather is damp heat, one should clear heat and di sinhibit damp, add Cang Zhu, Sang Pi, Fang Feng, Zhi Zi, and Huang Qin.

(4) In winter, the weather is wind cold, one should resolve the ex terior and move phlegm, add Ma Huang, Gui Zhi, Gan Jiang, Sheng Jiang, Ban Xia, and Fang Feng.

(5) for fire cough, add Qing Dai, Gua Lou, and Hai Shi.

(6) for food accumulation and phlegm, add Xiang Fu, Shan Zha, and Zhi Shi.

(7) for damp phlegm, eliminate Bei Mu and add Ban Xia, and Na n Xing.

(8) for dry phlegm, add Gua Lou, Zhi Mu, and Tian Men Dong.

(9) The cough in the forenoon belongs to stomach fire, one shoul d clear the stomach, add Shi Gao and Huang Lian.

(10) The cough in the afternoon belongs to yin vacuity, one shoul d nourish yin and descend water, add Chuan Xiong, Dang Gui Shao Yao, Shen g Di huang, Zhi Mu, Huang Bai, Mai Men Dong, Tian Men Dong, Zhu Li, and Jiang Zhi (juice of ginger).

(11) Cough in the dusk of the evening is related with fire floating i n the lung, this case cannot be treated with cool herbs. Wu Bei Zi, Wu Wei Zi, and He Zi should be used to restrain and descend the fire.

(12) Taxation cough with blood is often shown in the lung contrac ting heat evil, one should add Dang Gui Shao Yao, E Jiao, Tian Men Dong, Zhi Mu, Kuan Dong Hua, and Zi Yuan.

(13) Enduring cough indicates lung vacuity, add Ren Shen, Huang Qi. If there is lung heat, eliminate Ren Shen, and instead of it, use Sha Shen.

·**CHANNELS ENTERED** : The hand greater yin channel. [The lung]

·**Analysis of Formula** : (1) Xing Ren resolves the flesh, disperses cold, de scends qi, and moistens dry.

(2) Bei Mu clears fire, disperses binds, moistens the lung, and tra nsforms phlegm.

(3) Wu Wei Zi restrains the lung and quiets cough.

(4) Fu Ling eliminates damp and rectifies the spleen.

(5) Ju Hong moves qi.

(6) Gan Cao harmonizes the middle.

(7) Jie Geng clears the lung and disinhibits diaphragm. This conducts every herbs to ascend upward can open congestion and disperse the exterior.

6. 清肺飲
  ·總結：痰嗽
  ·組成：五味子, 桔梗, 橘紅, 茯苓, 貝母, 杏仁, 甘草
  ·主治：治痰溼氣逆而咳嗽.
  ·加減：(1)若春時傷風咳嗽, 鼻流清涕, 宜清解, 加薄荷, 防風, 紫蘇, 炒芩.

    (2)夏多火熱, 宜清降, 加桑皮, 麥冬, 黃芩, 知母, 石膏.

    (3)秋多溼熱, 宜清熱利溼, 加蒼朮, 桑皮, 防風, 栀, 芩.

    (4)冬多風寒, 宜解表行痰, 加麻黃, 桂枝, 乾薑, 生薑, 半夏, 防風.

    (5)火嗽加清黛, 栝蔞, 海石.

    (6)食積痰加香附, 山楂, 枳實.

    (7)溼痰除貝母, 加半夏, 南星.

    (8)燥痰加栝蔞, 知母, 天冬.

    (9)午前嗽屬胃火, 宜清胃, 加石膏, 黃連.

    (10)午後嗽屬陰虛, 宜滋陰降水, 加芎, 歸, 芍, 地, 知, 柏, 二冬, 竹瀝, 薑汁傳送.

    (11)黃昏嗽爲火浮于肺, 不可用涼藥, 宜五倍, 五味, 訶子, , 斂而降之.

    (12)勞嗽見血, 多是肺受熱邪, 宜加歸, 芍, 阿膠, 天冬, 知母, 款冬, 紫苑之類.

    (13)久嗽肺虛, 加參, 耆. 如肺熱, 去人參, 用沙參可也.
  ·歸經：此手太陰之藥, 治肺之通劑.
  ·方義：(1)杏仁解肌散寒, 降氣潤燥.

    (2)貝母清火散結, 潤肺化痰.

    (3)五味斂肺而寧嗽.

    (4)茯苓除濕而理脾.

(5)橘紅行氣.

(6)甘草和中.

(7)桔梗清肺利膈，載藥上浮，而又能開壅發表也.

7. Jin Fei Cao San. Inula Powder. 金沸草散

·**ACTIONS**： wind damage with cough

·**COMPOSITION**：Xuan Fu Hua, Qian Hu, Xi Xin, Jing Jie, Chi Fu Ling, Ban Xia, Gan Cao (mix fried)

·**INDICATIONS**：treats wind damage in the lung channel, headache, blurred vision, cough with copious phlegm.

·**MODIFICATIONS**：(1) for fullness and oppression, add Zhi Ke, Jie Geng.

(2) for heat, add Chai Hu, Huang Qin.

(3) for headache, add Chuan Xiong.

·**CHANNELS ENTERED**：The hand greater yin channel. [The lung]

·**Analysis of Formula**：(1) Phlegm is bound in the interior. Therefore Qian Hu and Xuan Fu Hua disperse phlegm and descend qi.

(2) Ban Xia dries phlegm and disperses counterfolw qi.

(3) Wind heat is congested in the upper part, Jing Jie is pungent and light, this promotes sweating and disperses wind.

(4) Gan Cao disperses and harmonizes the middle.

(5) Fu Ling moves water.

(6) Xi Xin warms the channel.

(7) Generally phlegm tends to be with fire and damp, therefore if qi is descended and damp is disinhibited, then the pattern spontaneously calm.

(8) Chi Fu Ling enters blood part and drains the fire of Bing and Ding.

·**Original Source**：Huo Ren

7. 金沸草散

·總結：傷風欬嗽

·組成：旋覆花, 前胡, 細辛, 荊芥, 赤茯苓, 半夏, 炙甘草

·主治：治肺經傷風, 頭目昏痛, 咳嗽多痰.

·加減：(1)如滿悶, 加枳殼, 桔梗.

366

(2)有熱加柴胡, 黃芩.

(3)頭痛加川芎.

·歸經：手太陰藥.

·方義：(1)痰涎內結, 前胡, 旋覆消痰而降氣.

(2)半夏燥痰而散逆.

(3)風熱上壅, 荊芥辛輕發汗而散風.

(4)甘草發散而和中.

(5)茯苓行水.

(6)細辛溫經.

(7)蓋痰必挾火而兼溼, 故下氣利溼而證自平.

(8)茯苓用赤者, 入血分而瀉丙丁也.

·煎服法：加薑, 棗煎.

·來源：活人

8. Bai Hua Gao. Lily Bulb and Tussilago Paste. 百花膏

·**ACTIONS**：phlegm cough

·**COMPOSITION**：Bai He, Kuan Dong Hua

·**INDICATIONS**：treats incessant panting and cough, or blood in the phlegm, this formula is more appropriate to vacuity people.

·**CHANNELS ENTERED**：The hand greater yin channel. [The lung]

·**Analysis of Formula**：Kuan Dong Hua drains heat, descends qi, clears blood, and eliminates phlegm. Bai He moistens the lung, quiets the heart, supplements the middle, and boosts qi. This formula is key medicinal to rectify cough.

·**RELATED FORMULA**：When Zi Yuan, Bai Bu Zi, and Wu Mei are added, this is called Jia Wei Bai Hua Gao. This treats same things.

·**Original Source**：Ji Sheng.

8. 百花膏

·總結：痰嗽

·組成：百合, 款冬花

·主治：治喘咳不已, 或痰中有血, 虛人尤宜.

·歸經：手太陰藥.

·方義：款冬瀉熱下氣, 清血除痰. 百花潤肺寧心, 補中益氣. 並為理嗽要藥.

367

·變化方：加紫苑，百部，烏梅，名「加味百花膏」．治同，煎服亦可．
·來源：濟生

9. San Xian Dan. Three Immortals Elixir. 三仙丹

·**ACTIONS**：qi phlegm
·**COMPOSITION**：Ban Xia, Nan Xing, Xiang Fu.
·**INDICATIONS**：treats qi stagnation in the middle stomach duct, inhibited phlegm-drool.
·**CHANNELS ENTERED**：The foot yang brightness and the hand and foot greater yin channels. [The stomach, lung and spleen].
·**Analysis of Formula**：(1) Ban Xia and Nan Xing dry phlegm in the lung and stomach.

(2) Xiang Fu disinhibits the qi of the triple burner. If one makes qi move, then phlegm moves.
·**Original Source**：Bai Yi Fang.

9. 三仙丹

·總結：氣痰
·組成：半夏麴，南星麴，香附．
·主治：治中脘氣滯，痰涎不利．
·歸經：足陽明，手足太陰藥．
·方義：(1)星，夏以燥肺胃之痰．
(2)香附以快三焦之氣，使氣行則痰行也．
·來源：百一方

10. Ban Xia Bai Zhu Tian Ma Tang. Pinellia, Atractylodes Macrocephala, and Gastrodia Decoction. 半夏天麻白术湯

·**ACTIONS**：phlegm reversal headache
·**COMPOSITION**：Ban Xia, Tian Ma, Ren Shen, Huang Qi, Cang Zhu, Bai Zhu, Fu Ling, Ze Xie, Shen Qu, Mai Ya, Chen Pi, Huang Bai, Gan Jiang
·**INDICATIONS**：treats internal damage of the spleen and stomach, dim

vision, dizziness, headache as like breaking, generalized heaviness as mountain, nausea, vexation and oppression, reversal cold of the limbs. This is called the foot greater yin phlegm reversal headache.

·**CHANNELS ENTERED**：The foot greater yin channel. [The spleen]

·**Analysis of Formula**：(1) In case of phlegm reversal headache, without Ban Xia, this cannot be eliminated.

(2) Dim vision and dizziness are caused by vacuous wind in the interior, without Tian Ma, this cannot be eliminated.

(3) Bai Zhu and Cang Zhu are bitter and warm, they can eliminate phlegm and also boost qi.

(4) Huang Qi and Ren Shen are sweet and warm. They can drain fire and also supplement the middle.

(5) Fu Ling and Ze Xie drain heat and abduct water.

(6) Chen Pi regulates qi and raises yang.

(7) Shen Qu disperses food and flushes stagnated qi in the stomach.

(8) Mai Ya transforms binds and assists Wu Ji [the spleen and stomach] to move.

(9) Gan Jiang is pungent and heat. This flushes cold in the middle.

(10) Huang Bai is bitter and cold, (washed with wine). This treats yin fire in the kidney which generates dry.

·**Original Source**：Li Dong Yuan

10. 半夏天麻白朮湯

·總結：痰厥頭痛

·組成：半夏，天麻，人參，黃耆，蒼朮，白朮，茯苓，澤瀉，神麴，麥芽，陳皮，黃柏，乾薑

·主治：治脾胃內傷，眼黑頭眩，頭痛如裂，身重如山，惡心煩悶，四肢厥冷，謂之足太陰痰厥頭痛.

·歸經：足太陰藥.

·方義：(1)痰厥頭痛，非半夏不能除.

(2)頭眩眼黑，虛風內作，非天麻不能除.

(3)二朮甘苦而溫，可以除痰，亦可以益氣.

(4)黃耆，人參甘溫，可以瀉火，亦可以補中.

(5)苓，瀉瀉熱導水.

369

(6)陳皮調氣升陽.

(7)神麴消食, 蕩胃中滯氣.

(8)麥芽化結, 助戊己運行.

(9)乾薑辛熱, 以滌中寒.

(10)黃柏苦寒, 酒洗, 以療少火在泉發躁也.

·來源：東垣

11. Fu Ling Wan. Poria Pill. 茯苓丸

·**ACTIONS**：collecting phlegm with forearm pain.

·**COMPOSITION**：Fu Ling, Feng Hua Xiao, Zhi Ke, Ban Xia

·**INDICATIONS**：treats phlegm collected in the middle stomach duct, pa in in the both forearms.

·**CHANNELS ENTERED**：The foot greater yin and yang brightness cha nnels. [The spleen and stomach]

·**Analysis of Formula**：(1) Fu Ling drains water.

(2) Hua Xiao softens hardness.

(3) Zhi Ke moves qi.

(4) Ban Xia dries damp.

(5) Sheng Jiang restrains the toxin of Ban Xia and eliminates phl egm. If one makes phlegm to move and qi to free, then forearm pain spontaneo usly stops.

·**Original Source**：Zhi Mi

11. 茯苓丸

·總結：停痰臂痛

·組成：茯苓, 風化硝, 枳殼, 半夏麴

·主治：治痰停中脘, 兩臂疼痛.

·歸經：足太陰, 陽明藥.

·方義：(1)茯苓滲水.

(2)化硝軟堅.

(3)枳殼行氣.

(4)半夏燥溼.

(5)生薑製半夏之毒而除痰, 使痰行氣通, 臂通自止矣.

·來源：指迷

12. Kong Xian Dan. Control Mucus Special Pill. 控涎丹

·**ACTIONS**：phlegm-drool

·**COMPOSITION**：Bai Jie Zi, Gan Sui, Da Ji

·**INDICATIONS**：(1) treats sudden pulling pain in the chest, back, the limbs, lumbus, nape, sinew, and bone, wandering pain, or cold impediment of the limbs, blocked qi and vessels.

(2) this treats phlegm and drool in the upper and lower of the chest and diaphragm. Do not be confused with paralysis.

·**MODIFICATIONS**：(1) for cold reverse, add Hu Jiao, Ding Xiang, Sheng Jiang, and Gui Zhi.

(2) for leg qi, add Bing Lang, Mu Gua, Song Zhi, and Juan Bai.

(3) for fright phlegm, add Zhu Sha and Quan Xie.

(4) for heat phlegm, add Pen Xiao.

(5) for fright qi causing lump, add Chuan Shan Jia, Bie Jia, Yan Hu Suo, and Peng Zhu.

·**CHANNELS ENTERED**：The hand and foot greater yang and yin channels. [The small intestine, bladder, lung, and spleen]

·**Original Source**：San Yin Fang

12. 控涎丹
·總結：痰涎
·組成：白芥子, 甘遂, 大戟
·主治：(1)治人忽患胸背手足腰項筋骨牽引鈎痛, 走易不定, 或手足冷痹, 氣脈不通.

(2)此乃痰涎在胸膈上下, 誤認癱瘓, 非也.

·加減：(1)寒厥加胡椒, 丁香, 薑, 桂.

(2)脚氣加檳榔, 木瓜, 松脂, 卷柏.

(3)驚痰加硃砂, 全蠍.

(4)熱痰加盆硝.

(5)驚氣成塊加穿山甲, 鱉甲, 延胡索, 蓬朮.

·歸經：手足太陽太陰藥.

·來源：三因方

13. San Zi Yang Qin Tang. Three-Seed Decoction to Nouris

h One's Parents. 三子養親湯

·**ACTIONS**：qi phlegm

·**COMPOSITION**：Zi Su Ye, Bai Jie Zi, Lai Fu Zi

·**INDICATIONS**：treats qi repletion and phlegm exuberance in old people, panting, fullness, and laziness to eat.

·**CHANNELS ENTERED**：The hand and foot greater yin channels. [The lung and spleen]

·**Analysis of Formula**：Bai Jie Zi eliminates phlegm, Zi Su Ye moves qi, and Lai Fu Zi disperses food. They move qi and sweep phlegm. When qi moves, fire descends and phlegm disperses.

13. 三子養親湯

·總結：氣痰

·組成：紫蘇子, 白芥子, 萊服子

·主治：治老人氣實痰盛, 喘滿懶食.

·歸經：手足太陰藥.

·方義：白芥子除痰, 紫蘇子行氣, 萊服子消食. 然皆行氣豁痰之藥, 氣行則火降而痰消矣.

14. Di Tan Tang. Phlegm-Flushing Decoction. 滌痰湯

·**ACTIONS**：wind phlegm

·**COMPOSITION**：Fu Ling, Ren Shen, Gan Cao, Ju Hong, Dan Nan Xing, Ban Xia, Zhu Ru, Zhi Shi, Shi Chang Pu

·**INDICATIONS**：treats wind strike, phlegm confounding the orifices of the heart, stiff tongue and impending speech.

·**CHANNELS ENTERED**：The hand lesser yin and the foot greater yin channels. [The heart and spleen]

·**Analysis of Formula**：(1) When the heart and spleen are insufficient, wind evil exploits this insufficiency and phlegm and fire block the channels and networks, therefore the root of tongue gets stiff and impending speech occurs.

(2)① Ren Shen, Fu Ling, and Gan Cao supplement the heart, boost the spleen, and drain fire.

②Chen Pi, Nan Xing, and Ban Xia disinhibit qi, dry damp, and eliminate phlegm.

372

③ Zhu Ru clears dries and opens depression.

④ Zhi Shi breaks phlegm and disinhibits diaphragm.

⑤ Shi Chang Pu opens orifice and frees the heart.

⑥ When phlegm disperses and fire descends, the chan nels get to free and the tongue gets soft.

·**Original Source**：Yan Shi

14. 滌痰湯

　·總結：風痰

　·組成：茯苓, 人參, 甘草, 橘紅, 膽星, 半夏, 竹如, 枳實, 菖蒲

　·主治：治中風痰迷心竅, 舌強不能言.

　·歸經：手少陰, 足太陰藥.

　·方義：(1)心脾不足, 風邪乘之, 而痰與火塞其經絡, 故舌本強而難語也.

　　　　　(2)①人參, 茯苓, 甘草一補心益脾而瀉火.

　　　　　　　②陳皮, 南星, 半夏一利氣燥濕而祛痰.

　　　　　　　③竹茹清燥開鬱.

　　　　　　　④枳實破痰利膈.

　　　　　　　⑤菖蒲開竅通心.

　　　　　　　⑥使痰消火降, 則經通而舌柔矣.

　·來源：嚴氏

15. Meng Shi Gun Tan Wan. Chlorite Phlegm- Rolling Pill. 礞石滾痰丸

·**ACTIONS**：stubborn and strange disease.

·**COMPOSITION**：Qing Meng Shi, Da Huang, Chen Xiang, Huang Qin

·**INDICATIONS**：treats replete heat and old phlegm, strange pattern and one hundred disease.

·**CHANNELS ENTERED**：The hand and foot greater yin and yang brig htness. [The lung, spleen, large intestine, and stomach]

·**Analysis of Formula**：(1) Meng Shi is quick and bold, this can attack old accumulation and latent and enduring phlegm.

(2) Da Huang flushes heat and eliminates repletion, this opens th e way to move downward.

373

(3) Chen Xiang can ascend and descend every qi, this reaches up ward to the heaven and downward a spring, this conducts every herbs, acting as courier.

(4) Huang Qin drains the lung and cools the heart, this calms fire skipping upward.

·**RELATED FORMULA**：(1) When Xuan Ming Fen and Zhu Sha are ad ded, this treats same things..

(2) When Da Huang and Huang Qin (respectively six liang) are r educed and Ju Hong and Ban Xia (respectively two liang), Gan Cao (one liang), Zhu Li, Jiang Zhi (juice of ginger) are added, this is called Zhu Li Da Tan Wan, treats same things.

·**Original Source**：Wan Yin Jun

15. 礞石滾痰丸

　·總結：頑病怪病

　·組成：青礞石，大黃，沉香，黃芩

　·主治：治實熱老痰，怪證百病.

　·歸經：手足太陰，陽明藥.

　·方義：(1)礞石剽悍之性，能攻陳積伏歷之痰.

　　　　　(2)大黃蕩熱去實，以開下行之路.

　　　　　(3)沉香能升降諸氣，上至天而下至泉，以導諸藥爲使也.

　　　　　(4)黃芩瀉肺涼心，以平上僭之火.

　·變化方：(1)本方加玄明粉一兩，硃砂爲衣，治同.

　　　　　(2)本方減大黃，黃芩各六兩，加橘紅，半夏各二兩，甘草一兩，竹瀝，薑汁爲丸，名「竹瀝達痰丸」，治同.

　·來源：王隱君

16. Niu Huang Wan. Cattle Gallstone Pill. 牛黃丸

·**ACTIONS**：wind epilepsy and fright phlegm

·**COMPOSITION**：Niu Huang, Fang Feng, Tian Ma, Jiang Can, Chan T ui, Bai Fu **Zi**, Dan Nan Xing, Quan Xie, She Xiang, Shui Yin, Da Zao, Sheng J iang, Jing Jie

·**INDICATIONS**：treats wind epilepsy with confounding and oppression of heart spirit, congested and exuberant phlegm and drool as like tidal water, co nvulsion and pulling of the limbs.

374

·**CHANNELS ENTERED**：The hand lesser yin and the foot greater and reverting yin channels. [The kidney, spleen, and liver]

·**Analysis of Formula**：Niu Huang clears the heart, resolves heat, opens orifices, and disinhibits phlegm. Tian Ma, Fang Feng, Nan Xing, and Quan Xie disperse with pungent. Jiang Can and Chan Tui clear and transform qi. Bai Fu is for head and face. They can track down liver wind and disperse phlegm binds. She Xiang frees orifice. Shui Yin extorts phlegm. Sheng Jiang and Jing Jie are used as channel conductor and to expel wind and move phlegm.

16. 牛黃丸

·總結：風癇驚痰

·組成：牛黃，防風，天麻，殭蠶，蟬蛻，白附子，膽星，金蠍，麝香，水銀，大棗，生薑，荊芥

·主治：治風癇迷悶，涎潮抽掣.

·歸經：手少陰，足太陰，厥陰藥.

·方義：牛黃清心，解熱開竅利痰. 天麻，防風，南星，全蠍辛散之味；殭蠶，蟬蛻清化之品；白附頭面之藥；皆能搜肝風而散痰結. 麝香通竅. 水銀劫痰. 引以薑，芥者，亦以逐風而行痰也.

·煎服法：煮棗肉和水銀五分，細研，入藥末爲丸. 荊芥薑湯下.

17. Chen Sha San. Cinnabar Powder. 辰砂散

·**ACTIONS**：wind phlegm and epilepsy

·**COMPOSITION**：Chen Sha, Zao Ren, Ru Xiang

·**INDICATIONS**：treats wind phlegm, all kinds of epilepsy, mania and withdrawal, and heart disease.

·**CHANNELS ENTERED**：The hand lesser yin channel. [The heart]

·**Analysis of Formula**：(1) Chen Sha settles the heart and drains heart fire.

(2) Zao Ren supplements the liver and gall bladder and quiets the heart.

(3) Ru Xiang enters the heart and disperses static blood.

·**Original Source**：Ling Yuan Fang

17. 辰砂散

·總結：風痰癲癇

·組成：辰砂，棗仁，乳香

375

·主治：治風痰諸癇, 癲狂心疾.

·歸經：手少陰藥.

·方義：(1)辰砂鎮心瀉心火.

(2)棗仁補肝膽而寧心.

(3)乳香入心散瘀血.

·來源：靈苑

18. Qing Zhou Bai Wan Zi. Qingzhou White Pill. 青州白丸子

·**ACTIONS**：wind phlegm.

·**COMPOSITION**：Chuan Wu, Bai Fu Zi, Ban Xia, Nan Xing

·**INDICATIONS**：(1) treats exuberant wind and phlegm, vomiting of drool and foam, deviated eye and mouth, paralysis, and fright wind of child.

(2) and exuberant phlegm with diarrhea.

·**CHANNELS ENTERED**：The foot reverting and greater yin channels. [The liver and spleen]

·**Analysis of Formula**：phlegm is engendered due to wind or cold or damp, therefore this formula is used

(1) Chuan Wu and Bai Fu are pungent and heat, they warm the channels and expel wind.

(2) Ban Xia and Nan Xing are pungent and warm, they dry damp and disperses cold.

18. 青州白丸子

·總結：風痰

·組成：川烏, 白附子, 半夏, 南星

·主治：(1)治風痰湧盛, 嘔吐涎沫, 口眼喎邪, 手足癱瘓, 小兒驚風.

(2)及痰盛泄瀉.

·歸經：足厥陰, 太陰藥.

·方義：痰之生也, 由風由寒由溼, 故用：

(1)川烏, 白附之辛熱, 以溫經逐風.

(2)半夏, 南星之辛溫, 以燥溼散寒.

376

19. Xing Xiang Tang. Arisaema and Saussurea Decoction. 星香散

·**ACTIONS**：wind phlegm

·**COMPOSITION**：Dan Nan Xing, Mu Xiang,

·**INDICATIONS**：treats wind stroke, exuberant phlegm, obesity without thirst.

·**CHANNELS ENTERED**：The foot reverting yin channel. [The liver]

·**Analysis of Formula**：(1) Nan Xing dries phlegm, being processed with cow's gall bladder kills the toxin of Nan Xing, and cow's gall bladder boosts the liver and gall bladder.

(2) Mu Xiang is used as assistant to move qi and disinhibit phlegm.

(3) Obesity without thirst indicates excessive damp, this should be treated with drying damp. Quan Xie can be added to disperse liver wind.

·**Another Side Formula**：or add Quan Xie.

19. 星香散
　·總結：風痰
　·組成：膽星, 木香
　·主治：治中風痰盛, 體肥不渴者.
　·歸經：足厥陰藥.
　·方義：(1)南星燥痰之品, 製以牛膽, 以殺其毒, 且膽有益肝膽之功.
　　　　(2)佐以木香, 取其行氣以利痰也.
　　　　(3)肥而不渴, 宜燥可知, 加全蠍者, 以散肝風也.
　·又附方：或加全蠍.

20. Chang Shan Yin. Dichroa Beverage. 常山飲

·**ACTIONS**：extort phlegm and interrupt malaria

·**COMPOSITION**：Chang Shan, Wu Mei, Cao Guo, Bei Mu, Bing Lang, Zhi Mu

·**INDICATIONS**：enduring malaria

·**CHANNELS ENTERED**：The foot lesser yang and greater yin channels. [The gall bladder and spleen]

·**Analysis of Formula**：(1) Somebody in ancient times says that without p

hlegm, malaria cannot occur. Chang Shan induces vomiting and moves water, a
nd eliminates old phlegm and accumulated rheum. Bing Lang descends qi and
breaks accumulation, this can disperse food and moves phlegm.

(2) When yin and yang are in disharmony, malaria occurs. Zhi M
u nourishes yin, this can treat the exuberant fire of yang brightness. Cao Guo is
pungent and heat, this can treats the exuberant cold of greater yin.

(3) Bei Mu clears fire, disperses binds, drains heat, and eliminate
s phlegm. The sour and astringency of Wu Mei restrains and contracts, and gen
erates the fluid and abates heat.

(4) This formula interrupts malaria.

·**Original Source**：Ju Fang

20. 常山飲
  ·總結：劫痰截瘧
  ·組成：常山，烏梅，草果，貝母，檳榔，知母
  ·主治：瘧久不已者，用此截之.
  ·歸經：足少陽，太陰藥.
  ·方義：(1)古云：「無痰不作瘧.」常山引吐行水，祛老痰積飲. 檳榔
下氣破積，能消食行痰.

(2)陰陽不和則瘧作. 知母滋陰，能治陽明獨勝之火. 草果辛
熱，能治太陰獨勝之寒.

(3)貝母清火散結，瀉熱除痰. 烏梅酸斂瘧收，生津退熱.

(4)合為截瘧之劑也.

·來源：局方

21. Jie Nue Qi Bao Yin. Malaria-Interrupting Seven-Jewel Beverage. 七寶飲

·**ACTIONS**：malaria phlegm

·**COMPOSITION**：Cao Guo, Bing Lang, Chen Pi, Qing Pi, Hou Po, Cha
ng Shan, Gan Cao

·**INDICATIONS**：(1) treats replete malaria that is enduring and incessant, a pulse
in inch that is string-like, slippery, floating and large.

(2) regardless of whether it is Gui malaria or food malaria, this tr
eats both of them.

·**CHANNELS ENTERED**：The foot lesser yang and greater yin. [The ga

378

ll bladder and spleen]

　　·**Analysis of Formula**：(1)① Cao Guo can disperse phlegm of fat meat an
d grain in greater yin.

　　　　　　　　　② Bing Lang can descend food, accumulation, phleg
m, and binds.

　　　　　　　　　③ Chen Pi disinhibits qi.

　　(2) Gan Cao enters the stomach to assistant Chang Shan which v
omits malaria phlegm.

　　·**Original Source**：Yi Jian

21. 截瘧七寶飲
　·總結：瘧痰
　·組成：草果, 檳榔, 陳皮, 青皮, 厚朴, 常山, 甘草
　·主治：(1)治實瘧久發不止, 寸口脈弦滑浮大者.
　　　　　(2)不問鬼瘧食瘧, 並皆治之.
　·歸經：足少陽, 太陰藥.
　·方義：(1)①草果—能消太陰膏粱之痰.
　　　　　　　②檳榔—能下食積痰結.
　　　　　　　③陳皮—利氣.
　　　　　(2)加甘草入胃, 佐常山以吐瘧痰也.
　·來源：易簡

Chapter 16. Dispersing and Abducting Formulas. 消導之劑

1. Ping Wei San. Calm the Stomach Powder. 平胃散

·**ACTIONS**：disinhibits damp and disperses fullness

·**COMPOSITION**：Chen Pi, Hou Po, Gan Cao (mix fried), Cang Zhu

·**INDICATIONS**：(1) treats damp retention in the spleen, phlegm and glomus in the diaphragm, retained food, fullness and oppression, retching and diarrhea.

(2) and miasmic toxin.

·**MODIFICATIONS**：(1) for food damage, add Shen Qu, Mai Ya, or Zhi Shi.

(2) for excessive damp, add Wu Ling San.

(3) for spleen fatigue and no thought of food, add Ren Shen and Huang Qi.

(4) for cold damage with headache, add Dan Dou Chi.

(5) for glomus and oppression, add Zhi Ke and Mu Xiang.

(6) for constipation, add Da Huang, Mang Xiao.

(7) for copious phlegm, add Ban Xia.

(8) for inhibited voiding of reddish urine, add Fu Ling and Ze Xie.

·**CHANNELS ENTERED**：The foot greater yin and yang brightness channels.

·**Analysis of Formula**：(1) Chen Pi is pungent and warm, disinhibits qi and moves phlegm.

(2) Hou Po is bitter and warn, eliminates damp and disperses fullness.

(3) Gan Cao controls the middle, can supplement and harmonize the middle. This is used in stir-bake with honey, acting as courier.

(4) Cang Zhu is pungent and harsh, dries damp and strengthens the spleen.

(5) This formula supplements in the middle of draining, and makes the spleen and stomach to get harmonious.

·**RELATED FORMULA**：(1) When Huo Xiang and Ban Xia are added, this is called Huo Xiang Ping Wei San, and this is also called Bu Huang Jin Zhe ng Qi San, treats the stomach cold with abdominal pain and vomiting, miasmic toxin, and damp malaria. When Ren Shen, Fu Ling, Cao Guo, Sheng Jiang, and Wu Mei are again added, this is called Ren Shen Yang Wei Tang, treats external contraction of wind and cold, internal damage engendering cold, retention phlegm with food, miasmic toxin, scourage epidemic, spleem damage due to food and drink, and malaria.

(2) When Er Chen Tang and Huo Xiang are added, this is called Chu Shi Tang, treats damp damage, abdominal pain, generalized heaviness, foot weakness, and sloppy stool or diarrhea. .

(3) When Gao Ben, Zhi Ke, and Jie Geng are added, this is called He Jie San, treats seasonal cold damage, headache, vexation and agitation, spontaneous sweating, cough, vomiting, and diarrhea.

(4) When Sang Bai Pi is added, this is called Dui Jin Yin Zi, treats the spleen and stomach contracting damp, abdominal distention, generalized heaviness, lack of appetite, aching limbs, and skin swelling.

(5) When Cang Zhu is eliminated and Mu Xiang, Cao Dou Kou, Gan Jiang, and Fu Ling are added, this is called Hou Po Wen Zhong Tang, treats the vacuous cold of the spleen and stomach, distention and fullness in the heart and abdomen, and cold invading the stomach in fall and winter with periodic pain.

(6) When Mai Ya and Shen qu are added, this is called Jia Wei Ping Wei San, treats retained food, acid regurgitation, and belching.

·**Original Source**：Ju Fang

1. 平胃散
　·總結：利溼散滿
　·組成：陳皮, 厚朴, 炙甘草, 蒼朮
　·主治：(1)治脾有停濕, 痰飲痞膈, 宿食不消, 滿悶嘔瀉.
　　　　　(2)及山嵐瘴霧, 不服水土.
　·加減：(1)傷食加神麴, 麥芽, 或枳實.
　　　　　(2)溼勝加五苓.
　　　　　(3)脾倦不思食加參, 耆.
　　　　　(4)傷寒頭痛加蔥豉, 取微汁.
　　　　　(5)痞悶加枳殼, 木香.
　　　　　(6)大便祕加大黃, 芒硝.
　　　　　(7)痰多加半夏.
　　　　　(8)小便赤澀加苓, 瀉.

·歸經：足太陰，陽明藥.

·方義：(1)陳皮—辛溫，利氣而行痰.

(2)厚朴—苦溫，除溼而散滿.

(3)甘草—中州主藥，能補能和，蜜炙爲使.

(4)蒼朮—辛烈，燥濕而強脾.

(5)泄中有補，務令溼土底于和平也.

·變化方：(1)本方加藿香，半夏，名「藿香平胃散」，又名「不換金正氣散」，治胃寒腹痛嘔吐，及瘴疫溼瘧. 再加人參，茯苓，草果，生薑，烏梅，名「人參養胃湯」，治外感風寒，內傷生冷，夾食停痰，嵐瘴瘟疫，或飲食傷脾，發爲痎瘧.

(2)本方合二陳，加藿香，名「除溼湯」，治傷溼腹痛，身重，足頓，大便溏瀉.

(3)本方加薰本，枳殼，桔梗，名「和解散」，治四時傷寒頭痛，煩燥自汗，咳嗽吐利.

(4)本方一兩，加桑白皮一兩，名「對金飲子」，治脾胃受溼，腹脹身重，飲食不進，肢痰膚腫.

(5)本方除蒼朮，加木香，草蔻，乾薑，茯苓，名「厚朴溫中湯」，治脾胃虛寒，心腹脹滿，及秋冬客寒犯胃，時作疼痛.

(6)本方加麥芽，炒麴，名「加味平胃散」，治宿食不消，吞酸噯臭.

·來源：局方

2. Zhi Zhu Wan. Immature Bitter Orange and Atractylodes Macrocephala Pills. 枳朮丸

·**ACTIONS**：fortifies the spleen and disperses food

·**COMPOSITION**：Bai Zhu, Zhi Shi

·**INDICATIONS**：disperses glomus and eliminate phlegm, fortifies the spleen and promotes eating.

·**CHANNELS ENTERED**：The foot greater yin and yang brightness channel.

·**Analysis of Formula**： Li Dong Yuan says that the sweet and warm of Bai Zhu supplements the source qi of the spleen and stomach, the bitter eliminates damp heat in the stomach and disinhibits blood between the lumbus and umbilicus. This is one time better than Zhi Shi in digesting food. The bitter and cold of Zhi Shi drains glomus and oppression in the stomach and digests food in th e stomach. This formula first supplements the vacuity and then digests food and drink, therefore the action of this formula is not harsh. He Ye is empty in the m iddle and blue color, this looks like Zhen Gua (震卦), in human this is related with lesser yang gall bladder which is the root of engendering transformation. F ood and drink enter the stomach, construction qi moves upward, this action is d one by the qi of lesser yang gall bladder. There is stomach qi, source qi, grain q i, and rising qi of gall bladder in the body, all of them are one kind. When food and medicinal are supplied with the qi of Bo He, how cannot stomach qi move upward? Boiled rice and Bai Zhu enrich and nourish the grain right qi together, supplement the stomach in order not to reach damage again.

·**RELATED FORMULA**：(1) When this formula is made into Decoction, this is called Zhi Chu Tang, treats water rheum, and large hardness below the h eart.

(2) When Ban Xia is added, this is called Ban Xia Zhi Zhu Wan, treats spleen damp, retained phlegm, and damage to cold food. For strangury, a dd Ze Xie (one liang).

(3) When Ju Pi(one liang) is added, this is called Ju Pi Zhi Zhu Wan, treats undigested food and drink, qi stagnation, and glomus and oppressio n.

(4) When Chen Pi and Ban Xia are added, this is called Ju Ban Z hi Zhu Wan, fortifies the spleen, disperses glomus, and transforms phlegm.

(5) When Mu Xiang (one liang) is added, this is called Mu Xiang Zhi Zhu Wan, treats qi stagnation, glomus, and fullness. Again when Sha Ren i s added, this is called Xiang Sha Zhi Zhu Wan, breaks stagnated qi, disperses f ood and drink, and strengthens the spleen and stomach. When Gan Jiang (five q ian) is added, this is called Mu Xiang Gan Jiang Zhi Zhu Wan, treats qi cold wi th the above. Again when Ren Shen and Chen Pi are added, this is called Mu X iang Ren Shen Gan Jiang Zhi Zhu Wan, opens the stomach and promotes eatin g.

(6) When Shen Qu and Mai Ya (respectively one liang) are adde d, this is called Qu Nie Zhi Zhu Wan, treats internal damage to food and drink, or diarrhea.

(7) When Huang Lian (stir-bake with wine), Huang Qin, Da Hua ng, Shen Qu (stir-bake), Ju Hong (respectively one liang) are added, this is call ed San Huang Zhi Zhu Wan, treats damage to meat, damp food, noodles, and s ome food with pungent, heat, and thick.

(8) When Fu Ling (five qian) and Gan Jiang (seven qian) are add ed, this is called Xiao Yin Wan, treats retained rheum, thoracic fullness, and ret

ching.

·**Original Source**：Jie Gu

2. 枳朮丸

　　·總結：健脾消食
　　·組成：白朮, 枳實
　　·主治：消痞除痰, 健脾進食.
　　·歸經：足太陰, 陽明藥.
　　·方義：李東垣曰：「白朮甘溫, 補脾胃之元氣, 其苦味除胃中溼熱, 利腰臍間血, 過于枳實剋化之藥一倍. 枳實苦寒, 泄胃中痞悶, 化胃中所傷, 是先補其虛, 而後化其傷, 則不峻矣. 荷葉中空色青, 形仰象震, 在人爲少陽膽生化之根蒂也；飲食入胃, 營氣上行, 卽少陽甲膽之氣也；胃氣元氣穀氣, 甲膽上升之氣一也；食藥感此氣化, 胃氣何由不上升乎？燒飯與白朮協力滋養穀氣, 補令胃厚, 不至再傷, 其利廣矣.」
　　·變化方：(1)本方作湯, 名「枳朮湯」, 治水飲心下堅大如盤, 邊如旋盤.

　　　　　　(2)本方加半夏一兩, 名「半夏枳朮丸」, 治脾溼停痰, 及傷冷食. 淋者加澤瀉一兩.

　　　　　　(3)本方加橘皮一兩, 名「橘皮枳朮丸」, 治飲食不消, 氣滯痞悶.

　　　　　　(4)本方加陳皮, 半夏, 名「橘半枳朮丸」, 健脾消痞化痰.

　　　　　　(5)本方加木香一兩, 名「木香枳朮丸」, 治氣滯痞滿. 再加砂仁, 名「香砂枳朮丸」, 破滯氣, 消飲食, 強脾胃. 如加乾薑五錢, 名「木香乾薑枳朮丸」, 兼治氣寒. 再加人參, 陳皮, 名「木香人參乾薑枳朮丸」, 開胃進食.

　　　　　　(6)本方加神麴, 麥芽各一兩, 名「麴蘗枳朮丸」, 治內傷飲食或泄瀉.

　　　　　　(7)本方加酒炒黃連, 黃芩, 大黃, 炒神麴, 橘紅各一兩, 名「三黃枳朮丸」, 治傷肉食溼麵辛熱味厚之物, 填塞悶亂不快.

　　　　　　(8)本方加茯苓五錢, 乾薑七錢, 名「消飲丸」, 治停飲胸滿嘔逆.
　　·來源：潔古

3. Bao He Wan. Preserve Harmony Pill from the Precious

Mirror. 保和丸

·**ACTIONS**： food damage and drink damage

·**COMPOSITION**：Chen Pi, Lian Qiao, Fu Ling, Shen Qu, Lai Fu Zi, Shan Zha, Ban Xia

·**INDICATIONS**：treats food accumulation, drink retention, abdominal pain, diarrhea, glomus and fullness, acid vomiting, accumulation and stagnation, aversion to eat, food malaria, and dysentery.

·**CHANNELS ENTERED**：The foot greater yin and yang brightness channel.

·**Analysis of Formula**：(1)① Chen Pi can descend and ascend, regulates the middle and rectifies qi.

② Enduring accumulation will be depressed and transform into heat, Lian Qiao disperses binds and clears heat.

③ Food damage tends to be combined with damp, Fu Ling supplements the spleen and drains damp.

④ Shen Qu is pungent and warm, can disperse accumulations of liquor, food, and putridity for long time.

⑤ Lai Fu Zi is pungent and sweet, descends qi and digests noodles.

⑥ Shan Zha is sour and warm and has the character of contracting. This can disperse oily food and fishes.

⑦ Mai Ya is salty and warm, disperses grain and softens hardness.

⑧ Ban Xia can warm and dry. This harmonizes the stomach and fortifies the spleen.

·**RELATED FORMULA**：(1) When Bai Zhu and Bai Shao Yao are added and Ban Xia, Lai Fu Zi, and Lian Qiao are eliminated, this is called Xiao Bao He Wan, assists the spleen to promote eating.   (2) When Bai Zhu (two liang) is added, this is called Da An Wan, or when Ren Shen is added, treats undigested food and drink, qi vacuity with mild evil.

(3) When Bai Zhu, Xiang Fu, Huang Qin, Huang Lian, Hou Po, and Zhi Shi are added, treats aggregation-accumulation, and lump gloumus.

(4) When Yue Ju Wan is combined, supports the spleen and opens depression.

3. 保和丸

·總結：傷食傷飲

·組成：陳皮, 連翹, 茯苓, 神麴, 萊服子, 山楂, 半夏

·主治：治食積飲停, 腹痛泄瀉, 痞滿吐酸, 積滯惡食, 食瘧下痢.

·歸經：足太陰, 陽明藥.

·方義：(1)①陳皮一能降能升, 調中而理氣.

②積久必鬱爲熱, 連翹散結而清熱.

③傷食必兼乎溼, 茯苓補脾而滲溼.

④神麴一辛溫蒸 之物, 能消酒食陳腐之積.

⑤菔子一辛甘下氣而製麵.

⑥山楂一酸溫收縮之性, 能消油膩腥羶之食.

⑦麥芽一鹹溫消穀而輭堅.

⑧半夏一能溫能燥, 和胃而健脾.

·變化方：(1) 本方加白朮, 白芍, 去半夏, 菔子, 連翹, 蒸餅糊丸, 名「小保和丸」, 助脾進食.

(2) 本方加白朮二兩, 名「大安丸」, 或加人參, 治飲食不消, 氣虛邪微.

(3) 本方加白朮, 香附, 黃芩, 黃連, 厚朴, 枳實, 治積聚痞塊.

(4) 本方合「越麴丸」, 扶脾開鬱.

4. Jian Pi Wan. Strengthen the Spleen Pills. 健脾丸

·**ACTIONS**：vacuous spleen and weak qi

·**COMPOSITION**：Chen Pi, Ren Shen, Bai Zhu, Shan Zha, Mai Ya, Zhi Shi

·**INDICATIONS**：treats vacuous spleen and weak qi, non-dispersion of food.

·**CHANNELS ENTERED**：The foot greater yin and yang brightness channels.

·**Analysis of Formula**：(1) The spleen and stomach hold the office of the granaries. When the stomach is vacuous, this is unable to take water and grain in, therefore there is no pleasure in eating. When the spleen is vacuous, this is unable to transform essence of water and grain, therefore there is accumulation. The reason of them is due to qi vacuity.

(2) Chen Pi disinhibits qi. Ren Shen and Bai Zhu supplement qi.

(3) When qi move, the spleen gets to be fortified and the stomac

h becomes strong.

(3) Shan Zha disperses meat type food, Mai Ya disperses grain type food. The spleen and stomach are insufficient, therefore the two herbs are used to assist them to transform food and drink.

(4) The force of Zhi Shi is harsh, this can disperse accumulation and transform glomus, and when this assists Ren Shen and Bai Zhu, the effect gets to fast but not to reach qi damage.

(5) When Spleen and Stomach get damaged, this should be treated with supplementing and boosting, when there is inability to transform food and drink, this should be treated with abductive dispersion, the combining of two methods are to fortify the spleen.

·**RELATED FORMULA**：(1) When Shan Zha and Mai Ya eliminated and Fu Ling and Gan Cao (mix fried) are added, this is called Yi Qi Jian Pi Wan, treats spleen vacuity and reduced eating.

(2) When Shan Zha, Mai Ya, and Chen Pi are eliminated and Dang Gui, Shao Yao, Chuan Xiong, Mai Men Dong, and Bai Zi Ren are added, this is called Yang Rong Jian Pi Wan, treats the insufficiency of spleen yin, food and drink which are hard to be transformed to nourish the flesh and skin.

(3) When Ren Shen, Zhi Shi, and Mai Ya are eliminated and Xiang Fu, Mu Xiang, Ban Xia, Fu Ling, Shen Qu, Huang Lian, Dang Gui, Shao Yao, and He Ye are added, this is called Li Qi Jian Pi Wan, treats the weakness of the spleen and stomach, enduring diarrhea and dysentery.

(4) When Ren Shen, Shan Zha, and Mai Ya are eliminated and Shen Qu, Chuan Xiong, and Xiang Fu are added, this is called Shu Yu Jian Pi Wan, treats the depression of spleen qi, non-dispersion of food and drink.

(5) When Shan Zha and Mai Ya are eliminated and Ban Xia, Dan Nan Xing, Ge Fen, Fu Ling, and Shen Qu are added, this is called Hua Tan Jian Pi Wan, treats internal damage with phlegm.

(6) When Ren Shen, Shan Zha, and Mai Ya are eliminated and Ban Xia, Shan Zhi Zi, and Huang Lian are added, this is called Qing Huo Jian Pi Wan, treats spleen vacuity with fire.

(7) When Ren Shen, Shan Zha, and Mai Ya are eliminated and Mu Xiang, Bing Lang, Hou Po, Ban Xia, and Gan Cao are added, this is called He Zhong Jian Pi Wan, treats stomach vacuity and no desire to eat despite hunger. Again when Ren Shen is added, this is called Miao Ying Wan, treats stomach vacuity, inability to eat, and constipation or diarrhea.

(8) When Shan Zha is eliminated and Ban Xia, Qing Pi, Mu Xiang, Sha Ren, Cao Dou Kou, Gan Jiang, Gan Cao (mix fried), Fu Ling, Zhu Ling

g, and Ze Xie are added, this is called Kuan Zhong Jin Shi Wan, supplements the spleen and stomach and promotes eating.

4. 健脾丸

　·總結：脾虛氣弱

　·組成：陳皮, 人參, 白朮, 山楂, 麥芽, 枳實

　·主治：治脾虛氣弱, 飲食不消.

　·歸經：足太陰, 陽明藥.

　·方義：(1)脾胃者倉廩之官, 胃虛則在則不能容受, 故不嗜食, 脾虛則不能運化, 故有積滯, 所以然者, 由氣虛也.

　　　　(2)陳皮利氣. 參, 朮補氣.

　　　　(3)氣運則脾健而胃強矣.

　　　　(3)山楂消肉食, 麥芽消穀食. 戊己不足, 故以二藥助之使化.

　　　　(4)枳實力猛, 能消積化痞, 佐以參, 朮, 則爲功更捷, 而又不致傷氣也.

　　　　(5)夫脾胃受傷, 則須補益, 飲食難化, 則宜消導, 合斯二者, 所以健脾也.

　·變化方：(1)本方去山楂, 麥芽, 加茯苓, 炙甘草, 名「益氣健脾丸」, 治脾虛食少.

　　　　(2)本方去山楂, 麥芽, 陳皮, 加當歸, 芍藥, 芎藭, 麥冬, 柏子仁, 名「養榮健脾丸」, 治脾陰不足, 飲食不爲肌膚.

　　　　(3)本方去人參, 枳實, 麥芽, 加香附, 木香, 半夏, 茯苓, 神麯, 黃連, 當歸, 芍藥, 荷葉燒飯丸, 名「理氣健脾丸」, 治脾胃虛弱, 久瀉久痢.

　　　　(4)本方去人參, 山楂, 麥芽, 加神麯, 川芎, 香附, 麯糊丸, 名「舒鬱健脾丸」, 治脾氣鬱滯, 飲食不消.

　　　　(5)本方去山楂, 麥芽, 加半夏, 膽星, 蛤粉, 茯苓, 神麯糊丸, 名「化痰健脾丸」, 治內傷挾痰.

　　　　(6)本方去人參, 山楂, 麥芽, 加半夏, 山梔, 黃連, 水丸, 名「清火健脾丸」, 治脾虛有火.

　　　　(7)本方去人參, 山楂, 麥芽, 加木香, 檳榔, 厚朴, 半夏, 甘草, 名「和中健脾丸」, 治胃虛飢不欲食. 再加人參, 名「妙應丸」, 治胃虛不能食, 臟腑或結或瀉.

　　　　(8)本方去山楂, 加半夏, 青皮, 木香, 砂仁, 草蔻, 乾薑, 炙甘草, 茯苓, 豬苓, 澤瀉, 蒸餅丸, 名「寬中進食丸」, 補脾胃, 進飲食.

5. Zhi Shi Xiao Pi Wan. Immature Bitter Orange Pill to Reduce Focal Distention. 枳實消痞丸

·**ACTIONS**：glomus and fullness

·**COMPOSITION**：Zhi Shi, Huang Lian, Ban Xia, Gan Jiang, Hou Po, Mai Ya, Ren Shen, Bai Zhu, Fu Ling, Gan Cao (mix fried)

·**INDICATIONS**：treats vacuous glomus below the heart, aversion to eat, fatigue, a pulse on the right bar that is string-like.

·**CHANNELS ENTERED**：The foot greater yin and yang brightness channels.

·**Analysis of Formula**：(1) Zhi Shi is bitter and sour, moves qi and breaks blood. Huang Lian is bitter and cold, drains heat and opens depression. And also this is sovereign herb of dispersing glomus.

(2) Hou Po is bitter and descends. This disperses damp and fullness, transforms food, and loosens intestines. Mai Ya is salty and warm. This assists stomach qi, softens hardness, and breaks binds. Ban Xia dries phlegm and damp and harmonizes the stomach. Gan Jiang eliminates malign blood and frees joints. The four herbs disperse and drain.

(3) Mai YA, Bai Zhu, Fu Ling, and Gan Cao are sweet and warm. They supplement the spleen. When qi is sufficient and the spleen moves, glomus spontaneously transforms. They assist the force of dispersing and draining and also secure the root in order not to damage true qi.

·**Original Source**：Li Dong Yuan

5. 枳實消痞丸

·總結：痞滿

·組成：枳實, 黃連, 半夏, 乾薑, 厚朴, 麥芽, 人參, 白朮, 茯苓, 炙甘草

·主治：治心下虛痞, 惡食懶倦, 右關脈弦.

·歸經：足太陰, 陽明藥.

·方義：(1)枳實苦酸, 行氣破血. 黃連苦寒, 瀉熱開鬱. 並消痞之君藥.

(2)厚朴苦降, 散濕滿而化食厚腸. 麥芽鹹溫, 助胃氣而輭堅破結. 半夏燥痰溼而和胃. 乾薑去惡血而通關. 皆所以散而瀉之也.

(3)麥, 朮苓, 草, 甘溫補脾, 使氣足脾運而痞自化, 既以助散瀉之力, 又以固本使不傷眞氣也.

·來源：東垣

6. Pi Qi Wan. Glomus Qi Pills. 痞氣丸

·**ACTIONS**：spleen accumulation

·**COMPOSITION**：Huang Lian, Hou Po, Sha Ren, Yin Chen, Fu Ling, Ze Xie, Gan Jiang, Rou Gui, Chuan Wu, Huang Qin, Chuan Jiao, Wu Zhu Yu, Ba Dou Shuang, Bai Zhu, Ren Shen

·**INDICATIONS**：treats spleen accumulation in the stomach duct, the size are like a plate, and which has not recovered for long time and causes loss of use of the limbs. Or jaundice, food and drink which are hard to be transformed into essence qi to nourish the flesh and skin.

·**CHANNELS ENTERED**：The foot greater yin and yang brightness channels.

·**Analysis of Formula**：(1) Huang Lian drains heat and dries damp. This treats glomus, acting as sovereign.

(2) Hou Po and Sha Ren move qi and disperse fullness.

(3) Yin Chen, Fu Ling, and Ze Xie disinhibit water to replete the spleen.

(4) Huang Qin clears the lung and nourishes yin.

(5) Chuan Jiao and Wu Zhu Yu dry the spleen and expel cold.

(6) Gan Jiang, Rou Gui, and Chuan Wu supplement life fire to engender spleen earth. And Gan Jiang and Rou Gui also can eliminate static blood and engender new blood.

(7) Ba Dou can disperse accumulation which is tangible.

(8) Ren Shen and Bai Zhu are added to supplement the original qi of the spleen, after the right qi gets exuberant, one can eliminate evil.

·**RELATED FORMULA**：(1) When Wu Zhu Yu, Bai Zhu, Fu Ling, Ze Xie, Yin Chen, Chuan Jiao, and Sha Ren are eliminated and Shi Chang Pu, Fu Shen, Dan Shen, and Hong Dou are added, this is called Fu Liang Wan, treats heart accumulation which arises from the umbilicus and reaches upward to below the heart, the size is as one of forearm, this causes vexation in the heart.

(2) When Wu Zhu Yu, Sha Ren, Rou Gui, Bai Zhu, Huang Qin, and Ze Xie are eliminated and Chai Hu, E Zhu, Zao Jiao, Kun Bu, and Gan Cao are added, this is called Fei Qi Wan, treats liver accumulation below the rib side. This has head and foot and causes persistent cough and malaria.

(3) When Wu Zhu Yu, Bai Zhu, Sha Ren, Huang Qin, Yin Chen, and Ze Xie are eliminated and Zi Wan, Jie Geng, Tian Men Dong, Bai Dou Kou, Chen Pi, Qing Pi, and San Leng are added, this is called Xi Ben Wan, treats lung accumulation below right rib side, this causes huddled aversion to cold and heat effusion, cough, panting, and lung welling abscess. In fall and winter, redu

390

ce the dose of Huang Lian.

　　(4) When Wu Zhu Yu, Bai Zhu, Sha Ren, Ren Shen, Gan Jiang, Chuan Jiao, Huang Qin, and Yin Chen are eliminated and Shi Chang Pu, Ding Xiang, Fu Zi, Ku Lian, Yan Hu Suo, Du Huo, Quan Xie are added, this is called Xi Tun Wan, treats kidney accumulation arising from lesser abdomen and reaching upward to below the heart. This feels like running piglet, there is fixed time or place when it occurs. This causes panting, cough, bone wilting, seven mounting (shan) in man, aggregation-accumulation and vaginal discharge in woman.

　　·**Original Source**：Li Dong Yuan

6. 痞氣丸

　·總結：脾積

　·組成：黃連、厚朴、砂仁、茵陳、茯苓、澤瀉、乾薑、桂、川烏、黃芩、川椒、吳茱萸、巴豆霜、白朮、人參

　·主治：治脾積在于胃脘，大如盤，久不愈，令人四肢不收，或發黃疸，飲食不爲肌膚.

　·歸經：足太陰，陽明藥也.

　·方義：(1)黃連—瀉熱燥溼，治痞君藥.

　　　　(2)厚朴，砂仁—行氣而散滿.

　　　　(3)茵陳，芩，瀉—利水以實脾.

　　　　(4)黃芩—清肺而養陰.

　　　　(5)椒，萸—燥脾而逐冷.

　　　　(6)薑，桂，川烏—補命火以生脾土；而薑，桂又能去瘀生新.

　　　　(7)巴豆—能消有形積滯.

　　　　(8)加參，朮者，以補脾元，然後可以祛邪也.

　·變化方：(1)本方除吳茱萸，白朮，茯苓，澤瀉，茵陳，川椒，砂仁，加菖蒲，茯神，丹參，紅豆，名「伏梁丸」，治心積起臍上至心下，大如臂，令人煩心.

　　　　(2)本方除吳茱萸，砂仁，桂，朮，黃芩，澤瀉，加柴胡，莪朮，皂角，昆布，甘草，名「肥氣丸」，治肝積在左脅下，有頭足，令人發咳疢瘧不已.

　　　　(3)本方除吳茱萸，白朮，砂仁，黃芩，茵陳，澤瀉，加紫菀，桔梗，天冬，白蔻，陳皮，青皮，三稜，名「息賁丸」，淡薑湯下，治肺積在右脅下，令人灑淅寒熱，咳喘發肺癰. 秋冬黃連減半.

　　　　(4)本方除吳茱萸，白朮，砂仁，人參，乾薑，川椒，黃芩，茵

391

陳, 加菖蒲, 丁香, 附子, 苦楝, 延胡索, 獨活, 全蠍, 名「賁豚丸」, 淡鹽湯下, 治腎積發于小腹上至心下, 若豚狀, 上下無時, 令人喘咳骨痿, 及男子七疝, 女子瘕聚帶下.

·來源：東垣

7. Ge Hua Jie Cheng San. Pueraria Flower Powder for Det oxification and Awakening. 葛花解醒湯

·**ACTIONS**：liquor accumulation

·**COMPOSITION**：Ge Hua, Fu Ling, Zhu Ling, Ze Xie, Sha Ren, Dou Kou, Qing Pi, Ju Hong, Mu Xiang, Gan Jiang, Ren Shen, Bai Zhu, Shen Qu

·**INDICATIONS**： mainly treats liquor accumulation, or vomiting, or diarrhea and blockage, headache, and inhibited urination.

·**CHANNELS ENTERED**：The hand and foot yang brightness.

·**Analysis of Formula**：(1) Excessive drinking, the toxin of damp-heat, accumulation in the intestines and the stomach.

(2) Ge Hua only enters yang brightness, this makes damp heat come out through the flesh. Dou Kou and Sha Ren disperse with pungent and resolve liquor, therefore act as sovereign.

Shen Qu resolves liquor and transforms food. Mu Xiang and Gan Jiang regulate qi and warm the middle. Qing Pi and Chen Pi eliminate phlegm and course stagnation. Fu Ling, Zhu Ling, and Ze Xie can expel damp heat through urine. This formula disperses heat-damp externally and internally.

(3) Overeating damages the middle qi, therefore Ren Shen and Bai Zhu are added to supplement the qi.

7. 葛花解醒湯

·總結：酒積

·組成：葛花, 茯苓, 豬苓, 澤瀉, 砂仁, 豆蔻, 青皮, 橘紅, 木香, 乾薑, 人參, 白朮, 神麴

·主治：專治酒積, 或嘔吐, 或泄瀉痞塞, 頭痛, 小便不利.

·歸經：手足陽明藥.

·方義：(1)過飲無度, 溼熱之毒積于腸胃.

(2)葛花獨入陽明, 令溼熱從肌肉而解. 豆蔻, 砂仁皆辛散解酒, 故以爲君.

神麴解酒而化食. 木香, 乾薑調氣而溫中. 青皮, 陳皮除痰

而疏滯. 二苓, 澤瀉能驅溼熱從小便出. 乃內外分消之劑.

(3)飲多則中氣傷, 故又加參, 朮以補其氣也.

8. Bie Jia Yin. Turtle Shell Drink. 鱉甲飲

·**ACTIONS**：mother of malaria (lump glomus occurring in malaria)

·**COMPOSITION**：Gan Cao, Chen Pi, Bing Lang, Hou Po, Bai Zhu, Bie Jia, Huang Qi, Chuan Xiong, Bai Shao Yao, Cao Dou Kou

·**INDICATIONS**：treats enduring malaria, and binds and lump in the abdomen, this is called mother of malaria (Nue Mu).

·**CHANNELS ENTERED**：The foot lesser yang, reverting yin, and greater yin channels. [The gall bladder, liver, and spleen]

·**Analysis of Formula**：(1) Enduring malaria is definitely due to spleen vacuity. Bai Zhu supplements spleen qi, Huang Qi supplements lung qi. When qi is sufficient and the spleen moves, accumulation is about to be dispersed.

(2) Chuan Xiong supplements the liver and move qi stagnation in the middle of blood, Shao Yao assists the spleen and disperses fire evil in the liver channel. They together harmonize the construction and qi of reverting yin. When construction and blood are regulated, yin and yang get harmonious.

(3) Bing Lang descends qi and attacks accumulation, Cao Dou Kou warms the stomach and eliminates cold, Hou Po breaks blood and disperses fullness, Chen Pi rectifies qi and disperses phlegm, Gan Cao harmonizes the middle and supplements earth.

(4) Bie Jia is salty and neutral, belongs to yin, the color is blue, enters the liver. This can boost yin, supplement vacuity, disperse heat, and dissipate binds, therefore this is sovereign medicinal to treat malaria.

·**Original Source**：Yan Shi

8. 鱉甲飲

·總結：瘧母

·組成：甘草, 陳皮, 檳榔, 厚朴, 白朮, 鱉甲, 黃耆, 芎藭, 白芍, 草蔻

·主治：治瘧久不愈, 腹中結塊, 名曰瘧母.

·歸經：足少陽, 厥陰, 太陰藥.

·方義：(1)久瘧必由脾虛, 白朮補脾氣, 黃耆補肺氣, 使氣足脾運, 方能磨積也.

393

⑵川芎補肝而行血中氣滯，芍藥助脾而散肝經火邪．二藥並和厥陰，榮氣榮血調則陰陽和矣．

　　⑶檳榔下氣而攻積，草蔻暖胃而祛寒，厚朴破血而散滿，陳皮理氣而消痰，甘草和中而補土．

　　⑷鼈甲鹹平屬陰，色青入肝，專能益陰補虛，消熱散結，故爲瘧之君藥也．

　·來源：嚴氏

Chapter 17. Contracting and Astringing Formulas. 收濇之劑

1. Chi Shi Zhi Yu Yu Liang Tang. Halloysitum and Limonite Decoction. 赤石脂禹餘糧湯

·**ACTIONS**：checks diarrhea.

·**COMPOSITION**：Chi Shi Zhi, Yu Yu Liang

·**INDICATIONS**：(1) treats that when in cold damage, a decoction medicine has been taken and there is incessant diarrhea and a hard glomus below the heart. Heart-Draining Decoction (xie xin tang) has already been taken, and then, because other medicinal are used to precipitate there is incessant diarrhea. The physician gives to rectify the center and the diarrhea increase in severity.

(2) Rectifying the center rectifies the center burner, but this diarrhea is in the lower burner, Chi Shi Zhi Yu Yu Liang Tang governs it.

(3) If the diarrhea persists, one should disinhibit the urine.

·**CHANNELS ENTERED**：The hand yang brightness channel.

·**Analysis of Formula**：The astringent can stem desertion and heaviness can reach the lower part. The astringent of Chi Shi Zhi and Yu Yu Liang check efflux desertion, the heaviness secures the lower burner, and the sweet boosts qi.

·**Original Source**：Zhong Jing

1. 赤石脂禹餘糧湯

·總結：止利

·組成：赤石脂, 禹餘糧

·主治：(1)治傷寒服湯藥下利不止, 心中痞硬, 服瀉心湯已, 復以他藥下之, 利不止, 醫以理中與之, 利益甚.

(2)理中者, 理中焦, 此利在下焦, 赤石脂禹餘糧湯主之.

(3)復利不止者, 當利其小便.

·歸經：手陽明藥.

·方義：濇可去脫, 重可達下. 石脂, 餘糧之濇以止脫, 重以固下, 甘以益氣.

·來源：仲景

2. Tao Hua Tang. Peach Blossom Decoction. 桃花湯

·**ACTIONS**：lesser yin diarrhea

·**COMPOSITION**：Chi Shi Zhi, Gan Jiang, Geng Mi

·**INDICATIONS**：treats that when in lesser yin disease that has lasted two or three days, for up to four or five days, there is abdominal pain, inhibited urination, and incessant diarrhea with pus and blood in the stool.

·**CHANNELS ENTERED**：The lesser yin channel.

·**Analysis of Formula**：Li Shi Zhen says that：

(1) Chi Shi Zhi is heavy and astringent. This enters the lower burner in blood part and stems desertion.

(2) Gan Jiang is pungent and warm. This warms the lower burner in qi part and supplements vacuity.

(3) Geng Mi is sweet and warm. This assists Chi Shi Zhi and Gan Jiang to moisten the intestines and stomach.

·**Original Source**：Zhong Jing

2. 桃花湯

·總結：少陰下利

·組成：赤石脂 乾薑 粳米

·主治：治少陰病二，三日至四五日，腹痛，小便不利，下利不止，便膿血者.

·歸經：足少陰藥

·方義：李時珍曰：

(1)赤石脂之重濇，入下焦血分而固脱.

(2)乾薑之辛溫，暖下焦氣分而補虛.

(3)粳米之甘溫，佐石脂，乾薑而潤腸胃也.

·來源：仲景

3. He Zi San. Cheubule Powder. 訶子散

·**ACTIONS**： diarrhea and prolapse of the rectum

·**COMPOSITION**： Ying Su Ke, He Zi, Gan Jiang, Ju Hong

·**INDICATIONS**：treats vacuity cold with diarrhea, non-transformation of food and drink, borborigmus, abdominal pain, prolapse of the rectum with pus and blood at any time.

·**CHANNELS ENTERED**：The hand and foot yang brightness channels.

·**Analysis of Formula**：(1) Ying Su Ke is sour, astringent, and mild cold. This secures the kidney and astringe the intestines.

(2) He Zi is sour, astringent, bitter, and warm. This contracts desertion and checks diarrhea.

(3) Gan Jiang is pungent and heat. This can expel cold and supplement yang.

(4) Chen Pi is pungent and warm. This can raise yang and regulate qi to stem qi desertion.

·**Original Source**：Li Dong Yuan

3. 訶子散
　·總結：泄瀉脫肛
　·組成：罌粟殼 訶子 乾薑 橘紅
　·主治：治虛寒泄瀉, 飲食不化, 腸鳴腹痛, 脫肛及作膿血, 日夜無度.
　·歸經：手足陽明藥
　·方義：(1)御米飲酸濇微寒, 固腎濇腸.
　　　　　(2)訶子酸濇苦溫, 收脫住瀉.
　　　　　(3)炮薑辛熱, 能逐冷補陽.
　　　　　(4)陳皮辛溫, 能升陽調氣, 以固氣脫, 亦可收形脫也.
　·來源：東垣

4. Zhen Ren Yang Zang Tang. True Man Decoction for Nourishing the Organs. 眞人養臟湯

·**ACTIONS**：diarrhea and prolapse of the rectum

·**COMPOSITION**：Ying Su Ke. He Zi. Rou Dou Kou. Mu Xiang. Rou Gui. Ren Shen. Bai Zhu. Dang Gui. Bai Shao Yao. Sheng Gan Cao

·**INDICATIONS**：(1) treats enduring diarrhea without pus and blood, vacuous cold with prolapse of the rectum.

(2) also treats dysentery with pus and blood, pain in the umbilicus and abdomen occurring at any time.

·**MODIFICATIONS**：for severe visceral cold, add Fu Zi

·**CHANNELS ENTERED**：The hand and foot yang brightness channels.

·**Analysis of Formula**：Prolapse of the rectum is due to vacuous cold, therefore this formula is used.

(1) Ren Shen, Huang Qi, and Gan Cao supplement the vacuity.

(2) Rou Gui and Rou Dou Kou eliminate the cold.

(3) Mu Xiang regulates the qi.

(4) Dang Gui moistens and harmonizes the blood.

(5) Shao Yao contracts with the sour.

(6) He Zi and Ying Su Ke check desertion with the astringent.

·another side formula：Dan Xi's Tuo Gang Fang (formula for prolapse of the rectum)：Ren Shen, Huang Qi, Dang Gui, Chuan Xiong, Sheng Ma.

·**Original Source**：Qian Fu

4. 眞人養臟湯

·總結：瀉痢脫肛

·組成：罌粟殼　訶子　肉豆蔻　木香　肉桂　人參　白术　當歸　白芍　生甘草

·主治：(1)治瀉痢日久，赤白已盡，虛寒脫肛.

　　　　(2)亦治下痢赤白，臍腹痛，日夜無度.

·加減：臟寒甚加附子

·歸經：手足陽明藥

·方義：脫肛由于虛寒，故用

　　　　(1)參，者，甘草以補其虛.

　　　　(2)肉桂，肉蔻以祛其寒.

　　　　(3)木香以調其氣.

　　　　(4)當歸潤以和血.

　　　　(5)芍藥酸以收斂.

　　　　(6)訶子，罌殼則濇以止脫也.

·附方：丹溪脫肛方：人參，黃者，當歸，川芎，升麻.

·來源：謙甫

5. Dang Gui Liu Huang Tang. Tangkuei and Six-Yellow De coction. 當歸六黃湯

·**ACTIONS**：blood sweating.

·**COMPOSITION**：Dang Gui, sheng Di Huang, Shu Di Huang, Huang Bai, Huang Lian, Huang Qin, Huang Qi

·**INDICATIONS**：treats yin vacuity with fire, night sweating, and heat ef

398

fusion.

·**CHANNELS ENTERED**：The hand lesser yin channel.

·**Analysis of Formula**：⑴ Night sweating is due to yin vacuity. Dang Gui, Shu Di Huang, and Sheng Di Huang nourish yin.

⑵ When sweating is due to fire depression, Huang Qin, Huang Bai, and Huang Lian drain fire.

⑶ When sweating is due to insecurity of the interstices, Huang Qi is doubled to secures the exterior.

5. 當歸六黃湯
　·總結：血汗
　·組成：當歸，生地黃，熟地黃，黃柏，黃連，黃芩，黃耆
　·主治：治陰虛有火，盜汗發熱.
　·歸經：手足少陰藥
　·方義：⑴盜汗由於陰虛，當歸，二地所以滋陰.
　　　　　⑵汗由火擾，黃芩，蘗，連所以瀉火.
　　　　　⑶汗由腠理不固，倍用黃耆，所以固表.

6. Mu Li San. Oyster Shell Powder. 牡蠣散

·**ACTIONS**：yang vacuity with spontaneous sweating
·**COMPOSITION**：Mu Li, Huang Qi, Ma Huang Gen, Fu Xiao Mai
·**INDICATIONS**：treats yang vacuity with spontaneous sweating.
·**CHANNELS ENTERED**：The hand greater yin and lesser yin channel.
·**Analysis of Formula**：Chen Lai Zhang：

⑴ Sweat is the humor of the heart, when there is fire in the heart, sweating is incessant. Mu Li and Fu Xiao Mai are salty and cool, they eliminate vexed heat and check sweating.

⑵ Yang is the defense of yin, when yang qi is vacuous, defense insecure. Huang Qi and Ma Huang Gen are sweet and warm. They wander the fleshy exterior and secure the defense.

6. 牡蠣散
　·總結：陽虛自汗
　·組成：牡蠣，黃耆，麻黃根，浮小麥

·主治：治陽虛自汗.

·歸經：此手太陰少陰藥

·方義：陳來章：

(1)汗爲心之液，心有火則汗不止，牡蠣，浮小麥之鹹涼，去煩熱而止汗.

(2)陽爲陰之衛，陽氣虛則衛不固，黃耆，麻黃根之甘溫，走肌表而固衛.

7. Bai Zi Ren Wan. Platycladus Seed Pills. 柏子仁丸

·ACTIONS：yin vacuity with night sweating

·COMPOSITION：Bai Zi Ren, Ren Shen, Bai Zhu, Da Zao, Ban Xia, Wu Wei Zi, Mu Li, Ma Huang Gen, Fu Xiao Mai

·INDICATIONS：treats yin vacuity with night sweating.

·CHANNELS ENTERED：The hand and foot greater yin and lesser yin channels.

·Analysis of Formula：Chen Lai Zhang says that when heart blood is vacuous, sweat issues when sleep.

(1) Bai Zi Ren is sweet, pungent, and neutral. This nourishes heart and quiets spirit, acting as sovereign.

(2) Mu Li and Fu Xiao Mai are salty and cool. They calm agitation and contract desertion, acting as minister.

(3) Wu Wei Zi contracts with sour and astringent, Ban Xia harmonizes the stomach and dries damp, acting as assistant.

(4) Ma Huang Gen only enters the fleshy exterior and conduct Ren Shen and Bai Zhu to secure defense qi, acting as courier.

7. 柏子仁丸

·總結：陰虛盜汗

·組成：柏子仁, 人參, 白朮, 大棗, 半夏, 五味子, 牡蠣, 麻黃根, 麥麩

·主治：治陰虛盜汗.

·歸經：此手足太陰少陰藥

·方義：陳來章：心血虛則睡而汗出.

(1)柏子仁之甘辛平, 養心寧神爲君.

(2)牡蠣, 麥麩之鹹涼, 靜躁收脫爲臣.

(3)五味酸歛濇收，半夏和胃燥溼爲佐.

(4)麻黄根專走肌表，引人參，白术以固衛氣爲使.

8. Fu Tu Dan. Poria and Cuscuta Elixir. 茯菟丹

·**ACTIONS**：seminal emission and white turbidity

·**COMPOSITION**：Fu Ling, Tu Si Zi, Wu Wei Zi, Shi Lian Rou, Shan Yao

·**INDICATIONS**：treats seminal emission, white turbidity, and wasting-thirst.

·**CHANNELS ENTERED**：The hand lesser yin channel.

·**Analysis of Formula**：(1) Tu Si Zi is pungent, sweet, harmonious, and neutral. This strengthens yin and boosts yang. This can treat cold semen and seminal emission.

(2) Wu Wei Zi enriches the kidney and engenders essence. Shi Lian Rou clears the heart and checks turbidity. Shan Yao fortifies the spleen and disinhibits damp. They astringe essence and secure qi.

(3) Fu Ling can free heart qi downward to the kidney, disinhibit urination without loss of qi, it is bland to drain kidney evil in the middle of supplementing the right qi.

·**Original Source**：Ju Fang

8. 茯菟丹

　·總結：遺精白濁

　·組成：茯苓，菟絲子，五味子，石蓮肉，山藥

　·主治：治遺精白濁，及强中消渴.

　·歸經：此手足少陰藥

　·方義：(1)菟絲辛甘和平，强陰益陽，能治精寒遺泄

　　　　(2)五味滋腎生精. 石蓮清心止濁. 山藥健脾利溼. 皆澀精固氣之品也.

　　　　(3)茯苓能通心氣於腎，利小便而不走氣，取其淡滲于補正中能泄腎邪也.

　·來源：局方

9. Zhi Zhuo Gu Ben Wan. Anti-Turbidity Root-Securing Pi

ll. 治濁固本丸

·ACTIONS：red and white turbidity

·**COMPOSITION**：Lian Xu, Huang Lian, Huang Bai, Yi Zhi Ren, Sha Ren, Ban Xia, Bai Fu Ling, Zhu Ling, Gan Cao

·**INDICATIONS**：treats that damp heat in the stomach which enters the bladder, causes incessant essence turbidity.

·**CHANNELS ENTERED**：The foot lesser yin, greater yang and yin channels.

·**Analysis of Formula**：(1) Essence turbidity tends to be damp-heat with phlegm.：Huang Lian drains heart fire, Huang Bai drains kidney fire, therefore they clear heat. Fu Ling and Zhu Ling disinhibit damp. Ban Xia eliminates phlegm.

(2) Damp-heat tends to be due to depression.：Sha Ren and Yi Zhi Ren are pungent and warm, they disinhibit qi, and also can secure the kidney and strengthen the spleen, therefore they are used to disperse stagnated qi, and they can restrain slightly the cold of Huang Lian and Huang Bai.

(3) Gan Cao disinhibits the middle and supplements earth.

(4) Only Lian Xu is astringent, this stems desertion.

9. 治濁固本丸

·總結：赤白濁

·組成：蓮鬚, 黃連, 黃柏, 益智仁, 縮砂仁, 半夏, 白茯苓, 豬苓, 甘草

·主治：治胃中溼熱, 滲入膀胱, 下濁不止.

·歸經：此足少陰太陽太陰藥

·方義：(1)精濁多由溼熱與痰：黃連瀉心火, 黃柏瀉腎火, 所以清熱. 二苓所以利溼. 半夏所以除痰.

(2)溼熱多由于鬱滯：砂仁, 益智辛溫利氣, 又能固腎強脾, 既以散留滯之氣, 且少濟連, 藥之寒.

(3)甘草利中而補土.

(4)惟蓮鬚之濇, 則所以固其脫也.

10. Shui Lu Er Xian Dan. Water and Earth Immortals Special Pill. 水陸二仙丹

·**ACTIONS**： essence turbidity

·**COMPOSITION**：Jin Ying Gao and Qian Shi

·**INDICATIONS**：treats seminal emission and white turbidity.

·**CHANNELS ENTERED**：The foot lesser yin channel.

·**Analysis of Formula**： The sweet of Jin Ying Gao and Qian Shi can boost essence, the moisture can nourish yin, and the astringent can check desertion.

·**Naming**： Qian Shi grows in water and Jin Ying Zi grows in mountain, therefore this is called Shui Lu Er Xian Dan (Water and Earth Immortals Special Pill).

10. 水陸二仙丹
　·總結：滑濁
　·組成：金櫻膏　芡實
　·主治：治遺精白濁.
　·歸經：此足少陰藥
　·方義：金櫻, 芡實, 甘能益精, 潤能滋陰, 澀能止脫.
　·命名：一生于水, 一生于山, 故名水陸二仙丹.

11. Jin Suo Gu Jing Wan. Golden Lock Essence-Securing Pill. 金鎖固精丸

·**ACTIONS**： seminal emission

·**COMPOSITION**：Sha Wan Ji Li, Qian Shi, Lian Xu, Long Gu, Mu Li, Lian Zi

·**INDICATIONS**：treats incessant seminal emission.

·**CHANNELS ENTERED**：The foot lesser yin channel.

·**Analysis of Formula**：(1) Ji Li supplements the kidney and boosts essence, Lian Zi makes the heart and kidney interact, Mu Li clears heat and supplements water, Qian Shi secures the kidney and supplements the spleen.

(2) The combination of Lian Xu and Long Gu astringes essence and secures to check seminal desertion.

11. 金鎖固精丸
　·總結：滑精
　·組成：沙菀蒺藜，芡實，蓮鬚，龍骨，牡蠣，蓮子
　·主治：治精滑不禁.
　·歸經：此足少陰藥
　·方義：⑴蒺藜補腎益精，蓮子交通心腎，牡蠣清熱補水，芡實固腎補
脾.

　　　　⑵合之蓮鬚，龍骨，皆濇精秘氣之品，以止滑脫也.

12. Ren Shen Chu Pi San. Gineng and Ailanthi Powder. 人 参樗皮散

·ACTIONS：visceral toxin and enduring dysentery.

·COMPOSITION：Ren Shen. Chu Gen Bai Pi

·INDICATIONS：treats visceral toxin with heat and blood, incessant end uring dysentery with pus and blood.

·CHANNELS ENTERED：The hand and foot yang brightness channel.

·Analysis of Formula：⑴ The sweet of Ren Shen supplements qi.

　　　　⑵ The bitter Chu Pi dries damp, the cold resolves heat, and the astringent contracts the desertion. This formula supplements vacuity and rises t he falling downward.

12. 人參樗皮散
　·總結：藏毒久痢
　·組成：人參　樗根白皮
　·主治：治臟毒挾熱下血，久痢膿血不止.
　·歸經：此手足陽明藥
　·方義：⑴人參之甘以補其氣，
　　　　⑵樗皮之苦以燥其溼，寒以解其熱，濇以收其脫. 使虛者補
而陷者升，亦劫劑也.

13. Sang Piao Xiao San. Mantis Egg-Case Powder. 桑螵蛸 散

·ACTIONS：frequent urination

404

·**COMPOSITION**：Sang Piao, Long Gu, Gui Ban, Dang Gui, Ren Shen, Shi Chang Pu, Fu Shen, Yuan Zhi

·**INDICATIONS**：(1) treats frequent urination and short voidings of scant urine.

(2) This formula can quiet sprite and ethereal soul, supplement heart qi, and treat forgetfulness.

·**CHANNELS ENTERED**：The foot lesser yin and the hand and foot greater yang channels.　·**Analysis of Formula**：(1) When the small intestine are vacuous, urination is frequent, therefore Sang Piao and Long Gu are used to secure it

(2) When the small intestine are heat, short voidings of scant urine occurs, therefore Dang Gui and Gui Ban are used to enrich it.

(3) Ren Shen supplements heart qi. Shi Chang Pu opens heart orifice. Fu Ling can free heart qi to kidney qi. Yuan Zhi can free kidney qi to heart qi. They can clear the heart and resolve heat.

The heart is connected with the small intestine, when the heart is supplemented, the small intestine is not vacuous, when the heart is cleared, the small intestine is not heat.

·**Original Source**：Kou Shi

13. 桑螵蛸散
　·總結：便數
　·組成：桑螵蛸，龍骨，龜板，當歸，人參，石菖蒲，茯神，遠志
　·主治：(1)治小便數而欠.

(2)能安神魂，補心氣，療健忘.
　·歸經：此足少陰手足太陽藥
　·方義：(1)虛則便數，故以螵蛸，龍骨固之.

(2)熱則便欠，故以當歸，龜板滋之.

(3)人參補心氣；菖蒲開心竅；茯苓能通心氣于腎；遠志能通腎氣于氣；並能清心解熱.

心者小腸之合也，心補則小腸不虛，心清則小腸不熱也.
　·來源：寇氏

Chapter 18. Worms-Killing Formulas. 殺蟲之劑

1. Wu Mei Wan. Mume Pills. 烏梅丸

·**ACTIONS**： roundworm reversal.

·**COMPOSITION**：Wu Mei, Xi Xin, Gui Zhi, Ren Shen, Fu Zi, Huang Bai, Huang Lian, Gan Jiang, Chuan Jiao, Dang Gui

·**INDICATIONS**：(1) treats that when in cold damage reverting yin pattern, there is cold reversal and vomiting of roundworm.

(2) also treats cough originated from the stomach, cough with retching, and longworm coming out when retching is severe.

(3) also treats enduring dysentery.

·**CHANNELS ENTERED**：The foot yang brightness and reverting yin channel.

·**Analysis of Formula**：(1) When roundworm is supplied with sour, this hides, therefore Wu Mei is used to make worm hide.

(2) When roundworm is supplied with bitter, this gets quiet, therefore Huang Lian and Huang Bia are used to quiet this.

(3) Roundworm gets stirred due to cold, therefore Gui Zhi and Fu Zi, Gan Jiang, and Chuan Jiao warm the viscera. And Xi Xin and Dang Gui moisten the Liver and Kidney.

(4) Ren Shen is used to assist the spleen. Wu Mei restrains the lung.

·**Original Source**：Zhong Jing

1. 烏梅丸

·總結：蚘厥

·組成：烏梅, 細辛, 桂枝, 人參, 附子, 黃柏, 黃連, 乾薑, 川椒, 當歸

·主治：(1)治傷寒厥陰證, 寒厥吐蚘.

(2)亦治胃腑發欬, 欬而嘔, 嘔甚則長蟲出.

(3)亦主久痢.

·歸經：此足陽明厥陰藥

·方義：(1)蚘得酸則伏, 故以烏梅之酸伏之.

(2)蚘得苦則安, 故以連, 藥之苦安之.

(3)蚘因寒而動，故以桂，附，薑，椒溫其中臟. 而以細辛，當歸潤其肝腎.

(4)人參用以助脾. 烏梅兼以歛肺.

·煎服法：苦酒浸烏梅一宿，去核，蒸熟和藥蜜丸.

·來源：仲景

2. Ji Xiao Wan. Effective Congregation Pill. 集效丸

·**ACTIONS**：worm pain.

·**COMPOSITION**：Da Huang, He Shi, Bing Lang, He Zi Pi, Yi Ti, Mu Xiang, Gan Jiang, Fu Zi

·**INDICATIONS**：treats abdominal pain due to worm biting the bowels, the pain is intermittent.

·**CHANNELS ENTERED**：The hand and foot yang brightness channels.

·**Analysis of Formula**：roundworm likes warmth, dislike sour, and is fear of bitter, therefore the heat of Gan Jiang and Fu Zi is used to warm it. The sour of Wu Mei and He Zi Pi is used to make it hide. The bitter of Da Huang, Bing Lang, Yi Ti, and He Shi is used to kill it. The pungent and warm of Mu Xiang normalize qi.

·**Original Source**：San Yin Fang

2. 集效丸

·總結：蟲痛

·組成：大黃，鶴蝨，檳榔，訶子皮，蕪荑，木香，乾薑，附子

·主治：治蟲嚙腹痛，作止有時，或耕起來往.

·歸經：此手足陽明藥

·方義：蟲喜溫惡酸而畏苦，故用薑，附之熱以溫之；烏梅，訶皮之酸以伏之；大黃，檳榔，蕪荑，鶴蝨之苦以殺之；木香辛溫，以順其氣也.

·來源：三因

3. Xiong Bing Wan. Realgar and Arecae Pills. 雄檳丸

·**ACTIONS**：worm pain

·**COMPOSITION**：Xiong Huang, Bing Lang, Bai Fan

·**INDICATIONS**：treats abdominal pain in the stomach, the pain is periodic without vomiting and diarrhea.

407

·**CHANNELS ENTERED**：The hand and foot yang brightness channel.

·**Analysis of Formula**：Xiong Huang is pungent and toxin, Bing Lang is bitter and tends to descend, bai fan is sour and astringent, all of them kill worm, therefore they are used together.

3. 雄檳丸
　·總結：蟲痛
　·組成：雄黃, 檳榔, 白礬
　·主治：治腹痛胃痛, 乾痛有時.
　·歸經：此手足陽明藥
　·方義：雄黃之辛毒, 檳榔之苦降, 白礬之酸澀, 皆殺蟲之品也, 故合用以治之.

4. Hua Chong Wan. Worm Transforming Pill. 化蟲丸

·**ACTIONS**：　all kinds of roundworms in the stomach duct.

·**COMPOSITION**：He Shi, Hu Fen, Ku Lian Gen, Bing Lang, Yi Ti, Shi Jun Zi, Ku Fan.

·**INDICATIONS**：treats a disease caused by all kinds of worm in the sto mach duct.

·**CHANNELS ENTERED**：The hand and foot yang brightness channels.

4. 化蟲丸
　·總結：腸胃諸蟲
　·組成：鶴蝨, 胡粉, 苦楝根, 檳榔, 蕪荑, 使君子, 枯礬
　·主治：治腸胃諸蟲爲患.
　·歸經：此手足陽明藥

5. Shi Jun Zi Wan. Quisqualis Pill. 使君子丸

·**ACTIONS**：worm accumulation

·**COMPOSITION**：Shi Jun Zi, Nan Xing, Bing Lang

·**INDICATIONS**：treats gu distention and abdominal pain, food taxation, jaundice, and predilection for strange food as herb leaf, raw grain, charcoal, an d earth.

·**CHANNELS ENTERED**：The hand and foot yang brightness channels.

·**Analysis of Formula**：Shi Jun Zi is sweet, Nan Xing is toxin, and Bing Lang is bitter, they can kill worms. They are used in stir-bake, because worm likes that.

5. 使君子丸
    ·總結：蟲積
    ·組成：使君子, 南星, 檳榔
    ·主治：治蟲脹腹痛, 及食勞發黃, 喜食茶米炭土等物.
    ·歸經：此手足陽明藥
    ·方義：使君子之甘, 南星之毒, 檳榔之苦, 皆能殺蟲.炒以諸物, 因其所嗜.

6. Ta Gan Wan. Otter's liver Pills. 獺肝丸

·**ACTIONS**：corpse transmission consumption

·**COMPOSITION**： Otter's liver

·**INDICATIONS**：treats demonic influx, corpse transmission consumption.

·**CHANNELS ENTERED**：The three yin channels.

·**Analysis of Formula**：Wu He Gao says that otter's liver treats demonic influx, why doses it treate that? If person is fear of people and tends to hide, and hide in day and come out at night, this is related with yin character, therefore otter's liver is used to treat yin disease. Here only the liver is used, the liver is related with reverting yin and stores ethereal soul.

·**Original Source**：Zhou Hou Fang

6. 獺肝丸
    ·總結：傳尸勞蟲
    ·組成：獺肝
    ·主治：治鬼疰傳尸勞瘵.
    ·歸經：此三陰藥
    ·方義：吳鶴皋曰：獺肝治鬼疰, 此何以故?凡物惡人而僻處, 晝伏而夜出者, 皆陰類也, 故假之以治陰疾. 獨用其肝者, 肝爲厥陰, 藏魂之臟也.
    ·來源：肘後

7. Xiao Ke and Sha Chong Fang. Wasting-Thirst and Killing Worm Formula. 殺蟲方

·**ACTIONS**：wasting-thirst with roundworm.

·**COMPOSITION**：Ku Lian Gen

·**INDICATIONS**：treats wasting-thirst with roundworm.

·**CHANNELS ENTERED**：The hand and foot yang brightness channels.

·**Analysis of Formula**：When in one pattern of wasting thirst if there is roundworm, this condition consumes essence and humor.

7. 消渴殺蟲方

　·總結：消渴有蟲

　·組成：苦楝根

　·主治：治消渴有蟲.

　·歸經：此陽明藥

　·方義：消渴一證, 有蟲耗其精液而成者.

Chapter 19. The Eyes Brightening Formulas. 明目之劑

1. Zi Yin Di Huang Wan. Rehmannia Pills to Nourish Yin. 滋陰地黃丸

·**ACTIONS**：nourishes yin and raises yang

·**COMPOSITION**：Shu Di Huang, Sheng Di Huang, Chai Hu, Huang Qin, Dang Gui, Tian Men Dong, Di Gu Pi, Wu Wei Zi, Huang Lian, Ren Shen, Gan Cao, Zhi Ke

·**INDICATIONS**：treats weak blood and vacuous qi, inability to nourish the heart, the effulgent exuberance of the heart fire, spontaneous repletion of liver fire, dilated pupils, and unclear vision.

·**CHANNELS ENTERED**：The hand and foot lesser yin and the foot reverting yin and lesser yang channels. [The heart, kidney, liver, and gall bladder]

·**Analysis of Formula**：(1) Shu Di Huang and Dang Gui tonify blood.

(2) Sheng Di Huang and Di Gu Pi cool blood.

(3) Huang Qin drains lung fire.

(4) Huang Lian drains liver fire.

(5) Tian Men Dong clears the lung and enriches the kidney.

(6) Chai Hu disperses the liver and raises yang.

(7) Wu Wei Zi contracts consumption and restrains disperses.

(8) Ren Shen and Gan Cao boost qi and supplement the middle.

(9) Zhi Ke disinhibits qi to move stagnation.

·**Original Source**：Li Dong Yuan

1. 滋陰地黃丸

·總結：滋陰升陽

·組成：熟地黃, 生地黃, 柴胡, 黃芩, 當歸, 天門冬, 地骨皮, 五味子, 黃連, 人參, 甘草, 枳殼

·主治：治血弱氣虛, 不能養心, 心火旺盛, 肝木自實, 瞳子散大, 視物不清.

·歸經：此手足少陰藥足厥陰少陽藥

·方義：(1)熟地, 當歸養血.

411

(2)生地, 地骨涼血.

(3)黃芩瀉肺火.

(4)黃連瀉肝火.

(5)天冬清肺而滋腎.

(6)柴胡散肝而升陽.

(7)五味收耗而斂散.

(8)人參, 甘草以益氣補中.

(9)枳殼以利氣行滯也.

·來源：東垣

2. Jia Jian Zhu Jing Wan. Modified Long Vistas Pills. 加減 駐景丸

·**ACTIONS**：supplements the live and kidney.

·**COMPOSITION**：Gou Qi Zi, Wu Wei Zi, Che Qian Zi, Chu Shi, Chuan Jiao, Shu Di Huang, Dang Gui, Tu Si Zi

·**INDICATIONS**：treats qi vacuity of the liver and kidney, blurred and dark eyes.   ·**MODIFICATIONS**：When Dang Gui, Wu Wei Zi, Chu Shi, and Chuan Jiao are eliminated, this is called Zhu Jing Wan, treats same things..

·**CHANNELS ENTERED**：The foot lesser yin and reverting yin.

·**Analysis of Formula**：(1) Shu Di Huang and Gou Qi supplement the liver and enrich the kidney.

(2) Tu Si Zi and Chu Shi boost essence and strengthen yin.

(3) Wu Wei Zi restrains consumption and assists metal water.

(4) Dang Gui harmonizes qi and blood and boosts the liver and spleen.

(5) Chuan Jiao supplements fire to expel the vacuous cold of the lower burner.

(6) Che Qian Zi disinhibits water and drains the evil heat of the liver and kidney.

·**Original Source**：Yi Jian

2. 加減駐景丸

·總結：補肝腎

·組成：枸杞子, 五味子, 車前子, 楮實, 川椒, 熟地黃, 當歸, 菟絲子

·主治：治肝腎氣虛, 兩目昏暗.
·加減：本方除當歸, 五味, 楮實, 川椒, 名駐景丸, 治同.
·歸經：此足少陰厥陰藥
·方義：(1)熟地, 枸杞補肝滋腎.
　　　　(2)菟絲, 楮實益精強陰.
　　　　(3)五味斂耗散而助金水.
　　　　(4)當歸和氣血而益肝脾.
　　　　(5)川椒補火, 以逐下焦虛寒.
　　　　(6)車前利水而瀉肝腎邪熱也.
·來源：易簡

3. Ding Zhi Wan. Mind-Stabilizing Pill. 定志丸

·**ACTIONS**： inability to see from far away

·**COMPOSITION**：Yuan Zhi, Shi Chang Pu, Ren Shen, Fu Ling

·**INDICATIONS**：(1) treats that one cannot see from far away but can see from near.

(2) Taking this formula from time to time boosts heart and strengthens mind. This can treat forgetfulness.

·**CHANNELS ENTERED**：The hand lesser yin channel. [The heart]

·**Analysis of Formula**：(1) Ren Shen supplements heart qi.

(2) Shi Chang Pu opens orifices of the heart.

(3) Fu Ling can make heart qi interact with the kidney.

(4) Yuan Zhi can free kidney qi to the heart.

(5) The color of Zhu Sha is red, this clears the liver and settles the heart.

·Another Side Formula：Zhang Zi He eliminates Shi Chang Pu and add Fu Shen, Bai Zi Ren, and Suan Zao Ren, this is also called Ding Zhi Wan. This stabilizes ethereal soul and calms fright.

·**Original Source**：Ju Fang

3. 定志丸
　·總結：不能遠視
　·組成：遠志, 石菖蒲, 人參, 茯苓
　·主治：(1)治目不能遠視, 而能近視者.

413

(2)常服益心強志，能療健忘．

·歸經：此手少陰藥

·方義：(1)人參補心氣．

(2)菖蒲開心竅．

(3)茯苓能交心氣于腎．

(4)遠志能通腎氣于心．

(5)硃砂色赤，清肝鎮心．

·又附方：張子和方無菖蒲，加茯神，柏子仁，酸棗仁，亦名定志丸，酒糊丸，薑湯下．定魂定驚．

·來源：局方

4. Di Zhi Wan. Rehmannia Root Pill. 地芝丸

·**ACTIONS**：inability to see from near.

·**COMPOSITION**：Sheng Di Huang, Tian Men Dong, Zhi Ke, Gan Ju Hua

·**INDICATIONS**：treats that one cannot see from near but can see from far away..

·**CHANNELS ENTERED**：The foot lesser yin channel [kidney]

·**Analysis of Formula**：(1) Sheng Di Huang cools blood and engenders blood.

(2) Tian Men Dong moistens the lung and enriches the kidney.

(3) Zhi Ke soothes intestines and eliminates stagnation.

(4) Ju Hua descends fire and eliminates wind.

·**Original Source**：Li Dong Yuan

4. 地芝丸

·總結：不能近視

·組成：生地黃，天冬，枳殼，甘菊花

·主治：治目能遠視，不能近視．

·歸經：此足少陰藥

·方義：(1)生地涼血生血．

(2)天冬潤肺滋腎．

(3)枳殼寬腸去滯．

(4)甘菊降火除風．

414

·來源：東垣

5. Ren Shen Yi Wei Tang. Stomach Boosting Decoction wit h Ginseng. 人參益胃湯

·**ACTIONS**：cataract

·**COMPOSITION**：Huang Qi, Ren Shen, Gan Cao, Bai Shao Yao, Huan g Bai, Man Jing Zi

·**INDICATIONS**：treats taxation, dietary irregularities, cataract, and eye disease.

·**CHANNELS ENTERED**：The foot greater yin and yang brightness. [T he spleen and stomach]

·**Analysis of Formula**：(1) Ren Shen, Huang Qi, and Gan Cao greatly sup plement the middle qi to strengthen the spleen and stomach.

(2) Man Jing Zi raises and clears yang and frees nine orifices.

(3) Bai Shao Yao enters reverting yin and harmonizes constructi on and blood.

(4) Huang Bai eliminates damp heat and enriches kidney water.

When essence qi is sufficient and clear yang raises, the viscera and bowels are harmonious and eye screen retreats.

·**RELATED FORMULA**：When Sheng Ma and Ge Gen are added, this i s called Yi Qi Cong Ming Tang.

5. 人參益胃湯

·總結：內障

·組成：黃耆, 人參, 甘草, 白芍藥, 黃柏, 蔓荊子

·主治：治勞役飲食不節, 內障目病.

·歸經：此足太陰陽明藥

·方義：(1)參, 耆, 甘草大補中氣, 以強脾胃.

(2)蔓荊升清陽而通九竅.

(3)白芍入厥陰而和榮血.

(4)黃柏除溼熱, 而滋腎水.

使精氣足而清陽升, 則臟腑和而障翳退矣.

·變化方：本方加升麻, 葛根, ...名益氣聰明湯

6. Xiao Feng Yang Xue Tang. Wind Dispersing Blood Nourishing Decoction. 消風養血湯

·**ACTIONS**：yang pattern with reddish swelling

·**COMPOSITION**：Jing Jie, Man Jing Zi, Ju Hua, Bai Zhi, Ma Huang, Fang Feng, Tao Ren, Hong Hua, Chuan Xiong, Dang Gui, Bai Shao Yao, Cao Jue Ming, Shi Jue Ming, Gan Cao

·**INDICATIONS**：treats sore red swollen eyes.

·**CHANNELS ENTERED**：The foot greater yang and reverting yin channels. [The bladder and liver]

·**Analysis of Formula**：(1) Jing Jie, Fang Feng, Ma Huang, Bai Zhi, Ju Hua, and Man Jing Zi are light, floating, and tend to ascend upward. They can disperse wind and dissipate heat

(2) Tao Ren, Hong Hua, Chuan Xiong, Dang Gui, and Shao yao disperse with pungent and contract with sour. They can tonify blood and eliminate stasis.

(3) Cao Jue Ming and Shi Jue Ming eliminate wind heat in the liver channel. They only treat eye disease.

(4) When stasis is eliminated and blood is activate, swelling gets dispersed. When wind is dispersed and heat is eliminated, pain gets to allay. And the eyes are the orifices of the liver. Tracking down wind and tonifying blood are to harmonize the liver.

(5) Gan Cao is added to moderate the liver and relieve pain.

6. 消風養血湯
　·總結：陽證赤腫
　·組成：荊芥, 蔓荊子, 菊花, 白芷, 麻黄, 防風, 桃仁, 紅花, 川芎, 當歸, 白芍, 草決明, 石決明, 甘草
　·主治：治目赤腫痛.
　·歸經：此足太陽藥厥陰藥
　·方義：(1)荊芥, 防風, 麻黄, 白芷, 甘菊, 蔓荊, 輕浮上升, 並能消風散熱
　　　　(2)桃仁, 紅花, 川芎, 歸, 芍, 辛散酸收, 並能養血去瘀.
　　　　(3)兩決明皆除肝經風熱, 專治目疾.
　　　　(4)瘀去血活則腫消, 風散熱除則痛止. 又目爲肝竅, 搜風養血, 皆以和肝.
　　　　(5)加甘草者, 亦以緩肝而止痛也.

7. Xi Gan San. Wash the Liver Powder. 洗肝散

·**ACTIONS**：wind toxin with red swelling

·**COMPOSITION**：Bo He, Qiang Huo, Fang Feng, Dang Gui, Chuan Xi ong, Da Huang, Zhi Zi, Gan Cao (mix fried)

·**INDICATIONS**：treats wind-toxin attacking upward, sudden red swelling, eye pain with difficulty to open, and copious eye discharge.

·**CHANNELS ENTERED**：The foot reverting yin and yang brightness. [The liver and stomach]

·**Analysis of Formula**：The liver belongs to wood and controls eyes. Wood has a desire to freely growing [likes to outthrust].

(1) Wind heat are depressed in the interior, therefore Bo He, Qiang Huo, and Fang Feng raise and disperses wind heat.

(2) The liver stores blood, therefore Dang Gui and Chuan Xiong are used to harmonize and nourish blood.

(3) Da Huang drains stomach fire and frees constipation.

(4) Zhi Zi descends heart fire and disinhibits urination.

(5) Gan Cao moderates liver qi and harmonizes the middle.

·**Original Source**：Ju Fang

7. 洗肝散
  ·總結：風毒赤腫
  ·組成：薄荷，羌活，防風，當歸，川芎，大黃，栀子，炙甘草
  ·主治：治風毒上攻，暴作赤腫，目痛難開，隱澀眵淚.
  ·歸經：此足厥陰陽明藥
  ·方義：肝屬木而主目，木喜條達，
        (1)風熱鬱于內，故用薄荷，羌，防，以升之散之.
        (2)肝藏血，故用當歸，川芎以和之養之.
        (3)大黃瀉胃火而通燥結.
        (4)栀子降心火而利小便.
        (5)甘草緩肝氣而和中州.
  ·來源：局方

8. Bu Gan San. Liver Supplementing Powder. 補肝散

·**ACTIONS**： liver vacuity with eye pain

417

·**COMPOSITION**：Xia Ku Cao, Xiang Fu

·**INDICATIONS**：(1) treats liver vacuity with eye pain, pain in the sinews and vessels, incessant cold eye discharge, photophobia, and fear of light.

(2) At night the pain gets severe, dripping of some medicinal with bitter and cold into eyes makes the pain worse..

·**CHANNELS ENTERED**：The foot reverting yin. [The liver]

·**Analysis of Formula**：(1) When Xia Ku Cao meets the summer solstice when yin begins to grow, this gets desiccated. This which supplied with pure yang qi, has an effect to supplement and nourish the blood and vessels of reverting yin. The pain gets severe at night so medicinal with bitter and cold are dripped into eyes, but the pain gets more severe, both night and cold are related with yin, Xia Ku Cao treats this, yang overcomes yin.

(2) Xiang Fu moves qi and disperses the liver, harmonizes the middle and resolves depression, pushes old and pulls new, therefore this is used as assistant.

·**Original Source**：Ju Fang

8. 補肝散
　·總結：肝虛目痛
　·組成：夏枯草, 香附
　·主治：(1)治肝虛目痛, 筋脈疼痛, 冷淚不止, 羞明怕日.
　　　　　(2)及夜則痛甚, 點苦寒之藥反劇.
　·歸經：此足厥陰藥
　·方義：(1)夏苦草遇夏至陰生則枯, 蓋稟純陽之氣, 有補養厥陰血脈之功. 夜痛及用苦寒藥反甚者, 夜與寒皆陰也, 夏枯草能治之者, 陽勝陰也.
　　　　　(2)香附行氣散肝, 和中解鬱, 推陳致新, 故用以爲佐.
　·來源：局方

9. Bo Yun Tui Yi Tang. Clearing-Cloud Eliminating-Eye screens Pills. 撥雲退翳丸

·**ACTIONS**：eye screens with wind heat

·**COMPOSITION**：Dang Gui, Chuan Xiong, Di Gu Pi, Bai Ji Li, Mi Meng Hua, Gan Ju Hua, Qiang Huo, Jing Jie, Mu Zei, Tian Hua Fen, Man Jing Zi, Bo He, Zhi Shi, Gan Cao, Chuan Jiao, Huang Lian, Chan Tui, Chan Tui

·**INDICATIONS**：treats eye screens with wind heat.

·**CHANNELS ENTERED**：The foot greater yang and reverting yin chan
nels. [The bladder and liver]

·**Analysis of Formula**：(1) Qiang Huo, Jing Jie, Man Jing Zi, and Bo He r
aises yang and disperse wind.

(2) Dang Gui and Chuan Xiong harmonize the liver and tonify bl
ood.

(3) Huang Lian, Di Gu Pi, and Tian Hua Fen clear fire heat.

(4) Zhi Shi break stagnated qi.

(5) Chuan Jiao warms the lower burner.

(6) Mu Zei and Chan Tui eliminate eye screens.

(7) Mi Meng Hua, Ji Li, and Ju Hua moisten the liver and supple
ment the kidney, drain fire and clear metal.

(8) Gan Cao supplements the middle to harmonize every channel.

·**Original Source**：Liu Chang Shi

9. 撥雲退翳丸
·總結：風熱障翳
·組成：當歸，川芎，地骨皮，白蒺藜，密蒙花，甘菊花，羌活，荊芥，
木賊，天花粉，蔓荊子，薄荷，枳實，甘草，川椒，黃連，蛇蛻，蟬蛻
·主治：治風熱障翳.
·歸經：此足太陽厥陰藥
·方義：(1)羌活，荊芥，蔓荊，薄荷，以升陽散風.
(2)當歸，川芎，以和肝養血.
(3)黃連，地骨，花粉，清火熱.
(4)枳實破滯氣.
(5)川椒溫下焦.
(6)木賊，蛇蛻，蟬蛻，以退翳.
(7)密蒙，蒺藜，甘菊，目家專藥，以潤肝補腎，瀉火清金.
(8)炙草補中以和諸藥也.
·來源：劉昌世

10. Shi Gao Qiang Huo San. Gypsum and Notopterygium P owder. 石膏羌活散

·**ACTIONS**：all kinds of eye disease

419

·**COMPOSITION**：Qiang Huo, Jing Jie, Bai Zhi, Gao Ben, Xi Xin, Chuan Xiong, Cang Zhu, Ju Hua, Mi Meng Hua, Bai Jie Zi, Ma Zi Ren, Mu Zei, Huang Qin, Shi Gao, Gan Cao

·**INDICATIONS**：treats dim vision of both eyes for long time, qi [vision] obstruction which is caused by internal and external damage, clouding due to wind heat, trichiasis, all kinds of eye disease.

·**CHANNELS ENTERED**：The foot greater yang, yang brightness, and reverting yin channels. [the bladder, stomach, and liver]

·**Analysis of Formula**：：⑴ Qiang Huo treats brain heat and head wind.

⑵ Gao Ben treats unbiased and hemilateral headache.

⑶ Bai Zhi clears head and eyes.

⑷ Chuan Xiong treats head wind.

⑸ Jing Jie treats sore in the eye.

⑹ Mi Meng Hua treats photophobia and fear of light.

⑺ Cang Zhu improves vision and warms water viscera.

⑻ Mu Zei eliminates sun screens. .

⑼ Ma Zi Ren makes curled eyebrows to be straightened.

⑽ Xi Xin and Bai Jie Zi raise up eyebrows which grows inward.

⑾ Huang Qin and Shi Gao clear the heart and abate heat.

⑿ Ju Hua descends fire and eliminates wind.

⒀ Gan Cao regulates and harmonizes every herbs.

·**Original Source**：Xuan Ming

10. 石膏羌活散
·總結：一切目疾
·組成：羌活, 荊芥, 白芷, 薰本, 細辛, 川芎, 蒼朮, 甘菊, 密蒙花, 白芥子, 麻子, 木賊, 黃芩, 石膏, 甘草
·主治：治久患雙目不明, 遠年近日, 內外氣障風昏, 拳毛倒睫, 一切目疾.
·歸經：此足太陽陽明厥陰藥
·方義：原文曰：⑴羌活治腦熱頭風.
⑵薰本治正偏頭痛.
⑶白芷清頭目.
⑷川芎療頭風.
⑸荊芥治目中生瘡.

420

(6)密蒙治羞明怕日.

(7)蒼朮明目暖水臟.

(8)木賊退障翳.

(9)麻子起拳毛.

(10)細辛, 菜子起倒睫.

(11)黃芩, 石膏洗心退熱.

(12)甘菊降火除風.

(13)甘草調和諸藥.

·來源：宣明

11. Fang Feng Yin Zi. Ledebouriella beverage. 防風飲子

·**ACTIONS**：trichiasis

·**COMPOSITION**：Huang Lian, Gan Cao, Ren Shen, Dang Gui, Ge Gen, Fang Feng, Xi Xin, Man Jing Zi.

·**INDICATIONS**：treats trichiasis

·**CHANNELS ENTERED**：The foot greater yin and yang brightness channel. [The spleen and stomach]

·**Analysis of Formula**：(1) Ren Shen and Gan Cao supplement qi.

(2) Dang Gui moistens blood.

(3) Huang Lian clears fire.

(4) Fang Feng and Ge Gen disperse wind heat.

(5) Xi Xin enter the lesser yin and moistens the kidney.

(6) Man Jing Zi runs to the head and face and raises yang.

·**RELATED FORMULA**：When Ren Shen, Dang Gui, and Huang Lian are eliminated and Huang Qi are added, this is called Shen Xiao Ming Mu Tang, treats the above pattern with marginal blepharitis, pain, incessant cold tear, and copious eye discharge.

11. 防風飲子

·總結：到睫拳毛

·組成：黃連 甘草 人參 當歸 葛根 防風 細辛 蔓荊子

·主治：治倒睫拳毛.

·歸經：此足太陰陽明藥

·方義：(1)參, 甘以補其氣.

421

(2)歸身以濡其血.

(3)黃連以清其火.

(4)防，葛以散風熱.

(5)細辛入少陰而潤腎.

(6)蔓荊走頭面而升陽.

·變化方：本方除人參，當歸黃連，加黃者…名神效明目湯，治前證兼赤爛昏痛，冷淚多眵.

12. Yang Gan Wan. Goat's Liver Pills. 羊肝丸

·**ACTIONS**：cataract

·**COMPOSITION**：Mu Zei, Ye Ming Sha, Chan Tui, Goat's Liver, Dang Gui

·**INDICATIONS**：treats eye disease and cataract.

·**CHANNELS ENTERED**：The foot reverting yin channel. [The liver].

·**Analysis of Formula**：(1) Mu Zei is light and is good at numbness, there fore this can pacify the liver, disperse heat, and eliminate eye screens.

(2) Chan Tui eats blood of worms, Ye Ming Sha has striped pattern eyes, therefore they can disperse malign blood in the eyes and improve vision.

(3) Chan Tui is good at casting the skin, therefore it can eliminate eye screens.

(4) Goat's Liver is used. The character of goat is related with fire, this can supplement qi and blood, and conduct every medicinal to enter the liver.

(5) Dang Gui can enter reverting yin, tonifies blood and harmonizes the liver.

·**Original Source**：Lei Yuan

12. 羊肝丸

·總結：內障

·組成：木賊，夜明砂，蟬蛻，羊肝，當歸

·主治：治目疾內障.

·歸經：此足厥陰藥也(肝).

·方義：(1)木賊：輕揚而善磨木，故能平肝散熱而去障.

(2)蚊食血之蟲，夜明砂皆蚊眼也，故能散目中惡血而明目.

(3)蟬性善蛻，故能退翳.

(4)用羊肝者，羊性屬火，取其氣血之屬，能補氣血，引諸藥
入肝以成功也.

(5)當歸能入厥陰，養血而和肝.

·來源：類苑

13. Tu Shi Tang. Hare's Droppings Decoction. 兔矢湯

·**ACTIONS**：sores and rashes entering the eyes.

·**COMPOSITION**： Hare's droppings.

·**INDICATIONS**：treats sores and rashes entering the eyes, dim vision, and eye screens.

·**CHANNELS ENTERED**：The foot reverting yin and yang brightness channels [the liver and stomach]

·**Analysis of Formula**：Hare is a spirit of bright moon, is supplied with metal qi, this droppings are called Ming Yue Sha, this can resolve toxin and kill worms, therefore this can improve vision, and also can treats taxation Gan.

13. 兔矢湯

·總結：瘡疹入眼

·組成：兔矢.

·主治：治瘡疹入眼，及昏暗障翳.

·歸經：此足厥陰陽明藥也(肝胃).

·方義：兔者明月之精，得金之氣，其矢名明月砂，能解毒殺蟲，故專
能明目，又可兼治勞疳也.

14. Er Bai Wei Cao Hua Gao. Two Hundreds Flavors of Leaf and Flower Paste. 二百味草花膏

·**ACTIONS**：red eye with pain and tear.

·**COMPOSITION**：Honey, wether's gall bladder

·**INDICATIONS**：treats red eye with tear, or pain or itch, inability to see at day, aversion to brightness at night.

·**CHANNELS ENTERED**：The foot lesser yang and reverting yin channels. [The liver and gall bladder]

·**Analysis of Formula**：(1) Wether's gall bladder is bitter and cold, boosts gall bladder and drains heat.

(2) Honey is sweet and moisture, supplements the middle and moderates the liver.

·**Original Source**：Zhao Qian

14. 二百味草花膏
   ·總結：赤痛流淚
   ·組成：蜂蜜, 羯羊膽
   ·主治：治目赤流淚, 或痛或癢, 晝不能視, 夜惡燈光.
   ·歸經：此足少陽厥陰藥也.
   ·方義：(1)羊膽苦寒, 益膽瀉熱.
           (2)蜂蜜甘潤, 補中緩肝.
   ·來源：趙謙

15. Dian An Fang. Eye Dropping Formula. 點眼方

·**ACTIONS**：yang pattern with eye disease.
·**COMPOSITION**：Huang Lian, breast milk (Ren Ni).
·**INDICATIONS**：treats one hundred disease in the eyes.
·**CHANNELS ENTERED**：The foot reverting yin channel. [The liver]
·**Analysis of Formula**：(1) Ben Cao Yan Yi says that in human, the heart governs blood, the liver stores blood, when eyes are supplied with blood, eyes can see. Generally water enters the channels and then the water transforms into blood.

(2) also says that blood in the upper part engenders breast milk and in the lower part menstruation, therefore one knows that breast milk is made from blood.

(3) Huang Lian is added to clear the fire of the heart and liver.
·**Original Source**：Dan Xi

15. 點眼方
   ·總結：陽證目疾
   ·組成：黃連, 人乳
   ·主治：治目中百病.
   ·歸經：此足厥陰藥也.

·方義：(1)衍義曰：「人心主血，肝藏血，目受血而能視，蓋水入于經，其血乃成.」

(2)又曰：「上則爲乳汁，下則爲月水，故知乳汁卽血也，用以點目，豈有不相宜者哉.」

(3)昂按：加黃連者，以清心肝之火也.

·來源：丹溪

16. Bai Dian Gao. One Hundred Dropping Paste. 百點膏

·**ACTIONS**：external obstruction of the eye.

·**COMPOSITION**：Rui Ren, Dang Gui, Fang Feng, Gan Cao, Huang Lian

·**INDICATIONS**：treats eye screen covering the pupil as like cloud.

·**CHANNELS ENTERED**：The foot reverting yin channel. [The liver]

·**Analysis of Formula**：(1) Rui Ren disperses wind, dissipates heat, boosts water, and engenders brightness.

(2) Dang Gui tonifies blood.

(3) Fang Feng disperses wind.

(4) Gan Cao harmonizes the middle.

(5) Huang Lian drains fire.

·**Original Source**：Li Dong Yuan

16. 百點膏

·總結：外翳

·組成：蕤仁, 當歸, 防風, 甘草, 黃連

·主治：治翳遮瞳人, 如雲氣障隔.

·歸經：此足厥陰藥也(肝)

·方義：(1)蕤仁：消風散熱, 益水生光.

(2)當歸：養血.

(3)防風：散風.

(4)甘草：和中.

(5)黃連：瀉火.

·來源：東垣

425

Chapter 20. Oral Formulas for Welling-Abscesses and Sores. 癰瘍之劑

1. Zhen Ren Huo Ming Yin. True Man Decoction to Revitalize Life. 眞人活命飲

·**ACTIONS**：disperses welling abscess and dissipates toxin.

·**COMPOSITION**：Bai Zhi, Bei Mu, Tian Hua Fen, Gan Cao, Dang Gui, Fang Feng, Chen Pi (eliminated white part), Mo Yao, Ru Xiang, Zao Jiao Ci, Chuan Shan Jia, and Jin Yin Hua

·**INDICATIONS**：all kind of welling abscess, flat abscess, swelling, toxin in initial stage.

·**CHANNELS ENTERED**：The foot yang brightness and reverting yin channels. [The stomach and liver]

·**Analysis of Formula**：(1) Jin Yin Hua disperses heat and resolves toxin, and is the holy medicion for welling abscess, therefore this acts as sovereign.

(2) Bai Zhi eliminates damp and removes wind, Tian Hua Fen clears phlegm and descends fire, they can expel pus and disperse swelling. Dang Gui harmonizes yin and activates blood. Chen Pi dries damp and moves qi. Fang Feng drains the lung and courses the liver. Bei Mu disinhibits phlegm and disperses binds. Gan Cao transforms toxin and harmonizes the middle, therefore acts as minister.

(3) Ru Xiang regulates qi, expulses interior, and protects the heart. Mo Yao dissipates stasis, disperses swelling and settles pain, therefore acts as assistant.

(4) Chuan Shan Jia which is good at running, can dissipate binds. Zao Jiao Ci is pungent and tends to disperse and is harsh. They is the main herbs for reverting yin and yang brightness, and can penetrate the channels and networks, reach directly to the place of the disease, pull down congestion and break hardness, therefore act as courier.

(5) Wine is boiled together, this makes the force of the other herbs to reach whole body and toxin evil dissipated.

1. 眞人活命飲
　·總結：消癰散毒
　·組成：白芷，貝母，天花粉，甘草節，當歸，防風，陳皮去白，沒藥，

426

乳香, 皂角刺, 穿山甲, 金銀花

　·主治：治一切癰疽腫毒初起未消者.

　·歸經：此足陽明厥陰藥也(胃肝).

　·方義：(1)金銀花散熱解毒, 癰疽聖藥, 故以爲君.

　　　　　(2)白芷除溼祛風, 花粉清痰降火；並能排膿消腫. 當歸和陰
而活血. 陳皮燥溼而行氣. 防風瀉肺疏肝. 貝母利痰散結. 甘草化毒和中.
故以爲臣.

　　　　　(3)乳香調氣, 托裏護心. 沒藥散瘀消腫定痛. 故以爲佐.

　　　　　(4)穿山甲善走能散. 皂角刺辛散剽銳. 皆厥陰陽明正藥, 能
貫穿經絡, 直達病所, 而潰癰破堅. 故以爲使.

　　　　　(5)加酒者, 欲其通行週身, 使無邪不散也.

2. Jin Yin Hua Jiu. Lonicera Flos Wine. 金銀花酒

　·**ACTIONS**：welling and flat abscess in initial stage.

　·**COMPOSITION**：Jin Yin Hua, Gan Cao

　·**INDICATIONS**：all kinds of welling and flat abscess and malign sore in any place, or lung and intestine welling abscess; this is effective when it is taken in initial stage.

　·**CHANNELS ENTERED**：The foot greater yin and yang brightness channels. [The spleen and stomach]

　·**Analysis of Formula**：(2) The cold of Jin Yin Hua can clear heat and resolve toxin, and the sweet can nourish blood and supplement vacuity, this is holy medicine for welling abscess and sore.

　　　　　(2) Gan Cao also supports the stomach and is good at resolving of toxin.

　·**RELATED FORMULA**：When Huang Qi and wine are added, this is called Hui Du Jin Yin HuaTang, treats pain and ulcer which color changes into purple with black.

2. 金銀花酒

　·總結：癰疽初起

　·組成：金銀花, 甘草

　·主治：治一切癰疽惡瘡, 不問發在何處, 或肺癰腸癰, 初起便服奇效.

　·歸經：此足太陰陽明藥也(脾胃).

　·方義：(2)金銀花：寒能清熱解毒, 甘能養血補虛, 爲癰瘡聖藥.

427

(2)甘草：亦扶胃解毒之上劑也.

·變化方：本方用金銀花，甘草，加黃耆，酒，重湯煮服，名回毒金銀花湯，治痛瘍色變紫黑者.

3. La Fan Wan. Wax and Alum Pills. 蠟礬丸

·**ACTIONS**：expulses the interior and protect the heart

·**COMPOSITION**：Huang La and Bai Fan

·**INDICATIONS**：all kinds of sore, welling abscess, and malign toxin. Initial taking of this pill leads to protect membrane and expulse the interior and prevent toxin from attacking the heart or damage from biting toxin of worm, snake, and dog.

·**CHANNELS ENTERED**：The hand lesser yin channel [the heart].

·**Analysis of Formula**：(1) The heart holds the office of monarch and does not contract evil easily, when one suffers from welling and flat abscess, and damage from biting of snake or dog, if the toxin attack upward to the heart, it is hard to survive.

(2) Huang La is sweet and warm, bai fan is sour and astringent, they can secure membrane and protect the heart, resolve toxin and settle pain, expulse the interior and expel pus, and let toxin qi not to attack interior.

·**RELATED FORMULA**：When Xiong Huang is added, this is called Xiong Huang Fan Wan, treats parasitic toxin and biting toxin of snake, dog, and worm.

·**Original Source**：Li Xun

3. 蠟礬丸

·總結：托裏護心

·組成：黃蠟，白礬

·主治：治一切瘡癰惡毒，先服此丸，護膜托裏，使毒不攻心，或爲毒蟲蛇犬所傷，並宜服之.

·歸經：此手少陰藥也(心).

·方義：(1)心爲君主，不易受邪，凡患癰疽及蛇犬所傷，毒上攻心，則命立傾矣.

(2)黃蠟甘溫，白礬酸澀，並能固膜護心，解毒定痛，托裏排膿，使毒氣不致內攻，故爲患諸證者所必用也.

·變化方：加雄黃，名雄黃礬丸，治蠱毒蛇犬蟲咬毒.

428

4. Tuo Li San. Drain the Interior Powder. 托裏散

·**ACTIONS**：drain interior

·**COMPOSITION**：Jin Yin Hua, Chi Shao, Dang Gui, Da Huang, Mang Xiao, Huang Qin, Mu Li, Lian Qiao, Tian Hua Fen, Zao Jiao Ci

·**INDICATIONS**：all kinds of malign sore, effusion of the back, clove sore, flat and swelling abscess, and Bian toxin [sore] in initial stage, the pulse that is string-like, surging, replete, and rapid, and severe swelling which is about to make pus.

·**CHANNELS ENTERED**：The foot yang brightness and reverting yin channels [the stomach and liver].

·**Analysis of Formula**：(1) Jin Yin Hua clears heat and resolves toxin. This is main herb for sore and welling abscess.

(2) Dang Gui and Chi Shao regulate Construction and blood.

(3) Da Huang and Mang Xiao flush stomach heat.

(4) Huang Qin drains and clears fire.

(5) Mu Li softens hard phlegm.

(6) Lian Qiao and Tian Hua Fen disperse binds and expel pus.

(7) Zao Jiao Ci is peaked and sharp. This directly reaches the place where the disease locates and makes sore and swelling abscess to disperse.

4. 托裏散

·總結：托裏內消

·組成：金銀花, 赤芍, 當歸, 大黃, 朴硝, 黃芩, 牡蠣, 連翹, 花粉, 皂角刺

·主治：治一切惡瘡, 發背疗疽便毒, 始發脈弦洪實數, 腫甚欲作膿者.

·歸經：此足陽明厥陰藥也(胃肝).

·方義：(1)金銀花：清熱解毒, 瘡癰主藥.

(2)當歸, 赤芍：調榮血.

(3)大黃, 芒硝：蕩胃熱.

(4)黃芩：瀉清火.

(5)牡蠣：輭堅痰.

(6)連翹, 花粉：散結排膿.

(7)角刺：鋒銳. 直達病所而潰散之也.

429

5. Jiu Ku Sheng Ling Dan Fang. Torment Relieving and Spirit Overcoming Pills. 救苦勝靈丹方

·**ACTIONS**：The foot lesser yang and yang brightness.

·**COMPOSITION**：Huang Qi, Lian Qiao, Lou Lu, Sheng Ma, Ge Gen, Mu Dan Pi, Dang Gui, Sheng Di Huang, Shu Di Huang, Bai Shao Yao, Fang Feng, Qiang Huo, Du Huo, Chai Hu, Niu Bang Zi, Ren Shen, Gan Cao, Rou Gui, Huang Lian, Huang Bai, Kun Bu, San Leng, E Zhu, Yi Zhi Ren, Mai Ya, Shen Qu, Hou Po·

·**INDICATIONS**：treats scrofula, saber lumps, and goiter which goes down from below or before the ear to neck and shoulder or enters Que Pen. These parts correspond to the channel of the hand and foot lesser yang. And also treats scrofula below neck or in Jia Che where the foot yang brightness takes evil from the heart and spleen.

·**MODIFICATIONS**：(1) if qi is not in normal, add Chen Pi and Mu Xiang.

(2) for fecal stoppage, add Da Huang (processed with wine).

(3) for blood dryness, add Tao Ren and Da Huang.

(4) for wind dryness, add Ma Zi Ren, Da Huang, Qin Jiao, and Zao Jiao Zi.

·**CHANNELS ENTERED**：The foot yang brightness and hand and foot lesser yang channels. [The stomach, San Jiao, and gall bladder].

·**Original Source**：Li Dong Yuan

5. 救苦勝靈丹方

·總結：少陽陽明經毒

·組成：黃耆, 連翹, 漏蘆, 升麻, 葛根, 丹皮, 當歸, 生地, 熟地, 白芍藥, 防風, 羌活, 獨活, 柴胡, 鼠粘子, 人參, 甘草, 肉桂, 黃連, 黃柏, 昆布, 三稜, 莪朮, 益智, 麥芽, 神麴, 厚朴

·主治：治療馬刀挾癭, 從耳下或耳後下頸至肩, 或入缺盆中, 乃手足少陽經分；其療癭在頸下或至頰車, 乃足陽明經分受心脾之邪而作也.

·加減：(1)如氣不順, 加陳皮, 木香.

(2)大便不通, 加酒製大黃.

(3)血燥, 加桃仁, 大黃.

(4)風燥加麻仁, 大黃, 秦艽, 皂角子.

·歸經：此足陽明手足少陽藥也(胃膽三焦).

·來源：東垣

6. San Zhong Kui Jian Tang. Disperse the Swelling and Bre ak the Hardness Decoction. 散腫潰堅湯

·**ACTIONS**：dissipates harndess and disperses swelling

·**COMPOSITION**：Chai Hu, Lian Qiao, Sheng Ma, Ge Gen, Gan Cao (mix fried), Tian Hua Fen, Jie Geng, Dang Gui Wei, Shao Yao, Kun Bu, San Le ng, E Zhu, Huang Qin, Huang Lian, Huang Bai, Zhi Mu, Long Dan Cao

·**INDICATIONS**：treats the above pattern. (scrofula, saber lumps, and go iter which goes down from below or before the ear to neck and shoulder or ente rs Que Pen. These parts correspond to the channel of the hand and foot lesser y ang. And also treats scrofula below neck or in Jia Che where the foot yang brig htness takes evil from the heart and spleen.)

·**CHANNELS ENTERED**：The hand and foot lesser yang and the foot y ang brightness channels. [The San Jiao, gall bladder and stomach]

·**Analysis of Formula**：(1) Chai Hu and Lian Qiao clear heat and disperse binds.

(2) Sheng Ma and Ge Gen resolve toxin and raise yang.

(3) Tian Hua Fen and Jie Geng clear the lung and expel pus.

(4) Dang Gui Wei and Shao Yao moisten the liver and activate b lood.

(5) Gan Cao harmonizes the middle and transforms toxin.

(6) Kun Bu disperses phlegm and breaks hardness.

(7) San Leng and E Zhu break blood and move qi.

(8) Huang Qin, Huang Bai, Huang Lian, Long Dan Cao, and Zhi Mu drain greatly the fire of San Jiao.

(9) Jie Geng also can make the other herbs ascend upward.

·**Original Source**：Li Dong Yuan

6. 散腫潰堅湯

·總結：消堅散腫

·組成：柴胡, 連翹, 升麻, 葛根, 炙甘草, 天花粉, 桔梗, 當歸尾, 芍藥, 昆布, 三稜, 廣朮, 黃芩, 黃連, 黃柏, 知母, 龍膽草

·主治：治同前證. (治療瘰馬刀挾瘿, 從耳下或耳後下頸至肩, 或入缺盆中, 乃手足少陽經分；其瘰瘿在頸下或至頰車, 乃足陽明經分受心脾之邪而作也. 今將三證合而治之.)

·歸經：此手足少陽足陽明藥也(三焦膽胃).

·方義：(1)柴胡, 連翹：清熱散結.

(2)升麻, 葛根：解毒升陽.

(3)花粉, 桔梗：清肺排膿.

(4)歸尾, 芍藥：潤肝活血.

(5)甘草：和中化毒.

(6)昆布：散痰潰堅.

(7)三稜, 莪朮：破血行氣.

(8)黃芩, 藥, 連, 龍膽, 知母：大瀉三焦之火.

(9)而桔梗又能載諸藥而上行也.

·來源：東垣

7. Fei Long Duo Ming Dan. 飛龍奪命丹

·**ACTIONS**：attacks toxin with toxin

·**COMPOSITION**：Ba Dou, Nao Sha, Tian Nan Xing, Huang Dan, Xiong Huang, Ban Mao, Xin Shi, She Xiang, Ru Xiang

·**INDICATIONS**：all kinds of clove sore, swelling, and welling and flat abscess, malign sore in initial stage, sunken hole with black, toxin qi which attacks interior.

·**CHANNELS ENTERED**：This frees and moves the twelve channels.

·**Analysis of Formula**：Toxin qi which attacks interior, sore and ulcer which have sunken black hole. Common medicinal cannot treat this.

(1) Ba Dou and Nao Sha are high toxicity and great heat, they can eliminate cold and transform accumulation.

(2) Nan Xing, Xiong Huang and Huang Dan are pungent and dry, they can kill toxin and break phlegm.

(3) Ban Mao and Chan Su are pungent, cold, and toxicity, they can draw out clove sore and swelling and precipitate something malign.

(4) Xin Shi is dry and harsh, eliminates phlegm.

(5) The aroma of She Xiang penetrates and frees orifice.

(6) Ru Xiang can make toxin qi come out to exterior in order not to reach to attack interior.

(7) Wine conducts herbs to move the channels and networks. And it is not toxic and does not drain.

7. 飛龍奪命丹

·總結：以毒攻毒
·組成：巴豆，硇砂，天南星，黃丹，雄黃，斑蝥，信石，麝香，乳香
·主治：治一切疔腫癰疽，惡瘡初發，或發而黑陷，毒氣內攻者．
·歸經：此十二經通行之藥也．
·方義：毒氣內攻，瘡瘍黑陷，非平劑所能勝．
　　(1)巴豆，硇砂：大毒大熱，能祛寒化積．
　　(2)南星，雄黃，黃丹：味辛性燥，能殺毒破痰．
　　(3)斑蝥，蟾酥：辛寒至毒，能拔疔腫，下惡物．
　　(4)信石：燥烈劫痰．
　　(5)麝香：香竄通竅．
　　(6)乳香：能使毒氣外出，不致內攻．
　　(7)引之以酒，使行經絡，無毒不瀉也．
　　此乃屬劑．所謂：「藥不瞑眩，厥疾不瘳」此類是也．

8. Xiong Huang Jie Du Wan. Realgar Piis to Relieve Toxin. 雄黃解毒丸

·ACTIONS：throat-entwining wind and impediment
·COMPOSITION：Xiong Huang, Ba Dou, Yu Jin
·INDICATIONS：urgent throat-entwining impediment
·CHANNELS ENTERED：The hand and foot lesser yin and lesser yang channels. [The heart, kidney, San Jiao, and gall bladder]
·Analysis of Formula：Wu He Gao says that if urgent throat-entwining impediment is treated moderately, death will occur. Xiong Huang can break bind qi. Yu Jin can disperse malign blood. Ba Dou can precipitate sticky drool. Dan Xi does not use drastic formulas all his life, this herb is inevitably used.
·Original Source：Dan Xi

8. 雄黃解毒丸
　·總結：纏喉風痺
　·組成：雄黃，巴豆，鬱金
　·主治：治纏喉急痺．
　·歸經：此手足少陰少陽藥也．
　·方義：吳鶴皋：「纏喉急痺，緩治則死．雄黃能破結氣．鬱金能散惡血．巴豆能下稠涎．丹溪生平不用屬劑，此蓋不得已而用者乎．」

433

·來源：丹溪

9. Zao Jiao Wan. Gleditsia fruit Pill. 皂角丸

·**COMPOSITION**：Zao Jiao

·**INDICATIONS**：lung abscess and cough with dyspnea, intermittent exp
ectorating of turbidity, and only sitting with insomnia.

·**CHANNELS ENTERED**：The hand greater yin channel [the lung].

·**Analysis of Formula**：喻嘉言 says that when the toxin of fire and heat
binds in the lung, these treatments of dispersing exterior, attacking interior, war
ming, and clearing are used, but there is no little response, this pills can be used.

·**RELATED FORMULA**：(1) Qian Jin Fang uses Gui Zhi Tang in which
Shao Yao is eliminated and Zao Jiao is added, this is called Gui Zhi Qu Shao Y
ao Jia Zao Jiao Tang, treats lung wilting with vomiting of saliva.

(2) When Ge Fen is added to this formula, this is called Zao Ha
Wan, treats wind evil in women that attacks breast and makes breast abscess. T
akes two qian every time with wine.

·**Original Source**：Jin Gui Yao Lue

9. 皂角丸

·組成：皂角

·主治：治肺癰欬逆上氣，時時唾濁，但坐不眠.

·歸經：此手太陰藥也(肺)

·方義：喻嘉言曰：「火熱之毒，結聚于肺，表之裏之，溫之清之，曾
不少應，堅而不可攻者，令服此丸，庶幾無堅不入，聿成洗蕩之功，不可以
藥之微賤而少之也.」

·變化方：(1)千金方用桂枝湯，去芍藥，加皂角，名桂枝去芍藥加皂角
湯，治肺痿吐沫.

(2)本方加蛤粉等分爲末，名皂蛤丸，治婦人風邪客于乳房，
而成乳癰. 每服二錢，酒下.

·來源：金匱

10. Tuo Li Shi Bu San. Drain the Interior and Supplement Ten Powder. 托裏十補散

·**ACTIONS**：resolves exterior and drains interior

·**COMPOSITION**：Chuan Xiong, Ren Shen, Bai Zhi, Jie Geng, Huang Qi, Gan Cao, Fang Feng, Dang Gui, Hou Po, Gui Xin

·**INDICATIONS**：welling abscess and sore in initial stage, evil in the high and pain in the lower, exuberant sore, emaciation, and the pulse that is weak.

·**CHANNELS ENTERED**：The hand and foot greater yin and the foot reverting yin and yang brightness channels. [The lung, spleen, liver, and stomach].

·**Analysis of Formula**：(1) Ren Shen and Huang Qi supplement qi. Chuan Xiong and Dang Gui activate blood. Gan Cao resolves toxin. Gui Zhi, Bai Zhi, and Jie Geng expel pus. Hou Po drains replete fullness. Fang Feng disperses wind evil.

(2) This formula is related with the herbs of exterior, interior, qi, and blood. This assists yang and drains interior.

·**RELATED FORMULA**：When Shao Yao, Lian Qiao, Mu Xiang, Ru Xiang, and Mo Yao are added, this is also called Tuo Li San, treats effusion of the back and clove sore.

·**Original Source**：Ju Fang

10. 托裏十補散
　·總結：解表托裏
　·組成：川芎，人參，白芷，桔梗，黃耆，甘草，防風，當歸，厚朴，桂心
　·主治：治癰瘡初發，或已發，邪高痛下，瘡盛形羸，脈無力者.
　·歸經：此手足太陰足厥陰陽明藥也.
　·方義：(1)參，耆補氣. 芎，歸活血. 甘草解毒. 桂枝，白芷，桔梗排膿. 厚朴瀉實滿. 防風散風邪.
　　　(2)爲表裏氣血之藥，共成助陽內托之功也.
　·變化方：本方加芍藥，連翹，木香，乳香，沒藥，亦名托裏散，治發背疔瘡.
　·來源：局方

11. Tuo Li Huang Qi Tang. Drain the Interior Decoction wi

th Astragalus.　托裏黃耆湯

·**ACTIONS**：supplements vacuity after open of sores.

·**COMPOSITION**：Huang Qi, Fu Ling, Ren Shen, Gui Xin, Dang Gui, Mai Men Dong, Wu Wei Zi子, Yuan Zhi

·**INDICATIONS**：every sore after open of sores, profuse pus with interior vacuity.

·**CHANNELS ENTERED**：The hand and foot greater yin and the foot yang brightness channels [the lung, spleen, and stomach].

·**Analysis of Formula**：(1) Ren Shen and Huang Qi supplement qi and secure Defense.

(2) Dang Gui and Gui Xin activate blood and generate the flesh.

(3) Fu Ling drains damp and fortifies the spleen.

(4) Mai Men Dong clears heat and supplements the lung.

(5) The pungent and dispersing of Yuan Zhi mainly rectifies welling and flat abscess.

(6) Wu Wei Zi is sour and warm, this is good at contracting of large swelling.

Dan Xi says that welling and flat abscess after open of sores should be treated with supplementing qi and blood and rectifying Spleen and Stomach, this is key point. If it is not treated as like that, in a few months or half year vacuity pattern will show and change into the other disease.

·**Original Source**：Sheng Ji Zong Ru

11. 托裏黃耆湯
　·總結：潰後補虛
　·組成：黃耆, 茯苓, 人參, 桂心, 當歸, 麥冬, 五味子, 遠志
　·主治：治諸瘡潰後, 膿多內虛.
　·歸經：此手足太陰足陽明藥也.
　·方義：(1)人參, 黃耆：補氣固衛.
　　　　(2)當歸, 桂心：活血生肌.
　　　　(3)茯苓：滲溼健脾.
　　　　(4)麥冬：清熱補肺.
　　　　(5)遠志：辛散, 專理癰疽.
　　　　(6)五味：酸溫, 善收腫大.
　　　丹溪曰：「癰疽潰後, 補氣血, 理脾胃, 實爲切要. 否則數

月半年之後，虛證仍見，轉成他病也.」

　　·煎服法：等分，每服五錢，食遠服.

　　·來源：總錄

12. Tuo Li Wen Zhong Tang. Dain the Interior and Warm the Middle Decocotion. 托裏溫中湯

·**ACTIONS**：sore and ulcer which are sunken inward.

·**COMPOSITION**：Ding Xiang, Qiang Huo, Yi Zhi Ren, Fu Zi, Gan Jiang, Chen Pi, Chen Xiang, Gan Cao (mix fried), Xiao Hui Xiang, Mu Xiang

·**INDICATIONS**：(1) sore and ulcer which are related with cold and change to sunken inward, pus which are clear and watery, the skin which are cool.

　　　　(2) glomus and fullness below the heart, borborigmus with cutting pain, and mild loose stool.

　　　　(3) retching as soon as eating, dyspnea with hiccup, inability to lie down, and intermittent occurring of dizziness.

·**CHANNELS ENTERED**：The foot yang brightness and three yin channels.

·**Analysis of Formula**：In Wei Sheng Bao Jian, Nei Jing says that excessive cold in the interior is treated with pungent and heat and is assisted with bitter and warm.

　　　　(1) Fu Zi and Gan Jiang are great pungent and heat, they warm the middle, disperse yang qi from interior to exterior, and acts as sovereign.

　　　　(2) Qiang Huo is bitter pungent and warm. It penetrates joints.

　　　　(3) Gan Cao (mix fried) warms and supplements the spleen and stomach, moves the channels and networks, and frees blood vessels. .

　　　　(4) When the stomach is cold, retching, vomiting, hiccup, and failing to descend food occur, Yi Zhi Ren, Chen Xiang, and Ding Xiang are great heat. They disperse cold evil and act as assistant.

　　　　(5) Sore qi attacking interior causes fullness, Mu Xiang, Xiao Hui Xiang, and Chen Pi are pungent, bitter, and warm. They treat glomus and disperse fullness, and act as courier.

·**Original Source**：Sun Yan He Fang

12. 托裏溫中湯

　　·總結：瘡瘍內陷

437

·組成：丁香，羌活，益智仁，附子，乾薑，陳皮，沈香，炙甘草，茴香，木香

　·主治：(1)治瘡瘍爲寒，變而內陷，膿出清稀，皮膚涼．

　　　　(2)心下痞滿，腸鳴切痛，大便微溏．

　　　　(3)食則嘔逆，氣短呃逆，不得安臥，時發昏憒．

　·歸經：此足陽明三陰藥也．

　·方義：衛生寶鑑曰：『經曰：「寒淫于內，治以辛熱，佐以苦溫．」

　　　　(1)附子，乾薑：大辛熱溫中，外發陽氣，自裏之表，爲君．

　　　　(2)羌活：味苦辛溫，透關節．

　　　　(3)炙甘草：溫補脾胃，行經絡，通血脈．

　　　　(4)胃寒則嘔吐呃逆，不下食，益智，沈香，丁香，大熱以散寒邪，爲佐．

　　　　(5)瘡氣內攻，聚而爲滿，木香，茴香，陳皮，辛苦溫，治痞散滿，爲使

　·來源：孫彥和

13. Zhi Tong Dang Gui Tang. Tangkuei Decoction to Relieve Pain. 止痛當歸湯

·**ACTIONS**：relieves pain

·**COMPOSITION**：Dang Gui, sheng Di Huang, Huang Qi, Ren Shen, Gan Cao (mix fried), Rou Gui, Shao Yao

·**INDICATIONS**：flat abscess of the brain and back, opens of sore with pain.

·**CHANNELS ENTERED**：The foot yang brightness and reverting yin channels.

·**Analysis of Formula**：(1) Dang Gui and Sheng Di Huang activate blood and cool blood.

　　　　(2) Ren Shen and Huang Qi boost qi and supplement the middle.

　　　　(3) Rou Gui resolves toxin and transforms pus.

　　　　(4) Shao Yao harmonizes the spleen and restrains yin with sour.

　　　　(5)Gan Cao supports the stomach. Sweet moderates and then pain spontaneously disappears.

·**Original Source**：Sheng Ji Zong Ru

13. 止痛當歸湯
　　·總結：止痛
　　·組成：當歸, 生地黃, 黃耆, 人參, 炙甘草, 官桂, 芍藥
　　·主治：治腦疽背疽, 穿潰疼痛.
　　·歸經：此足陽明厥陰藥也.
　　·方義：(1)當歸, 生地：活血涼血.
　　　　　　(2)人參, 黃耆：益氣補中.
　　　　　　(3)官桂：解毒化膿.
　　　　　　(4)芍藥：和脾, 酸以斂之.
　　　　　　(5)甘草：扶胃, 甘以緩之. 則痛自減矣.
　　·來源：總錄

14. Sheng Ji San. Flesh-Engendering Powder. 生肌散

·**ACTIONS**：closes sores and regenerates flesh

·**COMPOSITION**：Han Shui Shi, Hua Shi, Mi Tuo Seng, Hai Piao Xiao, Qian Fen, Ku Fan, Long Gu, Gan Yan Zhi.

·**INDICATIONS**：　closes sores and regenerates flesh.

·**CHANNELS ENTERED**：The yang brightness channels.

·**Analysis of Formula**：sore-opening which fails to close, owing to pus and water which disperse and overflow, thus ulceration occurs.

　　　　(1) Shi Gao and Hua Shi resolves flesh heat.

　　　　(2) Hai Piao Xiao, Mi Tuo Seng, and Qian Fen withdraw damp and dry pus.

　　　　(3) Long Gu and Ku Fan are good at contracting.

　　　　(4) Yan Zhi activates blood and resolves toxin.

　　　Therefore this formula can close sore and regenerate flesh.

·**Another Side Formula**：(1) Bing Lang, Ku Fan, Mi Tuo Seng, Huang Dan, Xue Jie, and Jing Fen, this is also called Sheng Ji San.

　　　　(2) In the formula of Zhang Zi He, ：Huang Lian, Mi Tuo Seng, Yan Zhi, Lu Dou Fen, Xiong Huang, and Jing Fen, this is also called Sheng Ji San, treats same things.

14. 生肌散
　　·總結：斂瘡長肉

439

·組成：寒水石，滑石，密陀僧，海螵蛸，定粉，枯礬，龍骨，乾胭脂

·主治：斂瘡長肉．

·歸經：此陽明藥也．

·方義：瘡口不斂，蓋因膿水散溢而潰爛也．

　　　　⑴石膏，滑石：解肌熱．

　　　　⑵螵蛸，陀僧，定粉：收溼燥膿．

　　　　⑶龍骨，枯礬：善收瀋．

　　　　⑷胭脂活血解毒．

　　　　故能斂瘡而生肉也．

·又附方：⑴檳榔，枯礬，陀僧，黃丹，血竭，輕粉，亦名生肌散．

　　　　⑵張子和方：黃連，密陀僧，胭脂，菉豆粉，雄黃，輕粉亦名

生肌散，治同．

·煎服法：共爲細末，摻瘡口上．

440

Chapter 21. Formulas for Menstruation and Childbirth. 經產之劑

1. Biao Shi Liu He Tang. Six Fold Decoction with Exterior Repletion. 表實六合湯

·**ACTIONS**： cold damage in pregnancy.

·**COMPOSITION**：Si Wu Tang(Dang Gui, Di Huang, Shao Yao, Chuan Xiong), Ma Huang, Xi Xin

·**INDICATIONS**：cold damage in pregnancy, headache, generalized hea viness, heat effusion, absence of sweating, the pulse which is tight, greater yan g channel disease.

·**CHANNELS ENTERED**：The foot greater yang channel.

·**Analysis of Formula**：(1) Generally when women suffers from cold dam age, the treat principle according to the six channels is same with man. But in c ase of pregnancy, quieting of fetus is mainly used. If there is medicine which at tacks the fetus, the medicine cannot be used.

(2) When Wang Hai Zang treats cold damage in pregnancy, he u sually uses Si Wu Tang as sovereign to nourish blood and quiet fetus, and the o ther residual signs of cold damage is treated with following common methods o f cold damage. .

(3) Ma Huang and Xi Xin promote sweating and resolve exterior, therefore they are used, this treats exterior repletion with absence of sweating.

·**RELATED FORMULA**：(1) Si Wu Tang (four liang) with Gui Zhi and Di Gu Pi (respectively seven qian), this is called Biao Xu Lie He Tang, treats c old damage in pregnancy, exterior vacuity spontaneous sweating, generalized h eat effusion, aversion to cold, the stiffness and pain of the head and nape, the p ulse that is floating and weak..

(2) Si Wu Tang (four liang) with Fang Feng and Cang Zhu (resp ectively seven qian), this is called Feng Shi Liu He Tang, treats cold damage in pregnancy, wind strike with damp qi, vexed pain in the limbs and joints, headac he, generalized heat effusion, and the pulse that is floating.

(3) Si Wu Tang (four liang) with Sheng Ma and Lian Qiao (respe ctively seven qian), this is called Sheng Ma Liu He Tang, treats that when in co ld damage of pregnancy after precipitation, the time has already passed the cha nnel and the disease has not recovered, and there is damp toxin with macula as shawl pattern.

(4) Si Wu Tang (four liang) with Chai Hu and Huang Qin (respe ctively seven qian), this is called Chai Hu Lie He Tang, treats cold damage in p regnancy, fullness and pain in the chest and rib-side, and the pulse that is string -like. This is lesser yang channel pattern.

(5) Si Wu Tang (four liang) with Da Huang (five qian), Tao Ren (ten mei, bran-fry), this is called Da Huang Liu He Tang, treats cold damage in pregnancy, constipation, reddish urine, abdominal fullness and distention, and t he pulse that is sunken and rapid. This is the original disease of greater yang an d yang brightness, precipitation is urgently required.

(6) Si Wu Tang (four liang) with Ren Shen, Wu Wei Zi (respecti vely five qian), this is called Ren Shen Liu He Tang, treats cold damage in preg nancy, incessant cough after promotion of sweating or precipitation.

(7) Si Wu Tang (four liang) with Hou Po and Zhi Shi (bran-fry, r espectively five qian), this is called Po Shi Liu He Tang, treats that after recove ring from cold damage in pregnancy, there is vacuous glomus, distention, and f ullness in the abdomen. This belongs to the original vacuous disease of yang br ightness.

(8) Si Wu Tang (four liang) with Zhi Zi and Huang Qin (respecti vely five qian), this is called Zhi Zi Liu He Tang, treats that when after promoti on of sweating or precipitation in cold damage in pregnancy, there is inability t o sleep.

(9) Si Wu Tang (four liang) with Shi Gao and Zhi Mu (respectiv ely five qian), this is called Shi Gao Liu He Tang, treats that when in cold dama ge in pregnancy, there is great thirst, vexation, and the pulse that is long and lar ge.

(10) Si Wu Tang (four liang) with Fu Ling and Ze Xie (respective ly five qian), this is called Fu Ling Liu He Tang, treats that when in cold damag e in pregnancy, there is inhibited urination. This belongs to the original disease of greater yang.

(11) Si Wu Tang (four liang) with E Jiao and Ai Ye (respectively five qian), this is called Jiao Ai Si Wu Tang, treats when in cold damage after p romotion of sweating or precipitation in pregnancy, there is incessant blood spo tting, detriment and stirred fetus qi.

(12) Si Wu Tang (four liang) with Fu Zi and Rou Gui (respectivel y five qian), this is called Fu Zi Liu He Tang, treats cold damage in pregnancy, contracture of the limbs, cool body with mild sweating, pain in the abdomen, th e pulse that is sunken and slow, this is lesser yin disease.

(13) Si Wu Tang (four liang) with Sheng Di Huang and Da Huang

442

(five qian), this is called Si Wu Da Huang Tang, treats cold damage blood amassment in pregnancy.

　　·Original Source：Wang Hai Zang

1. 表實六合湯
　　·總結：妊娠傷寒
　　·組成：四物湯(當歸, 地黃, 芍藥, 川芎), 麻黃, 細辛
　　·主治：治妊娠傷寒, 頭痛身熱, 無汗脈緊, 太陽經病.
　　·歸經：此足太陽藥也.
　　·方義：(1)凡婦人傷寒六經治例皆同. 有懷妊者, 則以安胎爲主. 藥中有犯胎者, 則不可用也.
　　　　　(2)海藏皆四物爲君, 養血安胎, 餘同傷寒例分證而治.
　　　　　(3)麻黃, 細辛, 發汗解表, 故加用之, 治表實無汗者.
　　·變化方：(1)四物四兩, 加桂枝, 地骨皮各七錢, 名表虛六合湯, 治妊娠傷寒, 表虛自汗, 身熱惡寒, 頭痛項強, 脈浮而弱.
　　　　　(2)四物四兩, 加防風, 蒼朮各七錢, 名風溼六合湯, 治妊娠傷寒, 中風溼氣, 肢節煩痛, 頭痛, 身熱, 脈浮.
　　　　　(3)四物四兩, 加升麻, 連翹各七錢, 名升麻六合湯, 治妊娠傷寒, 下後過經不愈, 溼毒發斑如錦紋者.
　　　　　(4)四物四兩, 加柴胡, 黃芩各七錢, 名柴胡六合湯, 治妊娠傷寒, 胸脇滿痛而脈弦, 少陽經證.
　　　　　(5)四物四兩, 加大黃五錢, 桃仁十枚, 麩炒, 名大黃六合湯, 治妊娠傷寒, 大便祕, 小便赤, 氣滿而脈沈數, 太陽陽明本病也, 急下之.
　　　　　(6)四物四兩, 加人參, 五味各五錢, 名人參六合湯, 治妊娠傷寒, 汗下後欬嗽不止.
　　　　　(7)四物四兩, 加厚朴, 枳實, 麩炒各五錢, 名朴實六合湯, 治妊娠傷寒後, 虛痞脹滿, 陽明本虛者.
　　　　　(8)四物四兩, 加梔子, 黃芩各五錢, 名梔子六合湯, 治妊娠傷寒汗下後, 不得眠.
　　　　　(9)四物四兩, 加石膏, 知母各五錢, 名石膏六合湯, 治妊娠傷寒, 大渴而煩, 脈長而大.
　　　　　(10)四物四兩, 加茯苓, 澤瀉各五錢, 名茯苓六合湯, 治妊娠傷寒, 小便不利, 太陽本病.
　　　　　(11)四物四兩, 加阿膠, 艾葉各五錢, 名膠艾四物湯, 治妊娠傷寒汗下後, 血漏不止, 損動胎氣者.

443

(12)四物四兩，加附子，肉桂各五錢，名附子六合湯，治妊娠傷寒，四肢拘急，身涼微汗，腹中痛，脈沈遲者，少陰病也.

(13)四物四兩，加生地，大黃和五錢，名四物大黃湯，治妊娠傷寒畜血證.

·來源：海藏

2. Jiao Ai Tang. Ass-Hide Gelatin and Mugwort Decoction. 膠艾湯

·**ACTIONS**：miscarriage and spotting

·**COMPOSITION**：E Jiao, Chuan Xiong, Gan Cao, Ai Ye, Dang Gui, Shao Yao, Gan Di Huang

·**INDICATIONS**：(1) spotting (persistent leakage of blood from the uterus), or incessant bleeding form the uterus after miscarriage.

(2) or bleeding from the uterus and abdominal pain during pregnancy, this is called placenta obstruction.

(3) (and also) detriment and damage of the thoroughfare and conception vessels, profuse menstruation, and persistent strangury.

·**MODIFICATIONS**：(1) Yan Shi treats stirring fetus with spotting from the uterus, lumbar pain, abdominal fullness, shortness of breath through adding Huang Qi.

(2) Qian Jin Yi treats falling dawn from high, the detriment and damage of five viscera with hematemesis, metal sore with the injury of the channels and flesh by adding Gan Jiang.

·**CHANNELS ENTERED**：The foot greater and reverting yin channels.

·**Analysis of Formula**：(1) Si Wu Tang tonifies blood.

(2) E Jiao boosts yin.

(3) Ai Ye supplements yang.

(4) Gan Cao is used to harmonize every herbs and the force of wine moves whole body, these actions make blood stay in the medians and nourish fetus, and then there will not the worry of spotting.

·Another Side Formula：(1) In another Jiao Ai Tang, Gan Jiang (three liang) is added.

(2) E Jiao (one jin), Ge Fen (stir-bake), Ai Ye (a few stem); this is also called Jiao Ai Tang, treats stirring fetus, pain in the lumbus and abdomen, or fetus qi which surging upward to the heart, bleeding from the uterus with ab

444

dominal pain.

(3) in Zhi Mi Fang, Qin Jiao is added.
·**Original Source**：Jin Gui Yao Lue

2. 膠艾湯
　·總結：半産漏下
　·組成：阿膠, 芎藭, 甘草, 艾葉, 當歸, 芍藥, 乾地黃
　·主治：(1)治婦人漏下, 或半産後下血不絶.
　　　　　(2)或妊娠下血, 腹痛爲胞阻.
　　　　　(3)亦治損傷衝任, 月水過多, 淋瀝不斷.
　·加減：(1)嚴氏治胎動經漏, 腰痛腹滿, 搶心短氣, 加黃耆.
　　　　　(2)千金翼治從高墬下, 損傷五臟吐血, 及金瘡經肉絶者, 加
乾薑.
　·歸經：此足太陰厥陰藥也.
　·方義：(1)四物：以養其血.
　　　　　(2)阿膠：以益其陰.
　　　　　(3)艾葉：以補其陽.
　　　　　(4)和以甘草, 行以酒勢, 使血能循經養胎, 則無漏下之患矣.
　·又附方：(1)一方加乾薑三兩.
　　　　　(2)阿膠一斤, 蛤粉炒, 艾葉數莖, 亦名膠艾湯, 治胎動不安,
腰腹疼痛, 或胎上搶心, 去血腹痛.
　　　　　(3)指迷方加秦芃.
　·來源：金匱

3. Gou Teng Tang. Uncaria Decoction. 鈎藤湯

·**ACTIONS**：convulsions and stirring fetus.
·**COMPOSITION**：Gou Teng, Jie Geng, Fu Shen, Ren Shen, Dang Gui,
Sang Ji Sheng
·**INDICATIONS**：convulsions and stirring fetus.
·**MODIFICATIONS**：(1) for wind heat, add Huang Qin, Zhi Zi, Chai Hu,
and Bai Zhu.

(2) for wind phlegm, add Ban Xia, Nan Xing, and Zhu Li.

(3) for prevalent wind, add Quan Xie and Jiang Can.
·**CHANNELS ENTERED**：The foot reverting yin channel.

·**Analysis of Formula**：⑴ The sweet and cold of Gou Teng eliminates he art heat and disperses liver wind.

⑵ The pungent and cool of Chai Hu and Jie Geng and the bitter and cold of Huang Qin and Zhi Zi pacify wind heat in lesser yang and reverting yin, when wind heat removes, convulsions stops.

⑶ Ren Shen and Fu Shen boost qi and quiet spirit.

⑷ Dang Gui and Sang Ji Sheng nourish blood and quiet fetus.

·**Original Source**：Fu Ren Da Quan Liang Fang

3. 鉤藤湯

·總結：瘛瘲胎動

·組成：鉤藤鉤，桔梗，茯神，人參，當歸，桑寄生

·主治：瘛瘲胎動不安.

·加減：⑴風熱加黃芩，梔子，柴胡，白朮.

⑵風痰加半夏，南星，竹瀝.

⑶風勝加全蠍，殭蠶.

·歸經：此足厥陰藥也.

·方義：⑴鉤藤之甘寒以除心熱，而散肝風.

⑵柴胡，桔梗之辛涼，黃芩，梔子之苦寒，以平陽厥陰之風熱，風熱去則瘛瘲止矣.

⑶人參，茯神以益氣而寧神.

⑷當歸，寄生以養血而安胎也.

·來源：良方

4. Ling Yang Jiao San. Antelope Horn Powder. 羚羊角散

·**ACTIONS**：eclampsia of pregnancy

·**COMPOSITION**：Ling Yang Jiao, Fang Feng, Du Huo, Fu Shen, Zao Ren, Chuan Xiong, Dang Gui, Xing Ren, Mu Xiang, Gan Cao, Yi Yi Ren

·**INDICATIONS**：Wind strike in pregnancy, phlegm and drool in the throat as the flowing tide, hanging eyes and clenched jaw, arched back rigidity, this is called eclampsia of pregnancy.

·**CHANNELS ENTERED**：The foot reverting yin channel.

·**Analysis of Formula**：⑴ The pungent and cool of Ling Yang Jiao pacifies liver fire.

⑵ The pungent and warm of Fang Feng and Du Huo disperse li

446

ver evil.

      (3) Fu Shen and Suan Zao Ren quiet spirit.

      (4) Dang Gui and Chuan Xiong activate blood.

      (5) Xing Ren and Mu Xiang disinhibit qi.

      (6) Yi Yi Ren and Gan Cao regulate the spleen.

·**Original Source**：Ben Shi Fang

4. 羚羊角散

  ·總結：子癇

  ·組成：羚羊角, 防風, 獨活, 茯神, 棗仁, 芎藭, 當歸, 杏仁, 木香, 甘草, 薏仁

  ·主治：治妊娠中風, 涎潮忽仆, 目弔口噤, 角弓反張, 名子癇.

  ·歸經：此足厥陰藥也.

  ·方義：(1)羚角之辛涼, 以平肝火.

        (2)防風, 獨活之辛溫, 以散肝邪.

        (3)茯神, 酸棗以寧神.

        (4)當歸, 川芎以活血.

        (5)杏仁, 木香以利氣.

        (6)薏仁, 甘草以調脾也.

  ·來源：本事方

5. Zi Su Ye Yin. Perilla Leaf Beverage. 紫蘇飲

·**ACTIONS**：pregnancy suspension

·**COMPOSITION**：Chuan Xiong, Dang Gui, Shao Yao, Su Ye, Chen Pi, Da Fu Pi, Ren Shen, Gan Cao

·**INDICATIONS**：unharmonious fetal qi which surges upward to the chest and abdomen, abdominal fullness and headache, the pain in the heart, abdomen, lumbus, and rip-side, this is called pregnancy suspension.

·**MODIFICATIONS**：for the pain in the heart and abdomen, add Mu Xiang and Yan Hu Suo.

·**CHANNELS ENTERED**：The hand and foot greater yin reverting yin channels.

·**Analysis of Formula**：Chen Lai Zhang says that Chuan Xiong, Dang Gui, and Shao Yao harmonize blood, Su Ye, Chen Pi, and Da Fu Pi normalize qi, when qi is in normal and blood is in harmony, fetus gets quiet. This formula dis

447

inhibits stagnant qi, and Ren Shen and Gan Cao nourish qi, normalizing of qi make evil qi which counterflow upward to normalize and nourishing of qi supplements and nourishing true qi.

·**Original Source**：Yan Shi

5. 紫蘇飲
　·總結：子懸
　·組成：芎藭，當歸，芍藥，蘇葉，陳皮，大腹皮，人參，甘草
　·主治：治胎氣不和，湊上胸腹，腹滿頭痛，心腹腰脅痛，名子懸.
　·加減：心腹痛者，加木香，延胡索.
　·歸經：此手足太陰厥陰藥也.
　·方義：陳來章曰：「芎，歸，芍藥以和其血，蘇，橘，大腹以順其氣，氣順血和則胎安矣. 既利其氣，復以人參，甘草養其氣者，順則順其邪逆之氣，養則養其冲和之氣也.」
　·煎服法：加薑煎，空心服.
　·來源：嚴氏

6. Tian Xian Teng San. Arisrolochia Stem Powder. 天仙藤散

·**ACTIONS**： pregnancy qi

·**COMPOSITION**： Tian Xian Teng, Xiang Fu, Wu Yao, Chen Pi, Gan Cao

·**INDICATIONS**： pregnancy qi

·**CHANNELS ENTERED**：The hand and foot greater yin channels.

·**Analysis of Formula**：(1) The bitter and warm of Tian Xian Teng courses qi and activates blood, and can resolve wind qi in blood.

(2) The pungent and warm of Xiang Fu, Wu Yao, and Chen Pi move stagnant qi.

(3) The pungent and warm of Zi Su Ye and Sheng Jiang courses exterior qi.

(4) The sweet of Gan Cao harmonizes the right qi.

(5) Mu Gua is added a little, eliminates damp heat, disinhibits sinew and bone, and regulates the construction and defense.

·**Original Source**：Chen Jing Chu Fang

6. 天仙藤散

　·總結：子氣

　·組成：天仙藤, 香附, 烏藥, 陳皮, 甘草

　·主治：治子氣.

　·歸經：此手足太陰藥也.

　·方義：(1)天仙藤之苦溫, 疏氣活血, 能解血中之風氣.

　　　　　(2)香附, 烏藥, 陳皮之辛溫, 以行鬱氣.

　　　　　(3)紫蘇, 生薑之辛溫, 以疏表氣.

　　　　　(4)甘草之甘緩, 以和正氣.

　　　　　(5)少加木瓜以除溼熱, 利筋骨, 調榮衛也.

　·來源：陳景初

7. Bai Zhu San. Atractylodes Macrocephala Powder. 白朮散

　·**ACTIONS**： pregnancy swelling

　·**COMPOSITION**：Bai Zhu, Da Fu Pi, Fu Ling Pi, Chen Pi, Jiang Pi

　·**INDICATIONS**： pregnancy swelling, vacuity floating as like water swelling form in the face, eye, limbs, and body.

　·**CHANNELS ENTERED**：The foot greater yang and greater yin channels.

　·**Analysis of Formula**：(1) Water disease should always be treated differently according to the location of the body. Jiang Pi and Ju Pi are pungent and they can disperse and make water to come out through pores. Da Fu Pi and Fu Ling Pi are bland and they can drain and make water to come out through urination.

　　　　　(2) Exuberance water is caused due to debilitated earth, therefore the sweet and warm of Bai Zhu are used to support spleen earth to build embankment to prevent flooding of water

　·Another Side Formula：(1) In Zhi Mi Fang, there is Sang Bai Pi without Bai Zhu.

　　　　　(2) Dan Xi eliminates Jiang Pi and Da Fu Pi and adds Chuan Xiong and Mu Tong to supplement the middle and conduct and move water qi.

　·**Original Source**：Quan Sheng Ji Mi Fan.

7. 白朮散

449

·總結：子腫
·組成：白朮, 大腹皮, 茯苓皮, 陳皮, 薑皮
·主治：治子腫, 面目肢體虛浮如水狀.
·歸經：此足太陽太陰藥也.
·方義：(1)水病常令上下分消：薑皮, 橘皮辛而能散, 使水從毛竅出. 腹皮, 苓皮淡而能泄, 使水從溺竅出.

(2)水盛由於土衰, 故用白朮之甘溫以扶脾土而隄防之, 不致泛溢也.

·又附方：(1)指迷方有桑白皮, 無白朮.

(2)丹溪除薑皮, 腹皮, 加川芎, 木通, 補中導行水氣.

·煎服法：爲末, 米飲下.
·來源：金生

8. Zhu Ye Tang. Lophatherum Decoction. 竹葉湯

·**ACTIONS**： pregnancy vexation

·**COMPOSITION**：Dan Zhu Ye, Mai Men Dong, Huang Qin, Fu Ling, Ren Shen

·**INDICATIONS**：When in pregnancy, if there is heart fright, timidity, and vexation and oppression for all day long, this is called pregnancy vexation.

·**MODIFICATIONS**：If there is phlegm, add Zhu Li.

·**CHANNELS ENTERED**：The hand greater and lesser yin channels. [The lung and heart]

·**Analysis of Formula**：(1) Zhu Ye clears vexation.

(2) Huang Qin disperse heat.

(3) Mai Men Dong cools the lung.

(4) Fu Ling quiets the heart.

(5) Ren Shen supplements vacuity. Heart vexation during pregnancy generally belongs to vacuity pattern.

·Another Side Formula：(1) In another Zhu Ye Tang, Fu Ling is used as sovereign without Ren Shen but with Fang Feng.

(2) In another Zhu Ye Tang, Ren Shen is eliminated and Fang Feng and Zhi Mu are added.

8. 竹葉湯

·總結：子煩
·組成：淡竹葉, 麥冬, 黃芩, 茯苓, 人參
·主治：治妊娠心驚膽怯, 終日煩悶, 名子煩.
·加減：如有痰者, 加竹瀝.
·歸經：此手太陰少陰藥也.
·方義：(1)竹葉：清煩.
　　　　(2)黃芩：消熱.
　　　　(3)麥冬：涼肺.
　　　　(4)茯苓：寧心.
　　　　(5)人參：補虛, 妊娠心煩, 固多虛也.
·又附方：(1)一方茯苓爲君, 無人參, 有防風.
　　　　(2)一方無人參, 有防風, 知母.

9. Zi Wan Tang. Aster Decoction. 紫菀湯

·**ACTIONS**：cough during pregnancy
·**COMPOSITION**：Gan Cao (mix fried), Zi Wan, Sang Bai Pi, Jie Geng, Xing Ren, Tian Men Dong, Zhu Ru
·**INDICATIONS**：　cough during pregnancy.
·**CHANNELS ENTERED**：The hand greater yin channel.
·**Analysis of Formula**：If cough during pregnancy is originated from fire evil, this should be treated with clearing fire and moistening the lung.

(1) Zi Wan and Zi Gan Cao are warm.

(2) The cool of Jie Geng and Sang Pi drains the lung.

(3) Xing Ren and Honey moisten the lung.

(4) The cold of Tian Men Dong and Zhu Ru clears the lung.

·**Original Source**：Fu Ren Da Quan Liang Fang

9. 紫菀湯
·總結：子嗽
·組成：炙甘草, 紫菀, 桑白皮, 桔梗, 杏仁, 天冬, 竹茹
·主治：治子嗽.
·歸經：此手太陰藥也.
·方義：子嗽由於火邪, 當以清火潤肺爲務.
　　　　(1)紫菀, 炙草之溫.

451

(2)桔梗，桑皮之涼以瀉之.

(3)杏仁，白蜜之澤，以潤之也.

(4)天冬，竹茹之寒以清之.

·煎服法：入蜜溫服.

·來源：良方

10. An Rong San. Quiet Construction Powder. 安榮散

·**ACTIONS**：strangury of pregnancy

·**COMPOSITION**：Mu Tong, Deng Xin Cao, Hua Shi, Ren Shen, Gan Cao, Mai Men Dong, Xi Xin, Dang Gui

·**INDICATIONS**：strangury of pregnancy, heart vexation and oppression.

·**CHANNELS ENTERED**：The hand greater yin, foot greater yang and lesser yin channels. [The spleen, bladder, and kidney]

·**Analysis of Formula**：Chen Lai Zhang says that vacuous heat should be supplemented, therefore the sweet of Ren Shen and Gan Cao is used. Strangury with oppression should be freed, therefore the draining of Mu Tong and Deng Xin Cao and the lubricating of Hua Shi are used. When the lung is dry, heaven qi is unable to descend, thus Mai Men Dong can clear this. When the kidney is dry, earth qi is unable to ascend, so Xi Xin can moisten this. When blood is dry, water way is unable to be moistened, Dang Gui can enrich this.

·**Original Source**：Ben Shi Fang

10. 安榮散

·總結：子淋

·組成：木通，燈草，滑石，人參，甘草，麥冬，細辛，當歸

·主治：治子淋，心煩悶亂.

·歸經：此手太陰足太陽少陰藥也.

·方義： 陳來章曰：「虛熱宜補，故用人參，甘草之甘. 淋悶宜通，故用木通，燈草之滲，滑石之滑. 肺燥則天氣不降，而麥冬能清之. 腎燥則地氣不升，而細辛能潤之. 血燥則溝瀆不濡，而當歸能滋之也.」

·來源：本事方

11. Shen Zhu Yin. Ginseng and Atractylodes Macrocephala Decoction. 參朮飲

·**ACTIONS**：shifted bladder

·**COMPOSITION**：Gan Cao (mix fried), Bai Zhu, Ren Shen, Dang Gui, Chuan Xiong, Shao Yao, Shu Di Huang, Ban Xia, Chen Pi

·**INDICATIONS**：shifted bladder in pregnancy.

·**CHANNELS ENTERED**：The foot greater and reverting yin channels.

·**Analysis of Formula**：Spleen vacuity should be supplemented with Si Jun Zi Tang. Blood vacuity should be supplemented with Si Wu Tang. Phlegm should be dispersed with Er Chen Tang. When making qi rise, then bladder spontaneously gets to be disinhibited.

·Another Side Formula：Dan Xi Shen Zhu Gao：Ren Shen, Bai Zhu, Huang Qi, Fu Ling, Chen Pi, Tao Ren, Gan Cao (mix fried), boils these herbs in Zhu Yang Bao Zhu Tang (the bladder of pig and sheep boiled in water), this treats strangury owing to bladder detriment after childbirth.

·**Original Source**：Dan Xi

11. 參朮飲

·總結：轉胞

·組成：炙甘草, 白朮, 人參, 當歸, 芎藭, 芍藥, 熟地黃, 半夏, 陳皮

·主治：治妊娠轉胞.

·歸經：此足太陰厥陰藥也.

·方義：脾虛補以四君. 血虛補以四物. 痰飲消以二陳. 使氣得升舉而胞自通也.

·又附方：丹溪參朮膏：人參, 白朮, 黃耆, 茯苓, 陳皮, 桃仁, 炙甘草用豬羊胞煮湯, 入藥煎服, 治產後胞損成淋瀝證.

·來源：丹溪

12. Hei Shen San. Black Spirit Powder. 黑神散

·**ACTIONS**：moves blood and aborts the fetus.

·**COMPOSITION**：Pu Huang, Hei Dou, Gui Xin, Gan Cao, Gan Jiang, Chi Shao, Shu Di Huang, Dang Gui Wei

·**INDICATIONS**：When after childbirth, there is persistent flow of lochia which causes surging pain, retention of the placenta, and death in utero.

·**CHANNELS ENTERED**：The foot greater and reverting yin channels. [The spleen and liver]

·**Analysis of Formula**：(1) The above pattern is generally due to blood stasis.

(2) Shu Di Huang, Dang Gui and Shao Yao nourish blood through moistening. Pu Huang and Hei Dou move blood through lubricating. The heat of Gui Xin and Gan Jiang breaks blood. Gan Cao is used to relax the right qi. Child's urine is used to disperse the stasis and counterflow. Wine is added to conduct other herbs to enter blood part and assist the force of herbs.

·**Original Source**：Ju Fang

12. 黑神散

·總結：行血下胎

·組成：蒲黃，黑豆，桂心，甘草，乾薑，赤芍，熟地黃，歸尾

·主治：治產後惡露不盡，攻衝作痛，及胞衣不下，胎死腹中.

·歸經：此足太陰厥陰藥也.

·方義：(1)前證皆因血瘀不行.

(2)熟地，歸，芍之潤以濡血. 蒲黃，黑豆之滑以行血. 桂心，乾薑之熱以破血. 用甘草者，緩其正氣. 用童便者，散其瘀逆. 加酒者，引入血分以助藥力也.

·來源：局方

13. Shi Xiao San. Sudden Smile Powder. 失笑散

·**ACTIONS**：blood pain.

·**COMPOSITION**：Pu Huang, Wu Ling Zhi

·**INDICATIONS**：retention of the lochia, pain in the pericardial network, or dead blood with abdominal pain.

·**CHANNELS ENTERED**：The hand and foot reverting yin channels.

·**Analysis of Formula**：The character of Pu Huang (raw) is lubricative and this moves blood. The qi of Wu Ling Zhi is dry and this disperses blood. Both of them can enter reverting yin and activate blood to relieve pain, therefore this power treats blood pain as like God.

·**RELATED FORMULA**：This formula (respectively one liang) with Mu Tong and Chi Shao (respectively five qian), this is called Tong Ling San, treats nine types of heart pain.

·**Original Source**：Ju Fang

13. 失笑散

　·總結：血痛

　·組成：蒲黃, 五靈脂

　·主治：治惡露不行, 心包絡痛, 或死血腹痛.

　·歸經：此手足厥陰藥也.

　·方義：生蒲黃性滑而行血. 五靈脂氣燥而散血. 皆能入厥陰而活血止痛, 故治血痛如神.

　·變化方：本方各一兩, 加木通, 赤芍各五錢, 每四錢入鹽少許服, 名通靈散, 治九種心痛.

　·來源：局方

14. Qing Hun San. Ethereal-Soul Clearing Powder. 清魂散

·**ACTIONS**：clouding and dizziness after childbirth.

·**COMPOSITION**：Jing Jie, Chuan Xiong, Ze Lan Ye, Ren Shen, Gan Cao (mix fried)

·**INDICATIONS**：treats that when lochia has already gone after childbirth, suddenly clouding and dizziness occurs.

·**CHANNELS ENTERED**：The foot reverting yin channel.

·**Analysis of Formula**：(1) The pathogen is wind evil which is contracted externally, therefore Jing Jie courses the wind.

(2) For the weakness of qi and blood, Chuan Xiong and Ze Lan nourish the blood, and Ren Shen and Gan Cao supplement the qi.

Then wind evil gets to be eliminated and qi and blood engender, and then spirit gets clear.

·**Original Source**：Yan Shi

14. 清魂散

　·總結：產後昏暈

　·組成：荊芥, 川芎, 澤蘭葉, 人參, 炙甘草

　·主治：治產後惡露已盡, 忽昏暈不知人.

　·歸經：此足厥陰藥也.

　·方義：(1)外感風邪, 故以荊芥疏其風.

455

(2)氣血虛弱, 故以芎藭, 澤蘭養其血, 人參, 甘草補其氣.
風邪去, 氣血生, 則神清矣.

·來源：嚴氏

15. Fan Hun Dan. Return Ethereal soul Pills. 返魂丹

·**ACTIONS**：regulates menstruation and disinhibits childbirth.
·**COMPOSITION**：Yi Mu Cao
·**INDICATIONS**：menstrual irregularities, red or white vaginal discharge, every disease after or before childbirth. \
·**MODIFICATIONS**：(1) if there is threatened abortion with abdominal pain, and incessant bloody discharge from one's vagina, then take this pills with Dang Gui Tang.

(2) if there is transverse growing, giving birth upside-down, and retention of the placenta, then take this pills with Chao Yan Tang (stir-fry salt decoction).

(3) if there is blood dizziness, thirst, and manic raving after child birth, ； or if there is wind strike, loss of voice, and clenched jaw after childbirth ； and blood binds with running pain, periodic aversion to cold and heat effusion, reddish complexion, and heart vexation ； or if there is nosebleed with black tongue and thirst, ； then takes this pills with child's urine with wine.

(4) for panting and cough, nausea with acid vomiting, and rip side pain with weakness of the limbs after childbirth, take this with wine.

(5) for blood with stool after childbirth, takes this with Zao Tang.

(6) for dysentery after childbirth, takes this with Mi Tang.

(7) for flooding and spotting after childbirth, takes this with Nuo Mi Tang.

(8) for vaginal discharge after childbirth, takes this with Jiao Ai Tang.

(9) for urinary and fecal stoppage, vexation and agitation, and bitter taste in the mouth after childbirth, takes this pills with Bo He Tang.

(10) taking this pills with child's urine after childbirth can quiet ethereal and corporeal soul, regulate channels and networks, and break blood pain.

(11) This pills can regulate menstruation, and also can make one with enduring subfertility pregnant.

456

·**CHANNELS ENTERED**：The hand and foot reverting yin channels.

·**Analysis of Formula**：Yi Mu Cao is good at dispersing water and moving blood, and this eliminates stasis, generates new blood, and disinhibits defecation and urination, therefore this is good herb for menstruation and childbirth, and also can alleviate deep-rooted boil and swelling and disperse welling abscess with hole.

15. 返魂丹

  ·總結：調經利產

  ·組成：益母草

  ·主治：治月經不調, 赤白帶下, 胎前產後一切諸病.

  ·加減：(1)如胎動腹痛, 下血不止, 當歸湯下.

        (2)橫生逆產, 胎衣不下, 炒鹽湯下.

        (3)產後血暈, 口渴狂言；產後中風, 失音口噤；及血結奔痛, 時發寒熱, 面赤心煩；或鼻衄舌黑口乾；並童便和酒下.

        (4)產後喘嗽, 惡心吐酸, 脇痛無力, 酒下.

        (5)產後瀉血, 棗湯下.

        (6)產後痢疾, 米湯下.

        (7)產後崩漏, 糯米湯下.

        (8)產後帶下, 膠艾湯下.

        (9)產後二便不通, 煩躁口苦, 薄荷湯下.

        (10)凡產後以童便化下一丸, 能安魂魄, 調經絡, 破血痛.

        (11)經不調者, 服之則調；久無子, 服之則孕.

  ·歸經：此手足厥陰藥也.

  ·方義：益母草功擅消水行血, 去瘀生新, 利大小便, 故為經產良藥；而又能消疔腫, 散孔癰也.

16. Dang Gui Yang Rou Tang. Tangkuei and Mutton Decoction. 當歸羊肉湯

·**ACTIONS**：childbirth taxatio

·**COMPOSITION**：Ren Shen, Huang Qi, Sheng Jiang, Dang Gui

·**INDICATIONS**：heat effusion and spontaneous sweating after childbirth, pain in the limbs and whole body, this is called childbirth taxation.

·**MODIFICATIONS**：(1) for persistent flow of lochia, add Gui Zhi.

457

(2) for profuse lochiorrhea, add Chuan Xiong.

(3) if there is cold, add Wu Zhu Yu.

·**CHANNELS ENTERED**：The hand and foot greater and reverting yin channels. [The lung, spleen, pericardium, and liver]

·**Analysis of Formula**：(1) Ren Shen and Huang Qi supplement qi and secure Defense.

(2) Dang Gui tonifies blood and regulates construction .

(3) Sheng Jiang is pungent and warm, this conducts qi herbs to enter qi part and generates new blood.

(4) Yang Rou (mutton) is sweet and heat, this supplements vacuity taxation.

·**RELATED FORMULA**：When Ren Shen and Huang Qi are eliminated, and Yang Rou (mutton), Sheng Jiang, and Dang Gui are used, this is called Dang Gui Sheng Jiang Yang Rou Tang, treats gripping pain in the abdomen after childbirth, cold abdominal colic with abdominal pain, and taxation vacuity and insufficiency.

16. 當歸羊肉湯

·總結：蓐勞

·組成：人參, 黃耆, 生薑, 當歸

·主治：治產後發熱自汗, 肢體疼痛, 名曰蓐勞.

·加減：(1)如惡露不盡, 加桂.

(2)惡露下, 外加川芎.

(3)有寒加吳茱萸.

·歸經：此手足太陰厥陰藥也.

·方義：(1)參, 耆：補氣而固衛.

(2)當歸：養血而調榮.

(3)生薑：辛溫, 引氣藥入氣分而生新血.

(4)羊肉：甘熱, 用氣血之屬以補虛勞, 熱退而汗收矣.

·變化方：本方除人參, 黃耆, 用羊肉, 薑, 歸, 名當歸生薑羊肉湯, 治產後腹中絞痛, 及寒疝腹痛, 勞虛不足.

17. Dang Gui San. Tangkuei Powder. 當歸散

·**ACTIONS**：tonifies blood and quiets fetus.

·**COMPOSITION**：Dang Gui, Chuan Xiong, Shao Yao, Bai Zhu, Huang

Qin

·**INDICATIONS**：women in pregnancy should often take this powder.

·**CHANNELS ENTERED**：The foot greater yin and reverting yin chann els, and the thoroughfare and conception vessels.

·**Analysis of Formula**：(1) When the blood of the thoroughfare and conce ption vessels is exuberant, women can nourish and quiet fetus. Chuan Xiong, D ang Gui and Shao Yao can nourish blood and boost the thoroughfare and conce ption vessels.

(2) Also women in pregnancy should be treated with clearing he at and cooling blood, if blood does not move frenetically, fetus gets quieted. Hu ang Qin which nourishes yin and removes [clears] yang, can eliminate stomach heat. Bai Zhu supplements the spleen and dries damp, and also eliminates stom ach heat. When the spleen and stomach are strong, they can transport and transf orm essence, and take juice [essence] which transforms into blood, and the bloo d nourishes fetus, and then there will be no worry of nausea and vomiting. Ther efore Dan Xi quiets fetus with Huang Qin and Bai Zhu which are considered as a holy medicine [for quieting fetus]

·**Original Source**：Jin Gui Yao Lue

17. 當歸散

·總結：養血安胎

·組成：當歸，川芎，芍藥，白朮，黃芩

·主治：婦人妊娠，宜常服之.

·歸經：此足太陰厥陰衝任藥也.

·方義：(1)衝任血盛，則能養胎而安胎. 芎，歸，芍藥，能養血而益衝任.

(2)又懷妊宜清熱涼血，血不妄行則胎安. 黃芩養陰退陽，能除胃熱. 白朮補脾燥溼，亦除胃熱. 脾胃健則能運化精微，取汁爲血以養胎，自無惡阻嘔逆之患矣. 故丹溪以黃芩，白朮爲安胎聖藥也.

·來源：金匱

18. Qi Gong Wan. Uterus Opening Pill. 啓宮丸

·**ACTIONS**：infertility of obese

·**COMPOSITION**：Chuan Xiong, Bai Zhu, Gan Cao, Fu Ling, Xiang Fu, Shen Qu, Ban Xia, Ju Hong

459

·**INDICATIONS**：fatty uterus with infertility.

·**Analysis of Formula**：The foot greater yin and reverting yin channels. [The spleen and liver]

·**RELATED FORMULA**：(1) Ju Hong, Ban Xia, and Bai Zhu dry damp by eliminating phlegm. Xiang Fu and Shen Qu rectify qi by dispersing stagnation. Chuan Xiong disperses congestion by activating blood. Then something congested gets to free and something blocked gets to open.

(2) Fu Ling and Gan Cao also eliminate damp, harmonize the middle, and assist right qi.

18. 啟宮丸

·總結：體肥不孕

·組成：芎藭, 白朮, 甘草, 茯苓, 香附, 神麴, 半夏麴, 橘紅

·主治：治子宮脂滿, 不能孕育.

·方義：此足太陰厥陰藥也.

·變化方：(1)橘, 半, 白朮, 燥溼以除其痰；香附, 神麴, 理氣以消其滯；川芎散鬱, 以活其血；則壅者通, 塞者啟矣.

(2)茯苓, 甘草, 亦以去溼和中, 助其生氣也.

19. Da Sheng San. Birth-Giving Powder. 達生散

·**ACTIONS**：breech birth

·**COMPOSITION**：Chen Pi, Da Fu Pi, Zi Su Ye, Bai Zhu, Ren Shen, Gan Cao (mix fried), Shao Yao, Dang Gui

·**INDICATIONS**：When in 8th of 9th month of pregnancy, taking dozens of dose of this formula makes women to have a safe delivery and strength.

·**MODIFICATIONS**：(1) sometimes add Zhi Ke and Sha Ren.

(2) sometimes in spring, Chuan Xiong is added, in summer, Huang Qin is added.

(3) or if there is another sign, modify according to the pattern.

·**CHANNELS ENTERED**：The foot greater yin and reverting yin channels.

·**Analysis of Formula**：(1) Dang Gui and Shao Yao boost blood. Ren Shen and Bai Zhu boost qi. Da Fu Pi, Chen Pi, Zi Su Ye, and Cong Ye course the congestion.

(2) If qi and blood are neither vacuity nor stagnate, there will be no worry of difficult delivery.

460

19. 達生散
   ·總結：易產
   ·組成：陳皮，大腹皮，紫蘇，白术，人參，炙甘草，芍藥，當歸
   ·主治：婦人妊娠八，九月，服數十劑，易生有力.
   ·加減：(1)或加枳殼，砂仁.
          (2)或春加川芎，夏加黃芩，冬加本方.
          (3)或有別證，以意消息.
   ·歸經：此足太陰厥陰藥也.
   ·方義：(1)當歸，芍藥以益其血. 人參，白术以益其氣. 腹皮，陳皮，紫蘇，蔥葉以疏其壅.
          (2)氣血不虛不滯，則臨產自無留難之患矣.
   ·來源：丹溪

20. Zhu Ti Tang. Pig's trotter Decoction. 豬蹄湯

  ·**ACTIONS**：promote lactation
  ·**COMPOSITION**： Zhu Ti (Pig's trotter), Tong Cao
  ·**INDICATIONS**：oligogalactia.
  ·**CHANNELS ENTERED**：The foot yang brightness channel.
  ·**Analysis of Formula**：(1) Zhu Ti is salty and can precipitate with moistness.
        (2) Tong Cao is bland and can free orifice.
  ·**Original Source**：Ling Yuan Fang

20. 豬蹄湯
   ·總結：通乳
   ·組成：豬蹄，通草
   ·主治：治乳少.
   ·歸經：此足陽明藥也.
   ·方義：(1)豬蹄鹹能潤下.
         (2)通草淡能通竅.
   ·來源：靈苑

21. Ren Shen Jing Jie San. Ginseng and Schizonepeta Powder. 人參荊芥散

·**ACTIONS**：blood-wind taxation

·**COMPOSITION**：Suan Zao Ren, Bai Zhu, Ren Shen, Gan Cao, Ling Yang Jiao, Chai Hu, Chuan Xiong, Zhi Ke, Dang Gui, Gui Xin, Bie Jia, Shu Di Huang, Jing Jie, Fang Feng

·**INDICATIONS**：blood-wind taxation.

·**CHANNELS ENTERED**：The foot greater and reverting yin, and the hand lesser yin channels. [The spleen, liver, and heart]

·**Analysis of Formula**：Chen Lai Zhang says that

(1) for vexation, fatigue, reduced eating, night sweating, and fearful throbbing, Ren Shen, Bai Zhu, Zi Gan Cao, Zao Ren supplement and contract qi.

(2) exuberant wood generates wind, Ling Yang Jiao and Chai Hu pacify that.

(3) pain, stagnation of blood and qi, and menstrual disorder are regulated by Chuan Xiong, Dang Gui, Gui Xin, and Zhi Ke.

(4) yin vacuity with heat effusion is enriched by Di Huang and Bie Jia.

(5) wind in the blood is dispersed by Jing Jie and Fang Feng.

·**Original Source**：Fu Ren Chan Yu Bao Qing Ji

21. 人參荊芥散

·總結：血風勞

·組成：酸棗仁, 白朮, 人參, 甘草, 羚羊角, 柴胡, 芎藭, 枳殼, 當歸, 桂心, 鼈甲, 熟地黃, 荊芥, 防風

·主治：治血風勞.

·歸經：此足太陰厥陰手少陰藥也.

·方義：陳來章曰

(1)煩怠食少, 盜汗心忡, 人參, 白朮, 炙草, 棗仁補而收之.

(2)木盛生風, 羚角, 柴胡平之.

(3)血氣痛滯, 月水不調, 芎藭, 當歸, 桂心, 枳殼調之.

(4)陰虛發熱, 地黃, 鼈甲滋之.

(5)血中之風, 荊芥, 防風散之.

·來源：婦寶

22. Bai Zi Ren Wan. Platycladus Seed Pills. 柏子仁丸

·**ACTIONS**：scant menstrual blood and menstrual block.

·**COMPOSITION**：Bai Zi Ren, Shu Di Huang, Niu Xi, Xu Duan, Juan Bai, Ze Lan

·**INDICATIONS**：pause in the middle of menstruation, scant menstrual blood, and debilitated spirit.

·**CHANNELS ENTERED**：The hand and foot lesser and reverting yin channel. [The heart, kidney, pericardium, and liver]

·**Analysis of Formula**：(1) Bai Zi Ren quiets spirit and nourishes the heart.

(2) Di Huang, Niu Xi, and Xu Duan supplement the liver and kidney and boost the thoroughfare and conception vessels

(3) Juan Bai and Ze Lan activate blood vessel and free menstrual block.

·**Original Source**：Fu Ren Da Quan Liang Fang

22. 柏子仁丸

·總結：血少經閉

·組成：柏子仁, 熟地黃, 牛膝, 續斷, 卷柏, 澤蘭

·主治：治經行復止, 血少神衰.

·歸經：此手足少陰厥陰藥也.

·方義：(1)柏子仁：安神而養心.

(2)地黃, 牛膝, 續斷：補肝腎而益衝任.

(3)卷柏, 澤蘭：活血脈而通經閉.

·來源：良方

23. Xiong Gui Liu Jun Zi Tang. Six-Gentlemen Decoction with Cnidium and Tangkuei. 芎歸六君子湯

·**ACTIONS**：delayed menstruation with phlegm obstruction

·**COMPOSITION**：Chuan Xiong, Dang Gui, Ren Shen, Bai Zhu, Fu Ling, Gan Cao, Ju Hong, Ban Xia

·**INDICATIONS**：delayed menstruation which is scant, the people tends to be obese constitution.

·**CHANNELS ENTERED**：The foot greater yin and reverting yin chann els.

·**Analysis of Formula**：⑴ Er Chen Tang in this formula treats phlegm stagnation.

⑵ Ren Shen and Bai Zhu supplement qi vacuity.

⑶ Chuan Xiong and Dang Gui activate menstrual blood.

23. 芎歸六君子湯
    ·總結：痰阻經遲
    ·組成：芎藭, 當歸, 人參, 白朮, 茯苓, 甘草, 橘紅, 半夏
    ·主治：治經水後期, 其來澁少, 形體肥盛.
    ·歸經：此足太陰厥陰藥也.
    ·方義：⑴二陳治其痰滯.
        ⑵參, 朮補其氣虛.
        ⑶芎, 歸活其經血.

24. Lian Fu Si Wu Tang. Four-Substance Decoction with Scutellaria and Cyperi. 連附四物湯

·**ACTIONS**：delayed menstruation with heat depression

·**COMPOSITION**：Si Wu Tang (Dang Gui, Di Huang, Shao Yao, Chuan Xiong) added with Xiang Fu and Huang Lian.

·**INDICATIONS**：delayed menstruation, colt which is purple and black.

·**CHANNELS ENTERED**：The hand lesser yin, and the hand and reverting yin channels. [The heart, pericardium, and liver]

·**Analysis of Formula**：⑴ Si Wu Tang boosts yin and tonifies blood.

⑵ with Huang Lian clears blood heat and with Xiang Fu moves stagnant qi.

·**RELATED FORMULA**：⑴ Si Wu Tang with Huang Qin and Bai Zhu treats profuse menstruation.

⑵ Si Wu Tang with Zhi Zi and Huang Lian is called Re Liu He Tang, with Gan Jiang and Fu Zi is called Han Liu He Tang, with Chen Pi and Hou Po is called Qi Liu He Tang, with Qiang Huo and Qin Jiao is called Feng Liu He Tang. They are usually used to women and menstrual disease, and after child birth.

·**Original Source**：Dan Xi

464

24. 連附四物湯

　·總結：熱鬱經遲

　·組成：四物湯(當歸，地黃，芍藥，川芎)，加香附，黃連

　·主治：治經水過期，紫黑成塊.

　·歸經：此手少陰手足厥陰藥也.

　·方義：(1)四物以益陰養血.

　　　　　(2)加黃連以清血熱，香附以行氣鬱.

　·變化方：(1)四物加芩朮湯，治經水過多.

　　　　　　(2)四物加梔，連，爲熱六合湯；加薑，附，爲寒六合湯；加陳，朴，爲氣六合湯；加羌，芄，爲風六合湯. 皆婦病與經產通用之藥也.

　·來源：丹溪

25. Gu Jing Wan. Stabilize the Menses Pill. 固經丸

　·**ACTIONS**：flooding and spotting with blood heat

　·**COMPOSITION**：Huang Qin, Xiang Fu, Huang Bai, Shao Yao, Chu Pi, Gui Ban

　·**INDICATIONS**：incessant menses, clot that is purple and black, spotting in the middle of flooding.

　·**CHANNELS ENTERED**：The foot lesser yin and reverting yin channels.

　·**Analysis of Formula**：Incessant profuse menstruation is because vacuous yin is unable to restrain the ministerial fire of the pericardium, therefore it skips the routine track. Spotting in the middle of flooding indicates vacuity with heat. Clot that is purple and black means that extreme fire is as like cold water.

　　　　(1) Huang Qin clears the fire in the upper burner.

　　　　(2) The pungent of Xiang Fu disperses congestion.

　　　　(3) Huang Bai drains the fire of the lower burner.

　　　　(4) Shao Yao and Gui Ban nourish yin and blood, all of them invigorate water to restrain yang exasperation.

　　　　(5) Chu Pi is astringent and checks flooding collapse.

　·**Original Source**：Fu Ren Da Quan Liang Fang

25. 固經丸

　·總結：血熱崩漏

465

·組成：黃芩, 香附, 黃柏, 芍藥, 樗皮, 龜板
·主治：治經行不止, 紫黑成塊, 及崩中漏下.
·歸經：此足少陰厥陰藥也.
·方義：經多不止者, 陰虛不足以制包絡之火, 故越其常度也. 崩中漏下者, 虛而挾熱也. 紫黑成塊者, 火極似水也.

  (1)黃芩：清上焦之火.
  (2)香附：辛以散鬱.
  (3)黃柏：瀉下焦之火.
  (4)芍藥, 龜板：滋陰而養血；皆壯水以制陽光也.
  (5)樗皮：濇以止脫.

26. Sheng Yang Ju Jung Tang. Raise the Yang and Lift the Menses Decoction. 升陽舉經湯

·**ACTIONS**：taxation damage, flooding and spotting
·**COMPOSITION**：Bu Zhong Yi Qi Tang added with Bai Shao Yao, (He i) Zhi Zi
·**INDICATIONS**：flooding and spotting, generalized heat effusion, spont aneous sweating, shortness of breath, fatigue and laziness to eat.
·**CHANNELS ENTERED**：The foot greater yin and yang brightness cha nnels.
·**Analysis of Formula**：Bu Zhong Yi Qi Tang boosts qi, raises yang, abat es heat, and contracts sweating. Shao Yao is added to harmonize blood and rest rain yin, (Hei) Zhi Zi clears heat and stanches bleeding.
·The other Sheng Yang Ju Jung Tang：in Li Dong Yuan's Lan Shi Mi Ca ng there is Huang Qi, Dang Gui, Bai Zhu, Qiang Huo, Fang Feng, Gao Ben, Du Huo, **Fu Zi**, Gan Cao, Ren Shen, Shu Di Huang, Chuan Xiong, Xi Xin, Tao Re n, Hong Hua, **Rou Gui**, Shao Yao. This treats incessant menses.
·**Original Source**：Li Dong Yuan

26. 升陽舉經湯
·總結：勞傷崩漏
·組成：補中益氣湯加白芍, 黑梔子
·主治：治崩漏, 身熱自汗, 短氣, 倦怠懶食.
·歸經：此足太陰陽明藥也.
·方義：補中湯以益氣升陽, 退熱收汗. 加芍藥以和血斂陰, 黑梔以清

熱止血.

·又附方：又東垣蘭室祕藏「升陽擧經湯」：黃者，當歸，白朮，羌活，防風，薰本，獨活，附子，甘草，人參，熟地，川芎，細辛，桃仁，紅花，肉桂，芍藥. 每服三錢，漸加至五錢. 治經水不止.

·來源：東垣

27. Ru Sheng San, Sagely Powder. 如聖散

·**ACTIONS**：checks flooding and spotting

·**COMPOSITION**：Wu Mei, Zong Lu, Hei Jiang (ginger which is fried to black)

·**INDICATIONS**：incessant flooding and spotting.

·**CHANNELS ENTERED**：The foot reverting yin channel.

·**Analysis of Formula**：(1) Astringent can stanch bleeding, therefore Zong Lu is used.

(2) Sour can restrain, therefore Wu Mei is used.

(3) Warm can keep the middle, therefore Gan Jiang is used.

Black can stanch bleeding (water can restrain fire), therefore calcination is used.

27. 如聖散

·總結：止崩漏

·組成：烏梅，樓櫚，黑薑

·主治：治崩漏不止.

·歸經：此足厥陰藥也.

·方義：(1)濇能止血，故用樓櫚.

(2)酸能收斂，故用烏梅.

(3)溫能守中，故用乾薑.

黑能止血，故並煅用.

·煎服法：爲末，每服二錢，烏海湯下.

28. Mu Dan Pi San. Moutan Powder. 牡丹皮散

·**ACTIONS**：blood accumulation

·**COMPOSITION**：Mu Dan Pi, Gui Xin, Niu Xi, Chi Shao Yao, Dang G

467

ui Wei, Yan Hu Suo, San Leng, E Zhu

　　·**INDICATIONS**：blood accumulation.

　　·**CHANNELS ENTERED**：The foot reverting yin channel.

　　·**Analysis of Formula**：(1) Gui Xin, Mu Dan Pi, Chi Shao, and Niu Xi move blood.

　　　　　(2) San Leng, E Zhu, Dang Gui Wei, and Yan Hu Suo move blood in qi stagnation and qi in blood stagnation.

　　　　　(3) When qi and blood flow well, binds is dissipated.

　　·**Original Source**：Fu Ren Da Quan Liang Fang

28. 牡丹皮散

　·總結：血瘕

　·組成：丹皮，桂心，牛膝，赤芍藥，歸尾，延胡索，三稜，莪朮

　·主治：治血瘕.

　·歸經：此足厥陰藥也.

　·方義：(1)桂心，丹皮，赤芍，牛膝：以行其血.

　　　　(2)三稜，莪朮，歸尾，延胡：以行其血中氣滯，氣中血滯.

　　　　(3)氣血週流，則結者散矣.

　·煎服法：水，酒各半煎.

　·來源：良方

29. Zheng Qi Tian Xiang San. Qi-Righting Lindera and Cyperus Powder. 正氣天香散

·**ACTIONS**：　qi stagnation and delayed menstruation

·**COMPOSITION**：Wu Yao, Chen Pi, Su Ye, Xiang Fu, Gan Jiang

·**INDICATIONS**：every kind of qi, qi surging upward to the heart, surging pain in the heart and chest, stabbing pain in the rib-side, and menstrual disorder.

·**CHANNELS ENTERED**：The hand greater yin and foot reverting yin channels. [The lung and liver]

·**Analysis of Formula**：(1) Wu Yao and Chen Pi enter only qi part to rectify qi. Xiang Fu and Zi Su Ye can enter blood part and move qi. Gan Jiang is used channel conductor to make the other herbs to enter qi part and also blood part.

　　　　(2) practitioner uses pungent and warm to resolve depression and

468

disperse the liver, then qi gets to be regulated and blood becomes harmonious, and then menstruation turns back to normal and spontaneously the pain and con gestion will disappear.

·**Original Source**：Xin Yin Gan Zhu Jing

29. 正氣天香散

    ·總結：氣滯經遲

    ·組成：烏藥, 陳皮, 蘇葉, 香附, 乾薑

    ·主治：治一切諸氣, 氣上湊心, 心胸攻築, 脇肋刺痛. 月水不調.

    ·歸經：此手太陰足厥陰藥也.

    ·方義：(1)烏藥, 陳皮, 專入氣分而理氣. 香附, 紫蘇, 能入血分而行氣. 引以乾薑, 使入氣分兼入血分.

        (2)用諸辛溫以解鬱散肝, 令氣調而血和, 則經行有常, 自無痛壅之患.

    ·來源：紺珠

30. Yi Qi San. Restrain Qi Powder. 抑氣散

·**ACTIONS**： more exuberant qi than blood in women.

·**COMPOSITION**：Fu Shen, Xiang Fu, Chen Pi, Gan Cao (mix fried)

·**INDICATIONS**：When in women, qi is mor exuberant than blood, this condition changes into and generates every pattern, such as dizziness, fullness i n the diaphragm.

·**CHANNELS ENTERED**：The hand greater yin and lesser yang channel s. [The lung and San Jiao]

·**Analysis of Formula**：(1) Nei Jing says that high rising is treated by repr ession. Xiang Fu can disperse congested qi, Chen Pi can regulate every kind of qi, Fu Shen can calm heart qi, and Gan Cao can moderate counterflow qi. If qi gets to be balanced, there is no harm.

    (2) If the congestion of qi is severe, one should choose a formula in Qi-Regulating Formulas, there is no need to be attached to this formula.

·**Original Source**：Yan Shi

30. 抑氣散

    ·總結：氣盛於血

    ·組成：茯神, 香附, 陳皮, 炙甘草

·主治：治婦人氣盛於血，變生諸證，頭暈膈滿.

·歸經：此手太陰少陽藥也.

·方義：(1)經曰：「高者抑之.」香附能散鬱氣， 陳皮能調諸氣， 茯神能安心氣，甘草能緩逆氣. 氣得其平，則無亢害之患矣.

(2)若鬱甚者，當於理氣門中諸方選用，不必泥此.

·來源：嚴氏

31. Gu Xia Wan. Stabilize the Diarrhea Pill. 固下丸

·**ACTIONS**：vaginal discharge with damp heat

·**COMPOSITION**：Chu Pi, Bai Shao Yao, Huang Bai, Liang Jiang

·**INDICATIONS**：red or white vaginal discharge.

·**CHANNELS ENTERED**：The foot lesser yin and reverting yin channel.

·**Analysis of Formula**：Chen Lai Zhang says that the bitter of Chu Pi dries damp, and the cold overcomes heat, and the astringent secures diarrhea, therefore this is used to red or white vaginal discharge with damp heat, acting as sovereign. The sour of Shao Yao restrains yin qi and contracts flooding downward, acting as minister. The heat of Liang Jiang disperses cold-damp, the cold of Huang Bai eliminates heat-damp, the two flavors of Liang Jiang and Huang Bai which are baked to black, stanch bleeding and secure collapse, acting as assistant and courier.

·**Original Source**：Zhang Zi He

31. 固下丸

·總結：溼熱帶下

·組成：樗皮，白芍，黃柏，良薑

·主治：治赤白帶下.

·歸經：此足少陰厥陰藥也.

·方義：陳來章曰：「樗皮苦燥溼，寒勝熱，濇固下，故赤白帶因於溼熱者，用之為君. 芍藥之酸，斂陰氣，收下溜為臣. 良薑之熱，以散寒溼；黃柏之寒，以祛熱溼；並炒黑以止血脫為佐使也.」

·來源：子和

470

32. Dang Gui Jian Wan. Dang Gui Decoction Wan. 當歸煎丸

·**ACTIONS**：vaginal discharge with vacuity heat

·**COMPOSITION**：Dang Gui, Xu Duan, E Jiao, Shu Di Huang, Bai Shao Yao, Chi Shao Yao, Mu Li, Di Yu

·**INDICATIONS**：red or white vaginal discharge, pain in the abdomen, inability to eat food, and marked emaciation.

·**CHANNELS ENTERED**：The foot lesser yin and reverting yin.

·**Analysis of Formula**：(1) Dang Gui, Shao Yao, Shu Di Huang, Xu Duan, and E Jiao supplement the liver and enrich the kidney to treat blood vacuity.

(2) Mu Li and Di Yu clear heat and contract collapse to check vaginal discharge.

(3) The sour and cold of Chi Shao can disperse malign blood and eliminate stasis to generate new blood, dispersing is a kind of contracting.

·**Original Source**：Yan Shi

32. 當歸煎丸
·總結：虛熱帶下
·組成：當歸，續斷，阿膠，熟地黃，白芍藥，赤芍藥，牡蠣，地榆
·主治：治赤白帶下，腹中痛，不飲食，羸瘦.
·歸經：此足少陰厥陰藥也.
·方義：(1)歸，芍，熟地，續斷，阿膠，補肝滋腎，以治血虛.
(2)牡蠣，地榆，清熱收脫，以止帶下.
(3)赤芍酸寒，能散惡血，去瘀所以生新，散之所以收之也.
·來源：嚴氏

33. Bai Zhi San. Angelicae dahuricae Powder. 白芷散

·**ACTIONS**：vaginal discharge due to wind-damp.

·**COMPOSITION**：Bai Zhi, Tai Fa (downy hair), Hai Piao Xiao

·**INDICATIONS**：treats red or white vaginal discharge, efflux desertion.

·**CHANNELS ENTERED**：The foot yang brightness, lesser yin, and reverting yin channels [the stomach, kidney, and liver].

·**Analysis of Formula**：(1) The pungent and warm of Bai Zhi dries damp and eliminates wind.

471

(2) Hair of the head is the surplus of the blood, supplements yin and disperses stasis, calcined to black can stanch bleeding.

(3) Hai Piao Xiao is salty and warm, contracts damp and harmonizes blood.

·**Original Source**：Fu Ren Da Quan Liang Fang

33. 白芷散

　·總結：風溼帶下

　·組成：白芷, 胎髮, 海螵蛸.

　·主治：治赤白帶滑脫不禁.

　·歸經：此足陽明少陰厥陰藥也.

　·方義：(1)白芷：辛溫燥溼而祛風.

　　　　　(2)髮者血之餘, 補陰消瘀, 煅黑又能止血也.

　　　　　(3)烏側鹹溫收溼而和血.

　·來源：良方

Bibliography

Craic mitchell, Feng ye, Nigel wiseman. SHANG HAN LUN ON COLD DAMAGE. Paradigm publication. 2004.

Dictionary of Chinese Medicine. Hunan Science &Technology Press.2006.

Huang Di Nei Jing Su Wen: An Annotated Translation of Huang Di's Inner Classic. University of California Press; CT. Paul U. Unschuld ed. Edition. 2011.

www.ingramcontent.com/pod-product-compliance
Lightning Source LLC
Chambersburg PA
CBHW080615190526
45169CB00009B/3192